Textbook on

PSYCHOLOGY

for Post Basic BSc Nursing

Textbook on

PSYCHOLOGY

for Post Basic BSc Nursing

I Clement
MA (Sociology) MA (Child Care and Education) MSc (Nursing)
PG Diploma in Hospital Administration
Principal
VSS College of Nursing
Bengaluru, Karnataka, India

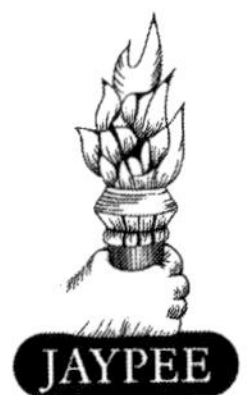

JAYPEE BROTHERS MEDICAL PUBLISHERS
The Health Sciences Publisher
New Delhi | London

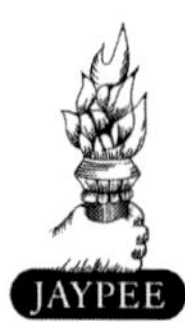

Jaypee Brothers Medical Publishers (P) Ltd

Headquarters
EMCA House
23/23-B, Ansari Road, Daryaganj
New Delhi - 110 002, India
Landline: +91-11-23272143, +91-11-23272703
+91-11-23282021, +91-11-23245672
E-mail: jaypee@jaypeebrothers.com

Corporate Office
4838/24, Ansari Road, Daryaganj
New Delhi - 110 002, India
Phone: +91-11-43574357
Fax: +91-11-43574314
E-mail: jaypee@jaypeebrothers.com

Overseas Office
J.P. Medical Ltd
83 Victoria Street, London
SW1H 0HW (UK)
Phone: +44 20 3170 8910
E-mail: info@jpmedpub.com

EU GPSR Authorised Representative
Logos Europe, 9 rue Nicolas Poussin
17000, La Rochelle, France
Phone: +33 (0) 6 67 93 73 78
E-mail: contact@logoseurope.eu

Website: www.jaypeebrothers.com
Website: www.jaypeedigital.com

Inquiries for bulk sales may be solicited at: jaypee@jaypeebrothers.com

Textbook on Psychology for Post Basic BSc Nursing

First Edition: **2014**

Reprint: **2026**

ISBN 978-93-5152-180-8

Printed at: Samrat Offset Pvt. Ltd.

Dedicated to

Professor PV Ramachandran
Chairman
Nursing Education
Sri Ramachandra University
Chennai, Tamil Nadu, India

PREFACE

Body and mind are the two sides of the same coin; they are inseparable, inter-related, interdependent and complex in nature. Each individual mind is unique. Understanding about mind and behavior is important for every nurse to get cooperation from each patient to provide a successful good quality care. Therefore, each nurse should learn the basics of psychology in order to empathize on the patients' problems, which helps the nurse to get better knowledge about patients' illness, and integrate, plan and implement the holistic care.

This book on psychology is framed with 21 chapters. Each chapter is illustrated in simple English and explained in points, which helps to grasp the contents from examination point of view. This book has all the required contents that meet the requirements of Indian Nursing Council, which are needed for Post Basic BSc nursing students. The students who travel through this book will definitely gain not only the knowledge about psychology but also develop good positive attitude towards understanding different kinds of behavior in human beings. Practicing the gained knowledge in appropriate areas also helps to gain good marks in examinations. This book can be used by all the nursing students and teachers as a reference book, since it has basics of psychology well explained.

I Clement

ACKNOWLEDGMENTS

I am thankful to the Lord Almighty, who strengthens me with abundant blessing through innumerable means and helping me in all accomplishments.

My heartfelt thanks are due to Shri Somanna, Chairman, VSS Group of Institutions, for his constant support and encouragement. I sincerely thank my teacher, BT Basavanthappa, Principal, Rajarajeshwari College of Nursing, Bengaluru, Karnataka, India.

Also, I thank PV Ramachandran, Chairman, Nursing Education, Sri Ramachandra University, Chennai, Tamil Nadu, India, a great philosopher and an internationally renowned teacher of nursing, who helped me in discovering the world of knowledge.

I am thankful to Ms Shylaja Somanna, Managing Director; Dr BS Arun and Dr BS Naveen, VSS Group of Institutions, for their support and encouragement.

I am also grateful to Dr Aswathnarayanan, Chairman, Padmashree Group of Institutions; Dr Bhagavan, Professor, Department of Surgery, Kempegowda Institute of Medical Sciences, Bengaluru, Karnataka, India; Dr TV Ramakrishnan, Professor of Anesthesiology and Head of Clinical Services, Department of Accident and Emergency Medicine, Sri Ramachandra University, Chennai, Tamil Nadu, India.

I convey my sincere thanks to my beloved parents, brothers, sisters and my wife Nisha Clement, for their continuous support and constant encouragement in each step of my life. I take this opportunity to thank my little ones, Cabin, Cynthia and Cavin. I also extend my thanks to beloved friend and brother, Mr Regi T Kurien.

My sincere thanks to Shri Jitendar P Vij (Group Chairman), Mr Ankit Vij (Managing Director), Mr Tarun Duneja (Director-Publishing), Mr KK Raman (Production Manager), Mr Venugopal V (Regional Manager, Bengaluru Branch), Mr Vasudev H (In Charge, Mangalore Branch), Mr Santhosh (Author Coordinator) and all staff of M/s Jaypee Brothers Medical Publishers (P) Ltd, New Delhi and Bengaluru Branch, for bringing out the excellent quality of the book.

CONTENTS

CHAPTER 1 Introduction to Psychology

LEARNING OBJECTIVES

1. To understand the operational definition of psychology.
2. To understand historical events in psychology.
3. To understand the concept and meaning of psychology.
4. To emphasize the psychological aspects, provide care, apply the same to save psychological problems in patients.
5. To study different types of schools and branches in psychology.
6. To understand and study psychological application in nursing.

INTRODUCTION

A sound mind is a sound body; man's mind should be healthy, brain and its functions are so complex, still there are many unrevealed facts about brain. Each person is unique; we cannot read the mind from outside, but can understand only through their activities and behaviors. As a nurse, we come across different kinds of people with divergent culture, taboos, ideas, customs, beliefs, religions, race, creeds, castes, etc. It will be difficult for the nurse to give care, communicate, unless/until she/he understands the mind of people, thoughts, ideas, psychological concepts. Once she/he learns, will empathize, understand and behave accordingly to gain the cooperation from the patient.

MEANING OF PSYCHOLOGY

The word 'psychology' is derived from two Greek words, 'psyche' and 'logos'. 'Psyche' means 'soul' and 'logos' means 'study of'.

Psychology is a scientific discipline in an extremely exciting field of knowledge. It continues to grow at an accelerating field pace each year and continues to provide answer to basic question about the human behavior. Psychology has enormous potential. It offers us the hope of both understanding and improving the quality of life. Psychological knowledge has been used in measuring intelligence, designing school curriculum, helping troubled marriages, controlling aggression, selling products and treating both the young and old with greater sensitivity and humanness.

DEFINITIONS

1. Psychology is defined as "a science of human and animal behavior."
2. Psychology is a science, which aims to give us better understanding and control of the behavior of the organism as a whole.
3. Psychology, as the scientific study of behavior, does not exclude mind and other internal process from the field of psychology; what a person does his/her behavior—is the outcome of the internal mental process.
4. Psychology is the science of human and animal behavior; it includes the applications of this science to human problems.
5. Psychology is the study of processes or activities of human in relation to his/her environment. —*Woodworth*
6. Psychology related to reaction to any and every situation of life. —*Skinner*
7. Psychology is the scientific study of the mind and its functions. —*Oxford dictionary*
8. Psychology is the scientific study of behavior and mental processes. Behavior includes all of our outward or overt actions and reactions, such as talking, facial expressions and movements. Mental processes refer to all the internal, covert activity of our minds, such as thinking, feeling and remembering. —*Ciccarelli and Meyer, 2006*

NATURE OF PSYCHOLOGY

1. Psychology deals with the mind and its working, and that the knowledge of psychology helps in reading other people's mind.

2. Psychology is concerned with behavior and while dealing with behavior, it extends to animal behavior.
3. Psychology possesses a well-organized theory, which is supported by the relevant psychological laws and principles.
4. Psychology has its applied aspects in the form of various branches of applied psychology like industrial, legal, clinical and educational psychology.
5. Psychology has established facts, principles and laws of the behavior in the subject; psychology enjoys universal applicability in practical life, other bodies of the knowledge and future researches in its own field.
6. Psychology as a science deals systematically with human behavior, with the motives, feelings, emotions, thoughts and actions of men and women.

Psychology as a Science

1. A science is a body of systemized knowledge that is gathered through careful observations and measurements of events in experimental setup by the scientist to produce the events being studied. Of course, all events studied by a scientist are not necessarily produced experimentally. At times, he/she has to observe the spontaneous events.
2. The psychologist do experiments and make observations, which others can repeat. They obtain data often in the form of quantitative measurements, which others can verify.
3. As a science, psychology is a systematic data from experiments and observations are essential, but from them to make some sense in helping us, understand events that must be organized in some way. Scientific theories are important tools for the organization of observed facts.
4. The most three essential requirements for a field of knowledge to be called science. Firstly, it deals with observable facts, secondly, science is not a mere collection or description of facts, it aims at the explanation of facts, thirdly, every science has its own methods, accordingly to these, a scientist has to choose a problem for investigation.
5. Measurement in psychology is often more difficult, than it is in science such as physics and chemistry, because many of the psychological studies cannot be measured directly by physical scales, e.g. emotion, intelligence and attitudes.

6. Psychology is related to many other sciences such as biological sciences, sociology, philosophy and psychiatry. Its scope is very wide, it has many branches such as general psychology, animal psychology, child psychology, abnormal psychology, clinical psychology and applied psychology.

Psychology as a Behavioral Science

1. Psychology deals with certain aspects of behavior as does anthropology, sociology, economics or political science. All these sciences concern themselves with a specific aspect of behavior.
2. Psychology deals with the general nature of behavior. It does not select a single aspect of behavior like the rest of the behavioral sciences. It pervades the entire range of behavior and the basic principles underlying it.
3. Psychology includes not only the conscious behavior and activities of human mind but also the subconscious and unconscious. Consequently, it covers not only the overt behavior but also the covert behavior involving all the inner experiences and mental processes.
4. An organism like a human being constantly behaves, so also the animals. Psychology as a science of behavior deals with these acts of the organism. The environment means the surroundings objects and circumstances. It may be physical or social in nature.
5. Overt behavior is the most obvious and outwardly expressed form of behavior. It is easily observable. Covert behavior is not so easily observable. The initial activities of feeling, thinking and the like are the examples of covert behavior, while the activities like walking, smiling, hitting, etc. are those overt behaviors.
6. Behavioral sciences are concerned with the observation and explanation of human behavior either in single individual or in groups. Psychology also inter-related with many other biological sciences.

Relation of Psychology with Other Fields of Study

Psychology and biological sciences: These studies gives light on their behavior and are closely related to the study of mental functions.

Psychology and sociology: These deal with the activities of a group of people taken as a whole. It studies traditions, customs, intuitions and other group of behaviors.

Psychology and philosophy: There is a close relationship between the two as both philosophy and psychology attempt to interpret human behavior.

Psychology and psychiatry: These deal with study, diagnosis and treatment of the mentally ill.

SCOPE OF PSYCHOLOGY

Psychology deals with all types of experience in society or private like all phases that emerge in the realism of human life. Psychology discusses the inner dynamics of behavior like motives and emotions. It concerns itself with individual differences in behavior and tries to find out the factors that explain these differences. It also deals with the study of abilities and aptitudes.

Psychologists have also devised appropriate tests for measuring these abilities and aptitudes in people. Psychology also considers the working of the sensory and response mechanism. It discusses the impact of the physical stimuli on sense organs. It also discusses and investigates the working of the sense organs, nervous system, muscles and glands. Social and community psychology deals with individual, family and group for the prevention of illness and promotion of health. It includes various types of group phenomenon like public opinion, propaganda, attitudes, beliefs and crowd behavior.

HISTORY OF PSYCHOLOGY

The subject psychology has a long past, but a short history. The meaning of this statement is simply that humankind has given thought to psychological questions for many centuries. The ancient philosophers wrote at length about psychology. However, psychology as an established and recognized science in universities and colleges, and is less than 100 years old. The date, when psychology became a field of study formally detached from philosophy is generally taken as 1879, the date when Wilhelm Wundt, the principal founder of experimental psychology established, the first psychological laboratory in Leipzig, Germany.

Brief Historical Background of Psychology

Karen Horney (1885–1952): Holistic psychology personality attributes as the result of the interaction between the person and environment.

Edith Jacobson (1897–1978): Object relation theorist. Infants experience of pleasure or displeasure as the core of the relationship with the mother.

Carl Gustav Jung (1875–1961): Analytical psychology. Collective unconscious as consisting of all human kinds.

Kernberg (1928): Borderline personality organization. Several defense mechanisms responsible for rapid alterations of transference.

Søren Kierkegaard (1813–1855): Philosophical theory. Behavior on the basis of response to stimuli.

Melanie Klein (1882–1960): Traditional psychoanalysis. Gratifying experiences reinforce basic trust.

Heinz Kohut (1913–1981): Theories of self-psychology. Patients become aware of their excessive needs for approval and self-gratification.

Jacques Lacan (1901–1981): Intrapsychic concepts of Freud. Primary process of thought is actually uncontrolled free flowing sequences of meaning.

Kurt Lewin (1890–1947): Field theory. Behavior becomes a function of the person and his environment.

Abraham Maslow (1908–1970): Self-actualization theory. The need to understand the totality of a person.

Adolf Meyer (1866–1959): Theory of psychobiology. He introduced the concept of common sense psychiatry disoriented behavior as reaction to genetic, physical, psychological, environmental and social stress.

Gardner Murphy (1895–1979): Parapsychology. He explained the essential stages of personality development such as stage of undifferentiated wholeness, stage of differentiation and stage of integration.

Henry Murray (1893–1988): Personology. It describes the study of human behavior. He focused on motivation, which is a need that is aroused by internal or external stimulation. He developed thematic apperception test (TAT).

Frederick S Perls (1893–1970): Gestalt theory. Behavior represents more than the sum of its parts.

Sandor Rado (1890–1972): Theories of adaptational dynamics disordered behavior by interfering with the organism's ability for self-regulation.

Otto Rank (1884–1957): Theory of birth trauma. The personality is divided into impulses, emotions and will.

Wilhelm Reich (1897–1957): Character armor. The personality that serve as a resistance to self-understanding and change. It is classified into four types; hysterical, compulsive, narcissistic and masochistic character.

Carl Rogers (1902–1987): Person centered theory of personality and psychotherapy. Personality not as a static entity composed of traits and patterns by as a dynamic phenomenon involving every changing communications, relationships and self-concepts.

Skinner BF (1904–1990): Operant learning. Personality was not different from the other behaviors or sets of behaviors; it required maintenance and strengthening.

Harry Stack Sullivan (1892–1949): The total configuration of personality traits is known as the self-system.

SCHOOLS OF PSYCHOLOGY

A 'school' of psychology is a group of individuals, who share a common vision about psychology. This includes a shared view of "How psychology should be defined? What its goals should be? What methods of research are appropriate?"

Structuralism

1. The aim of the school of psychology called structuralism was to analyze conscious experience into its sensory elements.
2. Wilhelm Wundt (1912) had subjects in his laboratory to introspect (look into their own minds) and report the sensory elements experiences such as hearing melodies, seeing paintings and tasting foods.
3. Structuralism did not receive its name from Wundt, but from its critics. Critics of Wundt's approach felt that Wundt was too interested in the static structure of the human mind and not its dynamic quality.

Functionalism

1. Functionalism, in contrast to structuralism, emphasized the changing and dynamic quality of consciousness.
2. The father of functionalism William James (1890) compared the human mind to a river always flowing and changing.
3. Functionalism as its name implies, asserts that consciousness has a function on aim. Functionalism provided an impetus for psychologists, who are interested in applying psychology to industry and education.

Behaviorism

1. Behaviorism came into being in the 1910s with the writings of John B Watson.
2. Watson (1919) claimed that the concept of consciousness was unnecessary for psychology. He thus, attacked at once both structuralism and functionalism.
3. The essential idea in behaviorism is that consciousness cannot be observed. It is completely private and personnel.
4. Watson suggested using more specific concepts such as habits or Pavlov's conditioning reflexes. Watson's aim has to transform psychology from quasi-philosophical study of the mind into valid 'science of behavior'.

Gestalt Psychology

1. Gestalt psychology came into being as a reaction against Wundt's structuralism. It came into prominence in Germany. Simultaneously, behaviorism was gaining attention in America.
2. During 1910s without being aware of one another's development. The father of Gestalt psychology is Max Wertheimer.
3. The essential point of Gestalt psychology is that, it is important to explain everything by analyzing it downward, by always reducing it something, i.e. presumably on a more basic level.

Psychoanalysis

1. The father of psychoanalysis is Sigmund Freud. His personal influence in psychology made itself known over a long period of time, beginning in the later part of the 19th century and ending in the 1930s.

2. Freud argued that motives, ideas and memories often exist in human personality outside of consciousness (awareness).
3. The human mind is like iceberg. The exposed tip represents consciousness. The large region below water level represents the unconscious domain of the mind. Freud argued that the unpleasant or painful ideas are repressed or pushed down into the unconscious.
4. Freud devised a technique called free association for making repressed material available to consciousness. Freud believed that if a neurotic patient could see into the nature of his conflicts, than those conflicts would lose most of their power to make the patient suffer.

Neo-freudian Theories

1. Several contemporary psychoanalysts like Karen Horney, Erich Fromm and Harry Stack Sullivan are all referred to as Neo-freudians.
2. Their theories of personality are essentially revisions of Freuds, while they differ from each other in many specific details and they are similar in that they all emphasized the role of culture in the development of personality rather than biological drives or instincts.
3. According to Harry Stack Sullivan, personality does not exist apart from interpersonal relations. In other words, there is no personality, unless one is interacting with others.

Humanistic Psychology

1. A single individual cannot be named as the father of humanistic psychology. The movement known as humanistic psychology did not become a powerful force in psychology until the 1960s.
2. Humanistic psychology sees the individual's task in life as the making of a series of conscious choices between constructive and destructive alternatives.
3. The humanistic psychology is also termed existential psychology or existential humanistic psychology.

BRANCHES OF PSYCHOLOGY

The science of psychology, since its foundation has grown into different levels, its application is widely used among; the other branches of pure psychology may be included experimental psychology, comparative psychology and physiological psychology. The branch of applied psychology includes clinical psychology, individual psychology, human psychology and educational psychology, etc.

Subfields of Psychology

Physiological Psychology

Physiological psychology is a branch, which experimentally investigates the physiological basis of behavior, including the anatomical structure and physiological processes, which are related to psychological events and mental functions. It often uses operative technique, investigating the functions of brain for instance, by removing portions of the brain tissue and noting the effect on behavior.

Experimental Psychology

1. Experimental psychology that studies the process of sensing, perceiving, learning and thinking about the mind.
2. It is the observation of concomitant variations and interpretation of the concomitance as cause and effects. In this method, a systematic controlled scientific methodology in the investigation of psychological phenomena is used.
3. The systematic presentation of the methodology and the results are usually within the context of a laboratory. The work of experimental psychology overlaps with that of the focus of biopsychology as well as that done by other types of psychologist.

Developmental Psychology

1. Developmental psychology deals with the changes in behavior that accompanies change in age from conception to death.
2. Since, behavior and abilities change most rapidly during the early years, child psychology has traditionally received the more attention from developmental psychologist.
3. Developmental psychology has both pure and applied aspects.

Social and Personality Psychology

1. Social psychology is the study of the individuals in the growth and relationship of group to one another. Thus, social psychology considers the psychological inter-relations of people forming families, crowds, societies and mobs and of the leader with his followers.
2. It includes the study of the formation of group attitudes and opinions. It is thus, forced into a consideration of social and national conflict or race prejudice and similar manifestation of the inter-relations of the conflicting needs of many individuals.
3. Personality psychology is concerned with individual people and administration of psychological tests extensively. The personality psychologist is interested in understanding the non-deviant or normal cases.

Clinical Psychology

1. Clinical psychology is the practical application of dynamic and normal psychology to the problem of human adjustments.
2. Clinical psychology is devoted to study, diagnosis and treat behavior disorders. It is the largest subfield of psychology.
3. A clinical psychology is well-trained in the etiology of causes, of the various forms of abnormal behavior such as psychoneurosis, psychosis, etc. and also trained in various methods of diagnosis of abnormal behavior through psychological testing.

Counseling Psychology

1. Counseling psychology is related to clinical psychology, but different in that the problem it deals with is generally of less serious in nature.
2. Personal, vocational and educational guidance are provided. Psychologists, who are well-versed in the different diagnosis and treatment of such minor behavior problems, are known as psychological counselors.
3. The counseling psychologist deals with individuals' milder emotional and personal problems. He also practices psychotherapy, as well as depending upon the severity of the problems.

School Psychology

1. The counseling psychologist who administers tests and guides individual students is generally called school psychologist.
2. The school psychologist is on specializing in problems associated with elementary and secondary, an educational system who utilizes psychological concepts and methods in programs or reactions, which attempt to improve learning conditions for students.

Industrial-organizational Psychology

1. Industrial-organizational psychology is concerned with the psychology of the workplace. Specifically, it considers issues such as productivity, job satisfaction and decision-making.
2. The first application of psychology to the problems of industries and organizations was the use of intelligence and aptitude tests in selecting employees.
3. Now, private and public organizations also apply psychology to problems of management and employee training, to supervision of personnel, to improving communication within the organizations, to counseling employees and to alleviating industrial conflict.

Consumer Psychology

1. Consumer psychology considers peoples buying habits and the effects of advertising on behavior.
2. Consumer psychologist to research on consumer attitude toward the company's product.
3. As a subfield of psychology, in this the psychology principles are applied to practical problems of consumer products.

Health Psychology

1. Health psychology explores the relationships between psychological factors and physical ailments or disease.
2. For instance, health psychologist are interested in long-term stress can affect physical health.
3. They are also concerned with identifying ways of promoting behavior related to good health or discouraging unhealthy behavior such as smoking.

Cross-cultural Psychology

1. Cross-cultural psychology investigates the similarities and differences in psychological functioning in various cultural and ethnic groups.
2. Psychologist specializing in cross-cultural issues investigates, the ways in which people in different culture attribute their academic successes or failures leading to differences in scholastic performance.

Forensic Psychology

1. Forensic psychology is another emerging specialty that works hand with the legal, court and connectional system.
2. Forensic psychologist assist police in a variety ways, from developing personality profiles of criminal offenders to helping law enforcement personnel understand problems like family conflict and substance abuse.
3. They may also assist judges and parole officers in making decisions about the disposition of convicted offenders.

METHODS OF PSYCHOLOGY

The scientific method is emphasized as the basis for investigation. The founding of Wundt's laboratory marked the beginning of the formal application of the scientific method to problems in psychology. This method is neither identified with any particular kind of equipment nor associated exclusively with specific research procedures.

Definition

Method is defined as a systematic procedure involved in the investigation of facts and concepts. It also uses special techniques in psychology such as, experimental method or the clinical method used to collect facts.

Methods

The methods used in psychology are as follows:

1. Descriptive techniques.
2. Introspection.
3. Case history method.
4. Naturalistic observation.

5. Survey.
6. Experimental method.
7. Rating scale and checklist.
8. Genetic or development method.

Descriptive Techniques

a. Introspective method, naturalistic observations, case history or case studies and survey can be clustered together as descriptive techniques.
b. These methods provide different way to describe behavior, without any attempt to interfere with the behavior under study.
c. Descriptive techniques can provide useful information about, how different techniques can provide useful information about how different events behaviors are related to each other.

Introspection

a. Introspection is one of the oldest methods used for investigating consciousness. It is a process of analyzing a conscious experience by reporting the sensory qualities of the stimuli that are expressed.
b. The word introspection means 'to look within'. In introspection, subjects were presented with a particular stimulus or task and asked to describe their mental state as thoroughly as possible.
c. This method is used to observe the individual, analyze and reports his own feelings, thought or all that passes in his mind during the course of a mental act or experience.
d. This method cannot be used by children or animals of mental defectives because, they cannot introspect. By the early 20th century, psychologist recognizes the inadequacies of introspection.

Case History Method

a. The detailed study of a single individual's behavior over an extended period of time is called case history or case study.
b. In a typical case study, the researcher presents a detailed description of the personality and behavioral characteristics of an individual.
c. The goal of this procedure is to provide a detailed description of person overtime as opposed to the naturalistic observation.

Naturalistic Observation

a. Naturalistic observation is a method within the descriptive research category on a topic. Just as the name states, phenomena of interest are systematically observed as they occur in nature.
b. The researcher observes behavior in its natural setting and systematically. The systematic observation means that, from the wide array of ongoing behavioral interaction, the researcher selects the focus and categories of his/her observations.
c. The systematic observation, means of the naturalistic observation method is probably, the oldest and in some ways most basic form of scientific research.

Surveys

a. Surveys study, large and small population of selecting representative samples chosen from the population to discover the relative incidence, distribution and inter-relation of psychological and sociological variables.
b. In survey research, the researcher simply collects data about psychological and sociological variables or characteristics of a sample that represents a known population in natural setting.
c. The survey research is concerned with conditions or relationships that exist, opinions that hold processes, which are going on, effects are evident or trends that are developing.
d. That survey research, which involves samples, is usually called 'sample survey'.

Experimental Method

a. The experimental method is the technique of discovering information by means of experimentation.
b. An experiment is a series of observations, carried out under controlled conditions for testing a hypothesis.
c. In using the experimental method, the researcher systematically manipulates one or more variables to determine how those variables affect behavior.
d. In an experiment, the variable that is manipulated is called independent variable, while the behavior that is measured is called dependent variable.
e. In the experiment method, the experimenter has complete control over the laboratory situation. The extraneous variances

are controlled. The measurements in a laboratory are more precise, because they are more with precision instruments.

Rating Scale and Checklist

a. There are commonly used devices of observing and evaluating personality of behavior traits. In rating scales, we rate on individual on the possession or absence of certain traits on a certain scale.
b. The measurement scale has 5 degree of the trait to be rated. This is a five-point scale. Some scales have 3 or 7 degree.
c. In a checklist examiners may be provided with a list of traits or qualities and may be asked to point out or checkup ones that applies to particular persons.

Genetic or Developmental Method

a. This method seeks to find out the causes of a complicated behavior in its simple beginning. It assumes that a full appreciation of each behavior patterns of an adult requires the study of simple behavior patterns.
b. This simple behavior pattern grows more complex gradually, as the individual grows in age. For example, if we are interested in understanding the learning behavior of an adult, we should begin with the learning behavior in his/her preadolescence and in the light of these, arrive at some conclusions about the learning behaviors in adulthood.

PSYCHOLOGICAL CONCEPTS OF NURSING

Psychology seeks to understand why people behave, think and feel the way they do, individually and in groups, in all areas of life include change behaviors to enhance well-being and quality of life. This can be seen to link very closely, with what nurses do. Nurses and psychologists seek to understand the health needs of the people they work with, but also to change their behaviors, thoughts and feelings to enhance the well-being of the person, not only at this moment but also for the future. At times, nurses need to provide very basic care for the people they work with, but they are always looking to develop the person's ability to be more independent in any area of their life.

Nursing Application Toward Psychological Concepts

1. The study of psychology will help the student nurse to appreciate the necessity for changing the environment or surroundings.
2. Psychology will help the nurse to understand, the close relationship between body, mind and spirit.
3. Psychology will help to understand other people; she will learn why others differ from her in their likes and dislikes, in their interests and abilities or in their reactions to others.

Nurses can use psychological research and theories to enhance their nursing practice and most nursing practice has a foundation in psychology, sociology or biology. Nursing now has developed its own unique body of knowledge, but other sciences can still enhance nurses' understanding and practice.

When the nursing field incorporates psychology, it begins to resemble a field called biopsychology. Biopsychology attempts to understand behavior through biological theories. Nursing already has a biological base and when a nurse attempts to understand patients beyond a biological level, biopsychology begins to emerge. The expansion of fields like biopsychology continues to be a key part in nursing and nurse training.

Nurses who want to integrate more psychology into their practice might choose to work as a psychiatric nurse, which may include taking care of suicidal patients, bipolar patients or patients with other forms of mental illness. In this field, an understanding of psychology is very important, as well as a solid medical background, since among psychiatrists and psychologists, the psychiatric nurse may be the only one with a general medical background. Nurses who want to focus on using even more psychology into their practice would have to pursue a master's degree and become a mental health nurse practitioner, who would be able to diagnose illness and prescribe medication and other treatments.

CONCLUSION

Psychology is a young science, a study of psychology can help to understand the self in better, understand other people, improve situations by helping others solve problems and understand the close relationship of body, mind and spirit.

Literary meaning of psychology is the science of mind. Some others have accepted it, as the science of consciousness. Both of these meanings are not the appropriate of psychology, as the modern psychology does not recognize mind and gives more importance to the mental processes or modes. According to modern concept, psychology is the study of human behavior. It includes stimulated behavior and internal mechanism. Psychology deals with the mind and its working and that the knowledge of psychology helps in reading other people's minds. Scope of psychology is very extensive. Behavior is associated with life and psychology with behavior. It studies all normal, abnormal, child, adult, man and animals and also compares them.

SUGGESTED READING

1. Anderson JR. Cognitive Psychology and its Implications, 5th edition. New York: Worth Publishers; 2000.
2. Banerjee JC. Fundamentals of Modern Psychology. Calcutta: Asia Publishing House; 1965.
3. Charles G Morris, Albert A Maisto. Understanding Psychology. New Jersey: Prentice Hall Inc; 2001.
4. Ciccarelli SK, Meyer GE. Psychology. Upper Saddle River. NJ: Prentice Hall; 2006. p. 4.
5. Clifford T Morgan. An Introduction to Psychology. New Delhi: Tata McGraw-Hill Publishing Co Ltd; 1978.
6. Gross R. Psychology: The Science of Mind and Behavior, 4th edition. London: Hodder and Stoughton; 2001.
7. Morgan, King. Introduction to Psychology. New Delhi: Tata McGraw-Hill Publishing Co Ltd; 1993.
8. Robert A Baron. Psychology. New Delhi: Prentice-Hall of India (P) Ltd; 2001.
9. Rogers CR. The necessary and sufficient conditions of therapeutic personality change. Journal of Consulting Psychology. 1957;21(2):95-103.
10. Rosenzweig MR, Breedlove SM, Watson NV. Biological Psychology, An Introduction to Behavioural and Cognitive Neuroscience, 4th edition. Sunderland, MA: Sinauer Associates, Inc; 2005. p. 137.

REVIEW QUESTIONS

1. Define psychology. Explain the nature of psychology.
2. Discuss psychology as a science.

3. Explain the scope of psychology.
4. Discuss in brief the history of psychology.
5. Describe the branches of psychology.
6. Explain the various methods of psychology.
7. Write short notes on introspection and experimental method.

CHAPTER 2 *Sensation, Attention and Perception*

LEARNING OBJECTIVES

1. Definitions.
2. Sensory process: normal and abnormal.
3. Attention and distraction: contributory factors.
4. Characteristics of perception: normal and abnormal.
5. To understand the meaning of perception.
6. To learn the differences between sensation and perception.
7. To understand the principles and organization of perception.
8. To explain the factors influencing perception.
9. To learn about extrasensory perception.
10. To understand the errors of perception.

SENSATION

A term sensation commonly used to refer to the subjective experience resulting from stimulation of a sense organ, for instance, a sensation of warm, taste and color. As a general scientific category, the study of sensation is the study of the operation of the senses. Sense receptors are the means by which information presented as one form of energy, for example, light is converted to information in the form used by the nervous system, i.e. impulses traveling along nerve fibers. Each sense has mechanisms and characteristics peculiar to itself, but all display the phenomena of absolute threshold, differential threshold and adaptation. Until sufficient stimulation impinges on a receptor, the presence of a stimulus cannot be detected. The quantity of stimulation required is known as the absolute threshold. Until a sufficient change occurs in some aspect of a stimulus, the change cannot be detected. The magnitude of the change required is called the differential threshold. Under steady stimulation, there is a decrease in sensitivity of the corresponding sense, as indicated by a shift in the absolute threshold and in the magnitude of sensation. After the stimulation ceases, sensitivity increases. An obvious example of visual adaptation occurs when one goes from bright to dim surroundings or vice versa.

Definitions

1. Sensations can be defined as the passive process of bringing information from the outside world into the body and to the brain. The process is passive in the sense that we do not have to be consciously engaging in a 'sensing' process.
2. Sensation is defined as the process by which our sensory receptors and nervous system receive and represent stimulus energies from our environment.

Meaning and Concepts

In psychology, sensation is the first stage in the biochemical and neurological events that begins with the impinging of a stimulus upon the receptor cells of a sensory organ, which then leads to perception, the mental state that is reflected in statements like "I see a uniformly blue wall."

A sensation that might lead to that statement could include the excitation of cone cells in the retina, spatially varying in the proportion of 'blue' and 'green' cone excitation due to portions of the wall receiving different proportions of yellowish artificial and bluish skylight. It is common for these variations to be compensated for, within the brain, so that the non-uniform sensation yields a perception of uniform color (Fig. 2.1).

Sensation is the process by which our senses gather information and send it to the brain. A large amount of information is being sensed at any one time such as room temperature, brightness of the lights, someone talking, a distant train or the smell of perfume. With all this information coming into our senses, the majority of our world never gets recognized. We do not notice radio waves, X-rays or the microscopic parasites crawling on our skin. We do not sense all the odors around us or taste every individual spice in our gourmet dinner. We only sense those things we are able to, since, we do not have the sense of smell like a bloodhound or the sense of sight like a hawk; our thresholds are different from these animals and often even from each other.

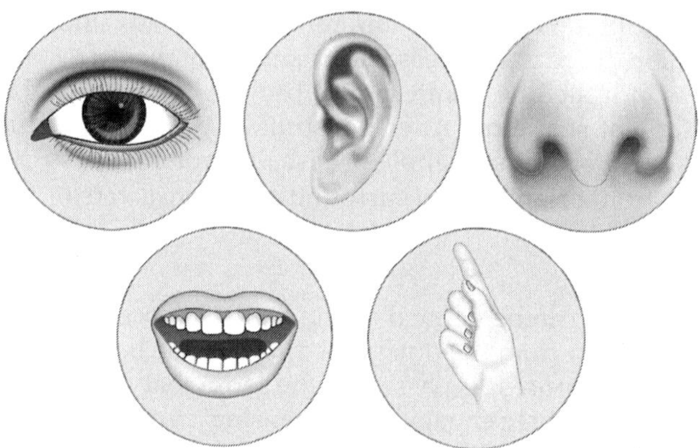

Fig. 2.1: Sense organs

Steps Involved in Sensation

There are four essential steps involved if stimulation has to lead to sensation (Floyd L Ruch, 1970). If any one of these four steps is missing, there will be no sensation at all.

1. *Stimulus:* It must be applied internally or externally. A stimulus is some kind of radiant, mechanical or other energy, which activates the receptors of the concerned sense organ.
2. *Receptor cell:* The stimulus must stir certain receptor cells or nerve endings into activity. Usually a receptor cell is activated only by a particular form of energy. For example, visual receptors are stimulated by light waves; auditory receptors are stimulated by sound waves and so on.
3. *Transmission of impulses:* The neural impulses released must travel from the receptor cells to brain through nerves.
4. *Sensory arousement:* Activity must be aroused in the sensory arouse of the brain, proceeding conscious sensations. Each sensory activity has its own special conscious sensations. Each sensory activity has its own special areas in the cerebrum or brain.

Classification

One convenient method of classifying sensations is to categorize them according to the location of the receptor. On this basis, receptors may be classified as exteroceptors, visceroceptors and proprioceptors.

1. Exteroceptors, which are located near the surface of the body, provide information about the external environment. They receive stimuli from outside the body and transmit sensations of hearing, sight, touch, pressure, temperature and pain on the skin.
2. Visceroceptors, which are located in blood vessels and viscera, provide information about the internal environment. This information arises within the body and may be felt as pain, taste, fatigue, hunger, thirst and nausea.
3. Proprioceptors, which are located in muscles, tendons and joints, allows us to feel sensations of position, movement, equilibrium and tension of muscles and joints through the stretching or movement of parts, where these receptors are located.

General Characteristics

The sensation, whether it is visual or auditory or gustatory or any other form, has certain fundamental characteristics common to all, some of them are given in the Table 2.1.

Table 2.1: Characteristics of sensation

Sl No	*Characteristics*	*Description*
1.	Stimulation	Sensation is a change brought about in us by a stimulus. We may call it as stimulation. It makes us aware of certain facts either in the world outside or within us. They come in the form of air waves, light waves or heat waves, etc.
2.	Intensity	Within each modality, sensations vary in intensity from low to high. Thus, we experience mild pain or severe pain. For sensation to be effective, it must possess some amount of intensity. It should not be very faint or very intense. For example, a very faint sound may not be heard or very faint light may not be seen. On the other hand, if it is very intense beyond certain limits it gives raise to some other experience than what it has to. For example, sound of very high intensity causes pain in the ear instead of causing the experience of sound.
3.	Limen	The point below which, a sensation has no effect is known as limen or lower limit. The point above which its effect is painful is known as upper limit. In between these two limits there is much sensory intensity.

Contd...

Contd...

Sl No	*Characteristics*	*Description*
4.	Threshold	The upper and lower limits are known as the threshold. The stimulus, which is below the threshold, causes no response. It is known as subliminal stimulus. Two or more subliminal stimuli, combining together, may produce a single strong reaction. This phenomenon is known as the summation of stimuli.
5.	Latency period	It is the time that lapses between the stimuli presented and the responses shown. The stimulus takes a certain length of time, i.e. roughly 0.005–0.1 second to arouse a sense organ. Than it takes time to arouse nerve fibers that lead to the brain. Further, the brain connections, the motor nerves and the muscles also take time to respond. Thus, there is bound to be lapse of time between the awareness of the sensation and consequent imitation of action. Usually the response and the stimulus appear to take place simultaneously, but there is always some lapse of time, which is known as latency period. This can be measured by reaction time apparatus.
6.	Duration	If a stimulus is to be effective, it must be presented for a certain length of time. It should be neither too short nor too long. If it is too short, it does not act upon the sense organ effectively and produce the desired sensation. If it is too long, the concentration sense organ either gets fatigue or their will be adopted in the sense organ and hence there will be no sensation and no response. For example, continuous presentation of an odor or sound for a long period causes negative adaptation and will not provoke the expected response.
7.	Extensity	Extensity refers to the amount of space that the stimulus occupies. In fact, many sensations will have extensity. Bigger stimulus occupies larger space and smaller stimulus occupies smaller areas. For example, hot water bath occupies larger space in the skin and a pinprick occupies smaller spaces in the skin. High intensity of sound occupies larger areas of the basilar membrane and low intensity occupies smaller area of the basilar membranes.
8.	Quality	Every sensation has quality in addition to quantity. The quality tells us the kind of sensation and the quantity refers to the amount of sensation. For example, two colors of same saturation value and brightness values may still differ in color. Similarly tones of different instruments, though they are equal in intensity and frequency of sound waves differ in their tonal quality, which is distinguishable.

Contd...

Contd...

Sl No	*Characteristics*	*Description*
9.	Absolute threshold	For any sensation to be aroused, the stimulus (light, sound, touch, etc.) must have a minimum intensity, called absolute threshold. The absolute threshold is different for each individuals; it also changes from time to time for the same person. Absolute threshold for the sense can be lower or higher in time of illness and fatigue. When we are much tried, our senses need fewer or greater stimuli to arouse them. A moderate sound may seem very loud, a weak light or small wrinkle in the sheet may irritate an ill person. Absolute threshold varies depending upon the individual's physical conditions under which the observations are made.
10.	Difference threshold	Just as there must be a certain minimum amount of stimulation to evoke a sensory experience, so there must also be certain magnitude of difference between two stimuli before one can be distinguished from the other. The minimum amount of stimulation necessary to tell two stimuli apart is known as the difference threshold.

Sense Organs and Their Functions

Visual Sense

The eye is the organ of vision. It has a complex structure consisting of a transparent lens that focusses light on the retina. The retina is covered with two basic types of light-sensitive cells—rods and cones. The cone cells are sensitive to color and are located in the part of the retina called the fovea, where the light is focused by the lens. The rod cells are not sensitive to color, but have greater sensitivity to light than the cone cells. These cells are located around the fovea and are responsible for peripheral vision and night vision. The eye is connected to the brain through the optic nerve. The point of this connection is called the 'blind spot' because it is insensitive to light. Experiments have shown that the back of the brain maps the visual input from the eyes (Fig. 2.2).

The brain combines the input of our two eyes into a single three-dimensional image. In addition, even though the image on the retina is upside-down because of the focusing action of the lens, the brain compensates and provides the right-side-up perception. Experiments have been done with subjects fitted with prisms that invert the images. The subjects go through an initial period of great confusion, but subsequently they perceive the images as right-side up.

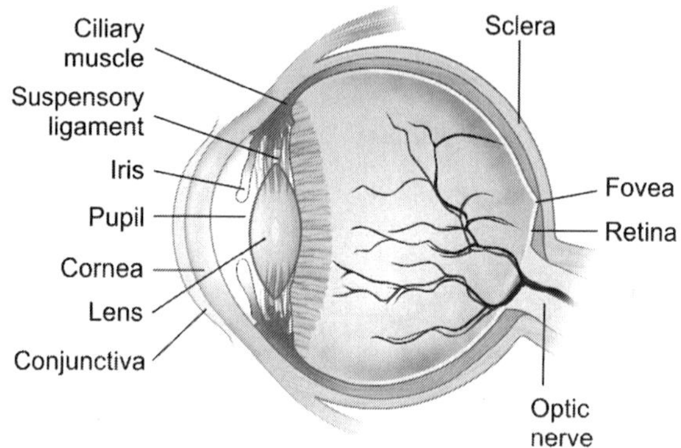

Fig. 2.2: Organ for vision (eyeball)

The range of perception of the eye is phenomenal. In the dark, a substance produced by the rod cells increases the sensitivity of the eye, so that it is possible to detect very dim light. In strong light, the iris contracts reducing the size of the aperture that admits light into the eye and a protective obscure substance reduces the exposure of the light-sensitive cells. The spectrum of light to which the eye is sensitive varies from the red to the violet. Lower electromagnetic frequencies in the infrared are sensed as heat, but cannot be seen. Higher frequencies in the ultraviolet and beyond cannot be seen either, but can be sensed as tingling of the skin or eyes depending on the frequency. The human eye is not sensitive to the polarization of light, i.e. light that oscillates on a specific plane. Bees, on the other hand, are sensitive to polarized light and have a visual range that extends into the ultraviolet. Some kinds of snakes have special infrared sensors that enable them to hunt in absolute darkness using only the heat emitted by their prey. Birds have a higher density of light-sensing cells than humans do in their retinas and therefore, have higher visual activity.

Hearing Sense

The ear is the organ of hearing. The outer ear protrudes away from the head and is cup-shaped to direct sounds toward the tympanic membrane, which transmits vibrations to the inner ear through a series of small bones in the middle ear called the malleus, incus and stapes. The inner ear or cochlea, is a spiral-shaped chamber covered internally by nerve fibers that react to the vibrations and transmit impulses to the brain via the auditory nerve. The brain combines the input of our two ears to determine the direction and distance of sounds (Fig. 2.3).

The inner ear has a vestibular system formed by three semicircular canals that are approximately at right angles to each other and responsible for the sense of balance and spatial orientation. The inner ear has chambers filled with a viscous fluid and small particles (otoliths) containing calcium carbonate. The movement of these particles over small hair cells in the inner ear sends signals to the brain that are interpreted as motion and acceleration.

The human ear can perceive frequencies from 16 cycles per second, which is a very deep bass, to 28,000 cycles per second, which is a very high pitch. Bats and dolphins can detect frequencies higher than 100,000 cycles per second. The human ear can detect pitch changes as small as 300th of 1 percent of the original frequency in some frequency ranges.

Some people have 'perfect pitch', which is the ability to map a tone precisely on the musical scale without reference to an external standard. It is estimated that less than 1 in 10,000 people have perfect pitch, but speakers of tonal languages like Vietnamese and

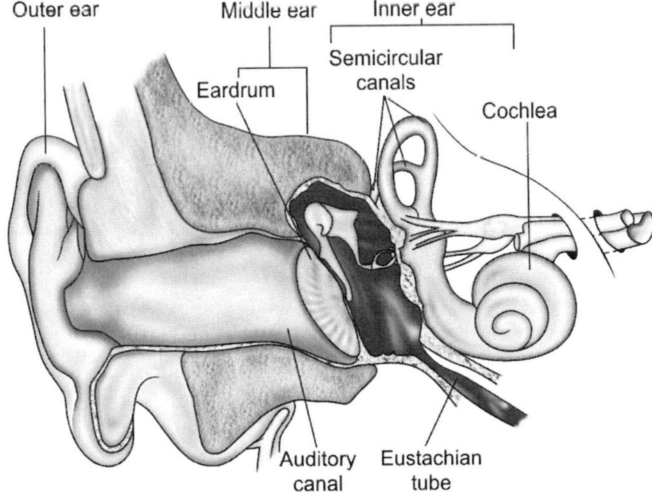

Fig. 2.3: Ear (hearing)

Mandarin show remarkably precise absolute pitch in reading out lists of words. It is because pitch is an essential feature in conveying the meaning of words in tone languages. The Eguchi method teaches perfect pitch to children starting before they are 4 years old. After the age of 7 years, the ability to recognize notes does not improve much.

Gustatory

Taste or gustation is the ability to detect sensory changes in the tongue through the use of taste buds, situated deep into the papillae. Interestingly, the sense of gustation has multiple sensory systems, which play an important role in helping to chew the food, sense the taste and help in swallowing. These include the taste buds, the sense of touch in the structures of the mouth and digestive system, chemical sensation of irritation in the trigeminal nerve system and unique receptors for sensing the properties of water located at the rear of the oral cavity (Fig. 2.4).

The receptors for taste called taste buds are situated chiefly in the tongue, but they are also located in the roof of the mouth and near the pharynx. They are able to detect four basic tastes: salt, sweet, bitter and sour.

The tongue also can detect a sensation called 'umami' from taste receptors sensitive to amino acids. Generally, the taste buds close to

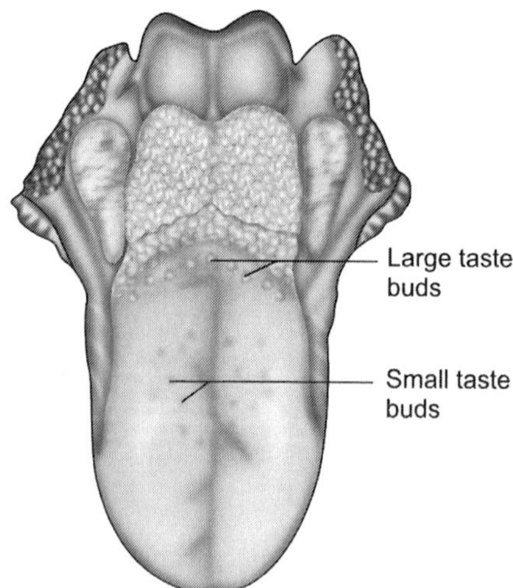

Fig. 2.4: Tongue (taste)

the tip of the tongue are sensitive to sweet tastes, whereas those in the back of the tongue are sensitive to bitter tastes. The taste buds on top and on the side of the tongue are sensitive to salty and sour tastes. At the base of each taste bud, there is a nerve, which sends the sensations to the brain. The sense of taste functions in coordination with the sense of smell. The number of taste buds varies substantially from individual to individual, but greater numbers increase sensitivity. Women, in general, have a greater number of taste buds than men. As in the case of color blindness, some people are insensitive to some tastes.

Olfactory

Smell or olfaction, is received by the olfactory bulb and the connection to the brain by the olfactory nerve, the first cranial nerve of the brain, just after the nasal turbinates of the nose warm, strain and filter the air (Fig. 2.5).

The nose is the organ responsible for the sense of smell. The cavity of the nose is lined with mucous membranes that have smell receptors connected to the olfactory nerve. The smells themselves consist of vapors of various substances. The smell receptors interact with the molecules of these vapors and transmit the sensations to

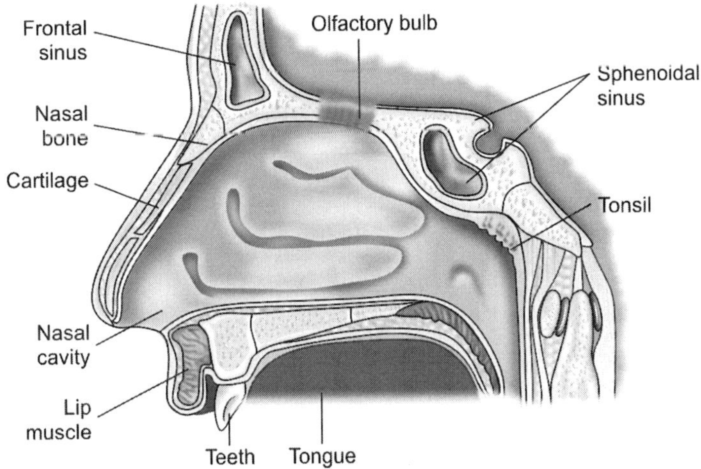

Fig. 2.5: Olfactory bulb (smell)

the brain. The nose also has a structure called the vomeronasal organ whose function has not been determined, but it is suspected of being sensitive to pheromones that influence the reproductive cycle. The smell receptors are sensitive to seven types of sensations that can be characterized as camphor, musk, flower, mint, ether, acrid and putrid. The sense of smell is sometimes temporarily lost when a person has a cold. Dogs have a sense of smell that is many times more sensitive than man's.

Skin (Touch)

The sense of touch is distributed throughout the body. Nerve endings in the skin and other parts of the body transmit sensations to the brain. Some parts of the body have a larger number of nerve endings and therefore, are more sensitive (Fig. 2.6).

Four kinds of touch sensations can be identified: Cold, heat, contact and pain. Hairs on the skin magnify the sensitivity and act as an early warning system for the body. The fingertips and the sexual organs have the greatest concentration of nerve endings.

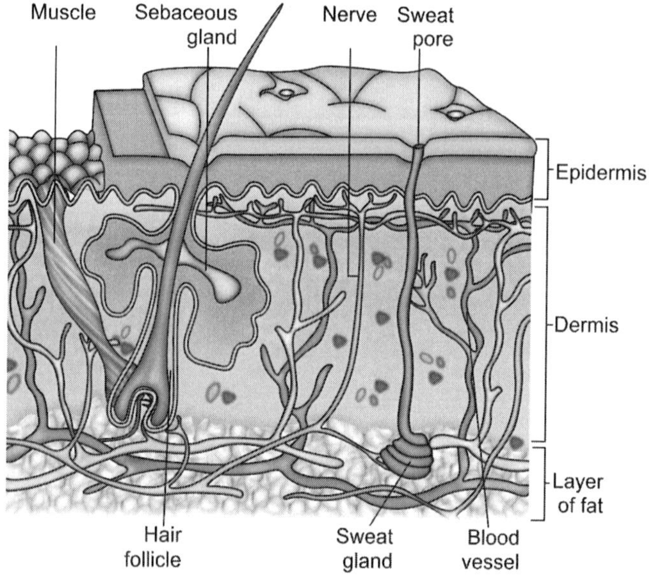

Fig. 2.6: Skin (touch)

The sexual organs have 'erogenous zones' that when stimulated start a series of endocrine reactions and motor responses resulting in orgasm.

Beyond the Five Sense Organs

In addition to sight, smell, taste, touch and hearing, humans also have awareness of balance (equilibrioception), pressure, temperature (thermoception), pain (nociception) and motion. All of which may involve the coordinated use of multiple sensory organs. The sense of balance is maintained by a complex interaction of visual inputs, the proprioceptive sensors (which are affected by gravity and stretch sensors found in muscles, skin and joints), the inner ear vestibular system and the central nervous system (CNS). Disturbances occurring in any part of the balance system or even within the brain's integration of inputs can cause the feeling of dizziness or unsteadiness.

Kinesthesia

Kinesthesia is the precise awareness of muscle and joint movement that allows us to coordinate our muscles when we walk, talk and use our hands. It is the sense of kinesthesia that enables us to touch the tip of our nose with our eyes closed or to know, which part of the body we should scratch when we itch.

Synesthesia

Some people experience a phenomenon called synesthesia in which one type of stimulation evokes the sensation of another. For example, the hearing of a sound may result in the sensation of the visualization of a color or a shape may be sensed as a smell. Synesthesia is hereditary and it is estimated that it occurs in 1 out of 1,000 individuals with variations of type and intensity. The most common forms of synesthesia link numbers or letters with colors.

Loss of Sensation

Many types of sense loss occur due to a dysfunctional sensation process, whether it is ineffective receptors, nerve damage or cerebral impairment. Unlike agnosia, these impairments are due to damages prior to the perception process.

Vision Loss

Degrees of vision loss vary dramatically, although, the International classification of disease (ICD-9) released in 1979 categorized them into three tiers: normal vision, low vision and blindness. Two significant causes of vision loss due to sensory failures include media opacity and optic nerve diseases, although hypoxia and retinal disease can also lead to blindness. Most causes of vision loss can cause varying degrees of damage, from total blindness to a negligible effect. Media opacity occurs in the presence of opacities in the eye media, distorting and/or blocking the image prior to contact with the photoreceptor cells. Vision loss due to media opacity often results despite correctly functioning retinal receptors. Optic nerve diseases such as optic neuritis or retrobulbar neuritis lead to dysfunction in the afferent nerve pathway—once the signal has been correctly transmitted from retinal photoreceptors.

Hearing Loss

Similarly to vision loss, hearing loss can vary from full or partial inability to detect some or all frequencies of sound, which can typically be heard by members of their species. For humans, this range is approximately 20 Hz to 20 kHz at ~6.5 dB, although a 10 dB correction is often allowed for the elderly. Primary causes of hearing loss due to an impaired sensory system include long-term exposure to environmental noise, which can damage the mechanoreceptors responsible for receiving sound vibrations as well as multiple diseases such as human immunodeficiency virus (HIV) or meningitis, which damage the cochlea and auditory nerve, respectively.

Anosmia

Primary causes of anosmia, a loss of smell—due to sensory damage involve the death of olfactory receptor neurons, often from nasal polyps or upper respiratory tract infections as well as damage to the olfactory nerve, often from hypothyroidism or physical trauma. Unfortunately, anosmia is strongly correlated with a loss of taste.

Somatosensory Loss

Insensitivity to somatosensory stimuli such as heat, cold, touch and pain, are most commonly a result of a more general physical impairment associated with paralysis. Damage to the spinal cord or other major nerve fiber may lead to a termination of both afferent and efferent signals to varying areas of the body, causing both a loss of touch and a loss of motor coordination. Other types of somatosensory loss include hereditary sensory and neuropathy (HSAN), which consists of ineffective afferent neurons with fully functioning efferent neurons; essentially, motor movement without somatosensation.

Ageusia

Taste loss can vary from true ageusia, a complete loss of taste/ to hypogeusia, a partial loss of taste to dysgeusia/a distortion or alteration of taste. The primary cause of ageusia involves damage to the lingual nerve, which receives the stimuli from taste buds for the front two-third of the tongue or the glossopharyngeal nerve, which acts similarly for the back third. Damage may be due to neurological disorders such as Bell's palsy or multiple sclerosis as well as infectious diseases such as meningoencephalopathy. Other causes include a vitamin B deficiency as well as taste bud death due to acidic/spicy foods, radiation and/or tobacco use.

Blind Spot

Blind spot is a small area in each eye, which is completely blind. The area is completely free from rods and cones and hence it is not sensitive to visualize stimulation. It is located in the place where the optic nerves leave the retina to the visual cortex.

ATTENTION

We are constantly being exposed to an extensive environment. Stimuli impinging upon us at a given moment are beyond exhaustive enlistment. It is a practical impossibility for a man to take note of all these stimuli collectively. Hence, he selects single stimuli or a few stimuli for observation. This purposive selection of stimuli for observation is called attention. During attention, there is a mobilization of various parts of the body muscles and sense organs toward the object of attention. That is why attention is often described as a process of adjustment of the entire body.

Meaning

1. Attention is the focusing of consciousness on a particular object or idea at a particular time, to the exclusion of all other objects or ideas.
2. Attention is a selective mental activity; it constantly shifts from one object to another or from one aspect of the situation to another. The process of attention involves motor adjustments on the part of the person who is attending.
3. Out of attention is controlled and directed by the intensity of the stimulus as well as a variation in intensity.
4. Attention is the chief characteristic of the conscious mind and is essential to acquiring knowledge.
5. The specific portion, which is selected for clear perception is called the focus of attention. Remaining part of the field is called the margin of attention.
6. Attention is not merely a cognitive function, but is essentially determined by emotional and conational factors of interest, attitude and striving.

Definitions

1. Attention is the process of getting an object or thought clearly before the mind. —*Ross*
2. Attention is the concentration of consciousness upon one object rather than upon another. —*Dumville*
3. Attention is being keenly alive to some specific factor in our environment. It is a preparatory adjustment for response. —*Morgan and Gilliland*

Importance

Attention is the focus of consciousness, which is compared with a stream that flows constantly. All our thoughts, sensation, ideas and experience constitute this stream of consciousness. Attention enables the individual to gain these experiences. It also involves specific physical adjustments. When we see an attentive class with pin-drop silence, we can have picture of such adjustments, which help attention. These physical adjustments are necessary for bringing out the importance of attention.

Firstly, attention increases efficiency. Woodworth shows the familiar instances of readiness or preparedness for action in the military command of 'attention' and the athletic call of 'ready'.

These signals bring about an increased state of motor readiness for responding very quickly to the instruction, 'go'!

Secondly, attention improves sensory discrimination. Like a bright searchlight, it shows the details of the landscape. All objects given attention are shown prominent or standout more prominently. They enter into the focus of consciousness and thus sensory discrimination is improved by attention.

Thirdly, attention is useful for acquisition of skill. The typist, the cyclist or the cricket player pays attention to the hands and movements, for coordination and control. When the skill is adequately developed, such attention is no longer required.

Lastly, attention is helpful for remembering. When attention is paid to certain specific areas or objects, concentration helps to know the details and retain them accurately. Other things, which are not properly attended, to be not remembered well and as such are forgotten as soon as possible.

Some Common Functions

1. Attention helps in bringing mental alertness and preparedness.
2. Attention helps in our awareness or consciousness of our environment.
3. It makes us better equipped for distinguishing or discriminating the object of attention from others.
4. Attention acts as a reinforcement of sensory process and help in the better organization of the perceptual field for the maximum clarity and understanding of the object or phenomenon.
5. Attention helps in providing proper deep concentration by focusing one's consciousness upon one object at a time rather than two.

Types

Non-volitional/Involuntary Attention

1. This type of attention is aroused without the play or will.
2. Non-volitional attention can be aroused by our instincts as also by our sentiments.
3. Here, we attend to an object or an idea without making any conscious efforts on our parts.
4. Example for involuntary attention is mother's attention toward her crying child, attention toward the members of the opposite sex, sudden loud noise, bright colors, etc.

5. Involuntary attention does not require any conscious effort on our part; we cannot ignore the stimulus because of its intensity.

Volitional or Voluntary Attention

1. Voluntary attention demands the conscious efforts on our part. A habit is a learned mode of behaving that is relatively fixed and it reliably occurs in certain situations. Frequent repetition or physiological exposure that shows itself in regularity of response acquires a behavior pattern.
2. Volitional attention is further subdivided into two categories: implicit volitional attention and explicit volitional attention.
3. Implicit volitional attention is single actor volition is sufficient to bring about attention.
4. Explicit volitional attention is obtained by repeated acts of will. One has to struggle hard for keeping one self-attentive. It requires strong will power, keen attention and strong motives for the accomplishment of the task.
5. Voluntary attention is not given wholeheartedly or spontaneously. It has been given on interesting objects—uninteresting lectures, difficult assignments, which have to be done at the time when you would like to be doing something else.

Habitual Attention

1. Habitual attend tinting occurs by nature, inclined to take special note of certain things since we have natural interest on them.
2. Our physiological makeup is such that, we are dragged toward them. Thus food, drinks, etc. are things in which we have natural interest.
3. Factors determining attention: Attention is a selective mental process by which attention to a particular stimulus is determined by a number of factors. We select one and give up others. It means there is something in the stimulus that makes us attend to them.

Factors Influencing Attention

Objective Factors

Intensity: It is a fact of our everyday experience that a louder sound attracts our attention easily. Similarly bright color is more effective than a lighter shade.

Size: Sometimes size also determines the selection of a stimulus. Bigger patch of color would certainly draw our attention more easily than a smaller patch of the same color even of brighter shade.

Repetition: Certain stimuli are seen to attract our attention only on the strength of their repetition. They may be neither intense nor large size. When we knock at the door, it is habitual to repeat the knocking. For example, we take very little notice of the continuous ticking of the clock in our room, the dripping of the tap in our bathroom.

Change: Although, we pay very little attention to the ticking of the clock, we may all of a sudden become aware of it, if it stops. Here, the factor that operates is change. Many fissions attract attention because of the change involved them.

Movement: Anything that moves has an attention value. Electronic signs are always made to move for attraction better attention. We often see infants attending not only to big and bright object but also to tiny insects that move.

Novelty: Attention is always aroused by something new. Some unfamiliar or strange object or a familiar one in some new setting catches attention.

Systematic forms: Among different things that arouse sensation, we may probably attend to those, which have definite systematic pattern or rhythm. A soft melodious tune may be easily heard in the midst of loud noises.

Subjective Factors

Interest: A person who is interested in a particular field attends to object related to that field. For example, one who is interested in gardening is attracted by a new kind of plant or a girl who is interested in dresses will promptly observe a novel pattern of dress.

Motive: Our inner motive and desires also determine to a great extent what we think we attend to. A sleeping mother may not be disturbed by the loud noises of traffic outside, but she may be easily aroused by even a faint cry of her baby. Appeal to certain important motives like self-assertion, security or sex are also observed to arouse quick attention.

Organic state: A person's organic state determines his attention. Thus, a hungry person is easily attracted by the flavor or sight of eatables.

Moods and attitudes: If one is in an angry mood, he is proving to notice even the minor mistake of others, but if he is in happy mood, he usually overlooks them. Similarly, attitudes toward people and object also determine attention.

Habits: These are enduring types of behavior, which becomes a part of a person. Habits are acquired over period in the object at a glance. For example, a person who has developed the habit of reading sports forever in a paper would look for the sports column in the newspaper.

Span of Attention

The maximum number of letters or number of figures that an individual can notice or apprehends at a glance is known as span of attention. According to this definition of attention, one can attend to only one stimulus or only one object at a glance. Therefore, what we call as span of attention is only a span of apprehension and what we measure in the laboratory is not even span of apprehension, but its reproduction.

1. One more interesting problem of attention is the span of attention, which is also called the span of apprehension. While defining attention, we have emphasized that in strict physiological sense only one object, idea or fact can be the center of consciousness at one particular moment and consequently we can attend to only one thing at time.
2. One of the oldest experiments in the physiological laboratory is concerned with determining how many separate items can thus, be apprehended in a single glance. Sir William Hamilton, in the year 1859, tried to perform experiments on the span of attention for the first time.
3. Experiments to study the span of visual attention are carried out with the help of an instrument known as tachistoscope. The apparatus tachistoscope gives a quick exposure of cards containing number of dots or other figures only for a fraction of second. The maximum number of dots or figures that an individual can discarnate correctly gives his span of attention.

There are individual differences, but usually four to five letters or numbers can be apprehended by an average individual.

4. The term span of attention may be defined in terms of the quality, size are extent to which the perceptual field of an individual can be effectively organized in order to enable him to attend a number of things in a given spell of short duration.

Objective and Subjective Factors

The span of an individual is determined by many objective and subjective factors:

1. Grouping and organization of the materials facilitate span of apprehension than scattering and disorganization.
2. Pre-exposure and postexposure field, if free from glare and other distractions, they facilitate span.
3. If the duration of exposure period is a little more than the optimum time, the span will be more and if it is less than the optimum time, the span will be less.
4. Optimum and constant interval between the ready signal and exposure of the material facilitate span.
5. Size of the stimulus, practice and meaning in the materials exposed add to the span.
6. Age, mental condition, memory images of materials observed, fatigue, familiarity and previous experience also affect the span of apprehension.

Shifting or Fluctuation of Attention

1. It is a fact of our experiences that we cannot attend to a certain stimulus for a longer time. Our attention oscillates among the stimuli around. Sometimes the center of our consciousness keeps on fluctuating from one stimulus to another or on the different parts of a stimulus; this is known as fluctuation of attention.
2. Fluctuation of attention also involves rapid change in the intensity of the attention. The intensity increases or decreases ranging between the paying of attention and no attention or at least of less attention.
3. While paying attention toward an object, event or phenomenon, it is not possible for us to hold it continuously with the same intensity for a longer duration. In course of time, the center of our consciousness either shifts from one stimulus to another

or from one part of the same stimulus to another part, this is called the shifting of our attention.

4. The phenomenon of fluctuation of attention was experimentally recorded for the first time by a psychologist named Urbantschitsch (1875). While testing the auditory sensation, he observed that the subject was not able to hear the tick continuously of an alarm clock kept at a distance.

Division of Attention

Division of attention means attending two tasks simultaneously, with equal attention and efficiency. We hear people telling that they can attend two tasks simultaneously with equal efficiency. They say that they read a novel and knit a sweater or listen to a radio program and knitting. As against this, studies have proved beyond doubt that one can attend only one task at a time. If anybody tries to attend two tasks at a time, the work suffers either in quality or in quantity or both.

1. The attention is divided between two tasks, if more than two tasks are attended and performed simultaneously, then the attention will have to be divided among those tasks.
2. Many researchers have tried to study the effect of the division of attention on the work product. It has been found that the work products suffer less if both the tasks are simpler, but in the case of difficult and similar tasks, the division of attempts proves disadvantages.

Sustained Attention

1. Sustained attention occurs if one desires to be successful in the operation of a task he/she has to begin with paying attention or concentrating his/her energies on the operation of that task. However, it is the beginning of a process and not the end.
2. After paying initial attention, care is to be taken to hold it for a long enough duration. The individual should be absolutely absorbed in handling the task, unmindful of anything else going on, without getting disturbed in the least.
3. One has to make serious and deliberate efforts for sustaining one's attention by taking care of all the factors responsible for

maintaining attention and eliminating or reducing the forces of distraction.

Distraction of Attention

1. Distraction may be defined as any stimulus whose presence interferes with the process of attention or draws away attention from the object, which we wish to attend.
2. Distraction represents a sort of interference with our attention. The source of distraction may be external (e.g. noise, improper lighting, uncomfortable seats, etc.) and internal (e.g. lack of motivation, emotional disturbances, ill health, boredom of fatigue, etc.).

PERCEPTION

Perception is the selection, organization and interpretation of sensory input. It involves giving meaning to sensations. Sensation refers to the immediate experiences that are generated by simple and isolated stimuli. Perception involves the organization and interpretation of these stimuli to give them meaning. For instance, in listening to a person who sings, we experience the qualities of loudness and pitch as sensations, while our ability to hear the sequence of sounds as a song is an act of perception. At the next level, if we understand and recognize the words of the song, our perception blends into 'cognition', a more complex interpretive process that involves memory and thought.

Meaning

1. Perception is the selection, organization and interpretation of sensory input. It involves giving meaning to sensations. In other words, it is the activity of selecting, organizing and interpreting sensations with one's previous experiences.
2. Perception is very essential to deal with the world around us as it influences our memory, thinking, reasoning emotions, etc. Our behavior is very much a reflection of how we react to an interpret stimuli from the world around us. The process of perception helps in becoming aware of objects, quality or relations by way of sense organs.

3. Perception is an intellectual and psychological process because it is a subjective process based on the different people, here they assume according to their environment and interpret accordingly to their own views.
4. Perception is the intellectual process through which a person selects the date from the environment, organizes it and obtains meaning from it. Sensations are the first stage of receiving stimuli; it is the experience we feel, when the receptors of the sense organs send impulses to specific areas of the brain. The activity of the organism is converting a sense impression into the awareness of some meaningful situation called perception.
5. Perception is a highly-individualized process that helps an organism, in organizing and interpreting one complex pattern of sensory stimulation for giving them, the necessary pattern meaning to initiate his/her behavioral responses.
6. It is a complex process, determined by both physiological and psychological characteristics of the organism.

Definitions

1. Perception is a process by which individual organize and interpret their sensory impressions in order to give meaning to their environment.
2. Perception is the appearance of things that is the focus on attention rather than objective reality.
3. Perception is the experience of objects, events or relationships obtained by extracting information from and interpreting sensations.
4. Perception is the organizing process by which it interprets our sensory input.
5. Perception is defined as all the processes involved in creating meaningful patterns out of a jumble of sensory impressions, which fall under the general category of perception.
6. Perception is an individual's awareness, aspects of behavior, for example, the way each person processes the raw data he/she receives from the environment, into meaningful patterns.
7. Perception is the intellectual process by which an individual screens, selects, organizes and interprets the stimuli in order to give meaning to their environment.

8. Perception can be defined as the active process of selecting, organizing and interpreting the information brought to the brain by the senses.

Nature of Perception

1. Perception is essentially a process rather than being a product or outcome of some psychological phenomenon.
2. Perception is the information extractor. Our sensory receptors are bombarded continuously by various stimuli present in our environment. Perception performs this duty by extracting relevant information out of a jumble of sensory impressions and converting them into some meaningful pattern.
3. Perception is the first event in the chain, which leads from the stimulus to action.
4. Perception is the act of interpreting a stimulus generated in the brain by one or more sense mechanism.
5. Perception is a mental process in which sensory cues and relevant past experiences organize together to give us meaningfulness to the perceived object.

Factors Influencing Perception

Sense organs: Perception depends upon sense impressions, which are related to the sense organ concerned with the specific stimulus. To perceive different auditory stimuli, auditory sense organ must be developed and it should function properly.

Brain function: Brain function provides various frames of references in organizing the previous experiences and sensory information, which helps in perception.

Motive: Our perception often depends upon our motives working at the given moment. When we are hungry, we perceive certain objects as eatables even though they are not eatables in reality.

Familiarity: Previous experiences are required to associate the sensory information, which helps in apprehension.

Set or readiness: It has been observed that what we see is influenced by what we are set to see. When we are in good mood, we do not perceive the mistakes of others very easily.

Values: When a person places a high premium on a stimulus, he tends to perceive it differently. In an experiment, children were asked to compare the size of a chip with the adjustable circle of a light. After a few brails, the children were told that the chips could be exchanged for a candy. Thus, the children were taught to value the chips higher than before. Then they were rewarded with candy for chips. Subsequently when the children were asked to compare the size of the chip with the circle of the light, most of them perceived the chips as longer than size of the circle.

Expectations: Anticipation influences one's perception. Sometimes one has a tendency to see what we expect to see. Thus, when subjects were shown a red light and asked to report the sign on a cardboard, most of them reported it as stop sign even though it was spelt as top.

Cognitive style: As a person matures, each one of us develops a way of dealing with the situation/environment, which is known as cognitive style. Cognitive styles could be viewed differently. One approach is field dependent and the other is field independent approach; in the former, the person sees the environment as a whole and does not delineate it into its parts. But in the latter, the person perceives the elements of the environment with its parts.

Personality: A person's personality influences the way he perceives. In two studies, healthy colleagues were compared to depressed patients or students with eating disorder in terms of their ability to identify words related to food. Persons with depression were able to identify adjectives related to depressed traits.

Culture: The culture background of a person influences the perception of a person. The way in which a person uses the cues depend on one's culture.

Inaccurate perceptions: Sometimes, our perceptions are inaccurate. We cannot make correct interpretations.

Differences Between Sensation and Perception

Normally sensation and perception are two sides of a same coin. We can only think of them separately, but cannot experience them separately. It is rather difficult to understand the differences between sensation and perception because the two are inseparable and always go together (Table 2.2).

1. Sensation is an experience that an individual will have, when the sensory area is stimulated by coded neural impulses (message), which are transmitted by the given sense organ to the concerned sensory area through the sensory nerves, when the sense organ is stimulated by either external or internal environment. Whereas perception is interpretation of the sensory experience by the association area of the cortex in collaboration with sensory area and in the background of the previous experience, present mental and physical status of the individual.
2. A sensation begins with the stimulation of the sense organ and ends with the interpretation of the sense experiences perception.
3. A sensation by itself cannot bring about the experience of an object, it is the psychological processes, which interprets the sensation, gives the knowledge of the object perception.
4. Pure sensation is a primary passive mental process, which is the resultant of the external stimulating energy, whereas perception is an active process of grouping and organizing the sensory experience and its interpretation in the background of previous experience.
5. A sensation by itself cannot give us complete and meaningful experience and it cannot independently lead to perception. In addition to sensation, a number of symbolic processes like images, memories, revival of previous experiences, etc. together cause perception. In short, the activity of converting a sense

Table 2.2: Differences between sensation and perception

Sl No	*Concepts*	*Sensation*	*Perception*
1.	Organization	Not organized	Organized
2.	Organs involved	Sense organs	The brain
3.	Meaningfulness	Meaningless	Meaningful
4.	Organs stimulated	Sense organs	It is selection, organization and interpretation of the sensory inputs
5.	Action	Rudimentary action	Perception is a much higher act

impression into awareness of some meaningful situation is called perception.

6. The sensory information merely provides raw data. The data then combined with previous information and with thought processes to create the world and then we actually experience perception.

Principles of Organization (Gestalt's Principles)

Figure and ground: Here the person divides the visual displays into figure and ground. In visual perception, the person keeps one as the figure object, while the other forms the ground (background) (Figs 2.7A to D).

Similarity: Objects of the same color, size and shape are perceived as a pattern. Here the dark colored dots are perceived as number two rather than a random array of dots (Fig. 2.7E).

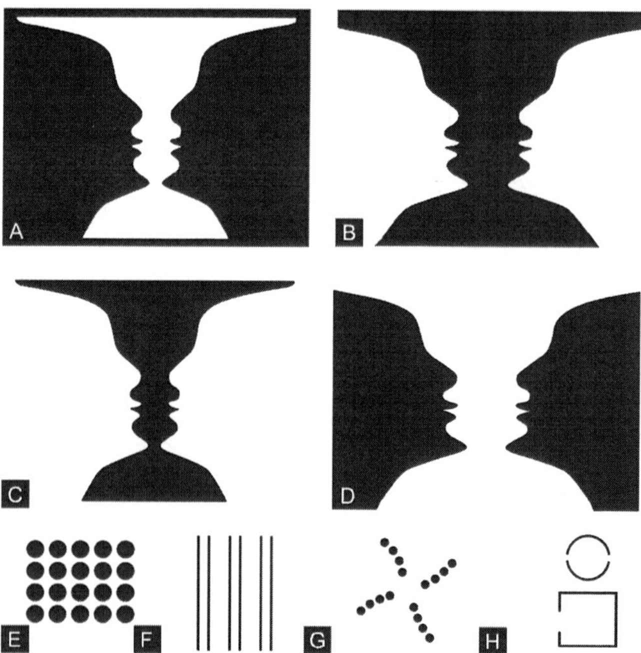

Figs 2.7A to H: Gestalt's principle. **A. and B.** Vases are seen compared to face; **C. and D.** Face is seen compared to vase; **E.** Similarity; **F.** Proximity; **G.** Continuity; **H.** Closure.

Closure: The tendency to perceive an incomplete object as a whole, complete object is known as the principle of closure. In the illustration, though the circle is not complete; one tends to perceive it as a circle (Fig. 2.7H).

Continuity: Objects that continue as a pattern or direction tend to be grouped together. In the illustration, one tends to perceive the dots as a straight line even though there is a break in the continuity (Fig. 2.7G).

Simplicity (proximity): The tendency to organize and perceive elements in the simplest possible way is known as the principle of simplicity (Fig. 2.7F).

Perception and Constancies

A tendency to experience a stable perception in spite of changing sensory input or changes in sensory information is known as perceptual constancy. This may apply to shape, size, brightness or color.

Shape constancy: The tendency to see an object in the same shape irrespective of the angle in which it is viewed is known as shape constancy. For example, familiar objects are seen as having the same shape though the retinal images may change for different angles.

Size constancy: The tendency to perceive objects in the same size regardless of the distance from which it is viewed. For example, a beautiful women standing at a distance of 20 feet looks the same, as she would be at a distance of 10 feet. Even though there is change in the retinal image.

Brightness constancy: The perception of brightness is the same even though the amount of light reaching the retina changes is known as brightness constancy. For example, the brightness of white paper remains same in sunlight or candle light.

Color constancy: The tendency to perceive objects, as retaining their color despite changes in sensory information is known as brightness constancy. For example, the red-colored Maruthi car looks red under streetlight as well as in the dark garage.

Depth perception: The process by which one interprets visual cues to know how near or far away the objects are is known as depth perception. There are two types of cues namely monocular and binocular that helps in depth perception. Monocular cues are the visual cues requiring one eye. Binocular cues are visual cues requiring both the eyes.

1. We cannot perceive and observe the objects correctly; sometimes our sense organs may be functioning defectively. For example, we are suffering from myopia, deafness or any other sensory defect.
2. Our receptors may not be stimulated adequately because the stimuli were not strong enough to stimulate them or the stimuli were rather vague and indefinite.
3. We may not perceive correctly because, we do not know what to perceive. In order that a student nurse should perceive correctly in the ward for proper nursing care, she needs to be guided by her instructor.
4. Our span of apprehension and attention is limited. If we try to apprehend more things than we can at a time, we are liable to have inaccurate perceptions.
5. Sometimes objects or figures are perceived with difficulty because they resemble their surroundings. The figure merges with the ground. For example, a white patch is difficult to detect on a white wall.
6. We are liable to perceive things wrongly if we are not in good health, sick people's perceptions, at times are not correct for this reason. Our sense organs cannot function adequately and correctly because of illness.

Common Sensory Abnormalities and Perceptual Disorders

The sensory disturbances of perceptions are given in Table 2.3.

Anesthesia

1. It implies complete absence/inability to respond to sensory (touch) sensation. It means a loss is absence of sensitivity.
2. Anesthesia may be caused by defective sense organs, effects or drugs or also by some emotional or functional factors. For example, we sometime do not notice a pen or a bunch of keys lying before us and make a frantic search of it. We are either emotionally disturbed or preoccupied with some other thoughts.

Table 2.3: Sensory disturbances of perceptions

Sl No	*Sensory disturbances*	*Description*
1.	Pain sensation	
	a. Analgesia	Absence of pain appreciation
	b. Hypoalgesia	Decrease of pain appreciation
	c. Hyperalgesia	Exaggeration of pain appreciation, which is often unpleasant
2.	Temperature sensation	
	a. Thermanalgesia	Absence of temperature appreciation
	b. Thermanesthesia	Decrease of temperature appreciation
	c. Thermohyperesthesia	Exaggeration of temperature sensation, which is often unpleasant
3.	Sensory abnormalities	
	a. Paresthesia	Abnormal sensation perceived without specific stimulation; they may be tactile, thermal or painful, episodic or constant
	b. Dysesthesia	Painful sensation elicited by painful cutaneous stimulus such as a light touch or gentle stroking over affected areas of the body
4.	Proprioceptive sensation (deep sensation)	
	a. Joint position sense (arthresthesia)	Absence of joint position sense
	b. Vibratory sense (pallesthesia)	Absence of vibratory sense
	c. Kinesthesia	Perception of muscular motion
5.	Cortical sensory function:	
	a. Astereognosis	Inability to recognize and identify objects by feeling them
	b. Graph anesthesia	Symbols written on the skin
	c. Topognosia	Inability to localize stimuli to parts of the body
	d. Sensory extinction	Inability to perceive a sensory stimulus when corresponding areas on the opposite side of the body are stimulated simultaneously

Hyperesthesia

It means excessive response to stimuli; sick people often shows this in their behavior. They react violently to noises or bright lights. When we are fatigue, we become hypersensitive to light, sound or to the weight of clothing and to odors.

Errors in Perception

It has been observed that we get the experience of objective reality through our perception. But perceptions are at time descriptive. They do not always give us the correct experience of facts that exist. Some erroneous illusive experience is the result of such descriptive perceptions. False perceptions occur when perceptual stimulus fails to correspond with the real stimulus in the environment. Two frequently occurring errors in perceptions are discussed under two different phenomena, namely illusion and hallucinations.

Illusion

Actually, we always evaluate the world around us with our perceptual habits that help us respond quickly and effectively to our normal environment. Sometimes our perceptual process may distort the images we receive, rather than correcting them with superficial changes in appearance.

An illusion is a mistaken perception of an object. In such cases the stimulus is, no doubt, present giving rise to definite sensory impulses, but, while interpreting the sensory impulses in the form of a meaningful experiences, fears or expectations.

Definitions: Illusion can be defined as:

1. Illusion is one such perceptual distortion, which may create bias in us, to distort reality; consequently, we make faulty interpretation of the environment.
2. An illusion is a wrong, inaccurate or mistaken perception of an existing sensory stimulus.

Nature: The nature can be explained as:

1. An illusion is a wrong perception, mistaking a rope for a snake, a tree for an animal and mistakes it for something that is not really exist there at that time.
2. Most of our illusions are visual and auditory, but others are also possible. Illusions are caused by inadequacies of our sense organs, which has to perceive it, misleading stimuli in the environment, our preconceived notions and expectancy.
3. These illusion are usually referred as any interpretation of sense information, psychologists usually distinguish illusions into two groups.

Causes: Optical illusions are caused by many factors; some causes are more predominant in some forms of illusions. In some other forms of illusion, some other causes are predominant; some illusion will have more than one cause. However, some of the causes of illusion are given below.

Similarity: If two objects are similar in appearance, illusion occurs more easily than others do. For example, it is natural to mistake a curled rope for snake due to similarity.

Expectancy: If we are waiting for a friend, every individual at a distance will be mistaken for a friend. While searching for a lost coin, every glittering is mistaken for the coin, which we are searching.

Physical causes: The mirror and the echo illusion are good examples for this. The former is due to reflection of light and the later is due to echo of sound. The mirrored objects seem to be behind the mirror because the light reaches our eyes from that direction. In the echo illusion, the echo seems to come from somebody across the lake because the sound actually reaches our ears from that direction.

Unanalyzed total impression: This is clear from Muller-Lyer illusion. Here, though we are supporting to perceive and estimate the actual length of the lines excluding the appendages, we will be compelled to perceive the total figure and thus overestimate or underestimate the lines. Thus, the unanalyzed total impression causes illusion.

Subjective factors: Such as habit and familiarity cause illusions, for example, cross two fingers and touch a marble or hold a pencil with the crossed part of both the fingers and you will feel two marbles or two pencils. Another example is proofreader's illusion.

Perceptual illusions: Causes are as follows:

1. Physical illusions occur because of the distortion of information. For example, when a portion of a stick is dipped in water there appears a bent to the stick. Many physical illusions are created by our natural tendency to view two-dimensional scenes as projections of three-dimensional realities.
2. Perceptual illusions occur because when the stimulus contains misleading cues that cause perceptions that are inaccurate or impossible.

Classification/Types

Moon illusions: Moon appears large near the horizon that it does later at night, when it is directly overhead. One explanation says that moon illusion depends on a visual constancy, i.e. when it is close to the horizon we have cues of distance and when it is overhead, we do not get any cues to distance.

Railroad or Ponzo illusion: In simple forms, Ponzo illusion consists of two gradually converging lines that give the impression of increasing depth in between, two crosswise parallel lines.

Horizontal/vertical illusions: Though both the horizontal and vertical lines are equal in length, the vertical line is perceived as longer than the horizontal.

Poggendorff illusion: A straight line appears to become slightly displaced as it passes through two parallel rectangles.

Zollner illusion: When two parallel lines are intersected by numerous short diagonal lines slanting in opposite direction, when the parallel lines are perceived as diverging. All these illusions originate from our perceptual processes, creating an internal representation based on inaccurate and misleading information caused by visual illusions.

Ponzo illusions: The geometrical illusions that a horizontal line appearing within the smaller end of a pair of divergent vertical lines is longer than an equal length line located at a point at which the vertical lines are farther apart.

Muller-Lyer illusion: It is a geometrical illusion where one line is longer than another equal length when the former has obtuse angles at both ends, while the later has acute angles at both ends.

Hallucination

Hallucination is a false perception that is idiosyncratic, not shared by others in the same situation. It is generally seen in some mental disorder like schizophrenia, alcoholic intoxication or drug abuse. Some people claim that their perceptions are quite vivid and life-like and they think them real. They may even become confused with reality. They are extreme forms of inaccurate observation. Such observations are usually associated with severe psychological disorders, but they occasionally occur among even non-mentally ill individuals as well.

Definitions: Are as follows:

1. Hallucinations are vivid sensory experiences that occur in the absence of external stimulus.
2. Hallucination is the imaginary perception; it is a gross error of perception of seeing objects that do not exist. This is an extreme form of inaccurate observation in which one sees or hears something that is not seen or heard by others around him.

Nature: It is explained below:

1. Hallucinations appear most frequently in the life of mentally disordered persons. The person hearing sounds that are false, seeing objects moving in a room are called hallucinations.
2. Hallucinations are deceptive perceptions and are at times caused purely because of our subjective makeup. The perception has no basis of a real sensory stimulus.
3. Hallucinations are found to be most common with auditory and visual perception. Hallucination is also caused due to certain organic condition such as damage of cerebral cortex or sense organs; certain drugs and alcohol can also produce hallucination.
4. Hallucinations are directly related to sensation; these can be classified into visual hallucination, auditory hallucination, taste hallucination, smell hallucination and cutaneous hallucination.

Differences Between Illusion and Hallucination

Though, illusions and hallucinations are common experiences; the high cadence of hallucination is more severe. It is a serious form of mental illness. Illusion and hallucination shows us that our perception depends to a large extend on subjective factors like set attitudes and inner needs (Box 2.1).

Hallucinations usually occur when individuals lose the capacity to differentiate between inner sensation and the outer environment. Both hallucination and illusion have an impact on behavior and distort our knowledge leading to many personal, social and psychological problems.

Extrasensory Perception

If there are so many influences upon perception other than those coming from the presented stimuli, are there perhaps perceptions that

Box 2.1: Differences between illusion and hallucination

Illusion
1. In illusion, there will always be one or more stimuli
2. Objective
3. Stimulus is present
4. Normal or universal
5. Mistaken perception
Hallucination
1. In hallucination, external stimulus is completely absent
2. Subjective
3. Stimulus is not present
4. Abnormal
5. False perception

require no sense organ stimulation whatsoever? The answer to this question is the source of a major controversy within contemporary psychology over the status of ESP. Parapsychology is the search for paranormal phenomena such as ESP and psychokinesis. Parapsychologists try to observe unexplainable phenomena. All other sciences have led us away from superstition and magical thinking, while parapsychology has tried to find a scientific basis for magical power and spirits.

Definition

Extrasensory perception is perception occurring independently of sight, hearing or other sensory processes. EPS also refers to telepathy, clairvoyance and precognition. It influencing of physical events by mental operations, are the source of controversy in contemporary psychology.

Characteristics

1. It is a most unstable ability, disappearing suddenly or gradually, often without recognized causes.
2. The ESP process is diametric in its function, encompassing more than a single object in its scope.
3. The ESP process is entirely unconscious, i.e. it is not thus far found reliability available to introspection in anyway or degree.

The extrasensory perception is variable and undependable effect upon performance in the tests.

4. The ESP does not seem to subject to development through use as other specific capacities.

Nature

1. The experiments go at work in accordance with the usual Niles of science and generally, disavow the connection between this work and spiritualism, supernaturalism, mediumistic phenomena and other occult effects.
2. Many psychologists who are not convinced would find it congenital to accept evidence that they found satisfactory.
3. The case for ESP is based largely on experiments in card-guessing trick in which, under various conditions, the subject attempts to guess the symbols on cards randomly arranged in packs.

Nurse's Role in Sensation, Attention and Perception

In caring the sick, nurse needs to remember the words of Plato, the treatments of a part should not be attempted without treatment of the entity. It emphasizes that wholeness of something is more than the sum of its parts because a part is meaningful only in the context of the whole (Table 2.4).

Table 2.4: Role of nurses in sensation and perception

Sl No	*Sensation*	*Description*
1.	Color	A sick person reacts to colors; there are some colors, which are soothing.
2.	Light	During illness, even moderate lighting may irritate and cause discomfort. For patients who need rest and sleep light can be subdued. For stimulation and encouragement, warm bright lights can be used.
3.	Noise	A sick person is very much averse to loud noises. Loud noises increase the patient's irritability. The nurse must avoid noises in the ward.
4.	Sensation	Patients with loss of skin sensation require special attention to provide further injuries to the skin, while treating or using treatments. Patients always should be handled gently and smoothly to avoid pain and discomfort.

Contd...

Contd...

Sl No	*Sensation*	*Description*
5.	Odor (smell)	In the ward or patients unit, the possible sources for bad odor are body eliminations, treatment procedures, dressings, drainages and medications. These must be controlled as much as possible by proper ventilation and prompt disposal of waste.
6.	Taste	The taste can be improved with good mouth care and well prepared, clean and fresh food served in an appetizing way.
	Perception	*Description*
7.	Perception of outside world	Our perception of the world outside is greatly affected by current state of mind. For example, we may feel particularly anxious when we tend to perceive our own different disturbed state of mind. A nurse needs to understand the role of sensation and attention in acquiring knowledge of environment, which depends to larger extent on the sensation received by the sense organs.
8.	Perception influences memory, thinking and emotions	Perception is essential to deal with the world around us as it influences our memory, thinking, reasoning and emotions, etc. A nurse should understand to interpret the whole environment and apply different types of perceptual skills to understand his/her patients. In caring the sick, nurse needs to remember the words of Plato, the treatment of a part should not be attempted without treatment of the entity. It emphasizes that wholeness of something is more than the sum of its parts because a part is meaningful only in the context of the whole.
9.	Provides positive outlook to sick	The perception of the nurse and that of the patient may be different in the hospital environment. The nurse is familiar with the hospital environment and also well accustomed. The nurse being a healthy and energetic person is working with a positive outlook and enthusiasm to help the patient.
10.	Helps to reduce the anxiety	The hospital may seem an alien and frightening environment to the patient. Because the new and unfamiliar hospital environment creates a lot of anxieties in the patient. It may influence the thought, behaviors and perceptual set of the patient. Emotional maturity is also another important factor influencing a person's perception of sensory data.

Contd...

Contd...

	Perception	*Description*
11.	Promotes coping	A nurse should share the worries, fears and emotions of the sick and help them to solve them. As a nursing student, he/she must learn to assess all factors with accuracy and efficiency.

CONCLUSION

The physical and social environments with their inherent nature draw our attention to them. When any stimulus is attended by the respective sense organ, it releases natural impulses. The encoded information about in the form of natural impulses constitutes sensation. Interpretation of sense impression is perception. Thus these functions are interrelated. They provide knowledge of the environment, so that the organism can act appropriately to adjust to the environment. Therefore, to understand behavior we have to know their interrelated functions.

SUGGESTED READING

1. Ann ZJ. Basic Psychology for Nurses. Chennai: BI Publications Pvt Ltd; 2003.
2. Bhatia BD, Margaretta C. Elements of Psychology and Mental Hygiene for Nurses in India. Chennai: Orient Longman; 2005.
3. Clifford MT, Richard KA. Introduction to Psychology, 7th edition. New Delhi: Tata McGraw-Hill Publishing Company Limited; 2004.
4. Clement I. Psychosocial Foundation of Nursing, 1st edition. New Delhi: Jaypee Brothers Medical Publishers (P) Ltd; 2010.
5. Hilgard RE, Atkinson CR. Introduction to Psychology, 6th edition. New Delhi: Oxford and IBH Publishing Co Pvt Ltd; 1975.
6. Jocob A. Psychology for Graduate Nurses, 4th edition. New Delhi: Jaypee Brothers Medical Publishers (P) Ltd; 2007.
7. Khan MA. Psychology for Nurses in India, New Delhi: Academic Publications; 2004.
8. Mangal SK. General Psychology. New Delhi: Sterling Publishers Pvt Ltd; 2006.
9. Thompson RF. Introduction to Psychology. New Delhi: Haper and Row; 1975.

REVIEW QUESTIONS

1. Define sensation. Explain the meaning of sensation.
2. Enumerate the steps involved in sensation.
3. Explain the general characteristics of sensation.
4. Discuss the sense organs. Explain the functions and loss of function of sense organs.
5. Define attention. Explain the importance and classifications of attention.
6. Discuss the factors influencing attention.
7. Explain span of attention, shifting or influctations of attention.
8. Describe division of attention.
9. Define perception. Explain the factors influencing perception.
10. Explain the differences between sensation and perception.
11. Discuss and describe illusion and hallucination.
12. Define extrasensory perception. Explain the characteristics of extrasensory perception.
13. Explain the roles and responsibilities of a nurse in sensory attention and perception.

CHAPTER 3

Motivation

LEARNING OBJECTIVES

1. To learn definitions and nature of motivation.
2. To understand biological and social motives.
3. To understand frustration and conflicts.
4. To learn self-actualization.

INTRODUCTION

1. The human behavior is controlled, directed and modified through certain motives. When a person is hungry and is searching for food or constructing a house or mating or learning new skills, he/she will always be able to trace some elements, which will guide their activities and behavior in the lights of success or failures.
2. Motivation is that force, which impels or incites individual's action, determines the individual's direction of action and the rate of action. When the individual gets any motives, he/she experiences a tension and disequilibrium and become restless. The activities are then initiated. The individual feels a push to behave in a certain direction.

MEANING

1. Motivation is something, which prompts, compels and energizes an individual to act or behave in a particular fashion at a particular time for attaining some specific goal or purpose.

2. The term 'motivation' has been derived from the word 'motive'. A motive is an inner state that activates, energizes or moves an individual and channelizes the behavior toward the goal.
3. Motivation is the art of understanding these motives and satisfying them to direct and sustain behavior toward the accomplishment of organizational goal.
4. Motivation is concerned with how behavior starts, is energized, sustained, directed and stopped. As motivation is the process of inspiring and impelling people to take required actions by providing stimuli, that satisfy their needs and motives.
5. Motivation is the complex of forces, which propel an individual into action and keep them at work. It reflects the will to work.
6. Motivation is defined as the process that initiates, guides and maintains goal-oriented behaviors. Motivation causes one to act, such as getting a glass of water to reduce thirst or reading a book to gain knowledge.

DEFINITIONS

1. Motivation means a process of stimulating people to action, to accomplish desired goals. It refers to the way in which urges, drives, desires, aspirations, stirrings or needs direct control or explain the behavior of human being. —*Scott*
2. Motivation is an inspirational process, which impels the members of the team to pull their weight effectively, to give their loyalty to the group, to carry out properly the tasks that they have accepted and generally to play an effective part in the job that the group has undertaken. —*Brech*
3. Motivation is the willingness to exert high levels of efforts toward organizational goals, conditioned by the effort's ability to satisfy some individual needs. —*Stephen P Robbins*
4. Motivation refers to the degree of readiness of an organism to pursue some designated goals, to imply the determination of the nature and laws of the focus including the degree of readiness. —*Encyclopedia*

NATURE OF MOTIVATION

Motivation is the force that initiates, guides and maintains goal-oriented behaviors. It is what causes one to take action, whether to grab a snack to reduce hunger or enroll in college to earn a degree. The forces that lie beneath the motivation can be grouped as biological, social, emotional or cognitive in nature.

1. Motivation is a psychological concept. It is concerned with the intrinsic forces operating within an individual, which impel to act or not to act in a particular way.
2. Motivation is a dynamic and continuous process as it deals with human being, which is an ever changing entity modifying itself every moment.
3. Motivation is a complex and difficult function. Every person adopts a different approach to satisfy the needs and one particular need may cause different behavior from different people.
4. Motivation is a circular process. Feeling of an unsatisfied need causes tension and an individual takes action (drive) to reduce this tension.
5. Motivation is different from satisfaction. Motivation is the process of stimulating an individual or a group to take desired action.
6. Motivation is the product of anticipated value from a given course of action and the perceived probability that the action will lead to these values.

MOTIVATION PROCESS

The motivational processes (Fig. 3.1) are the steps taken to get moti vated. It is a process, that when followed produces incredible results. It is amazing that, what the people do when they are properly motivated and getting properly motivated, is a matter of following the motivational process. Like any other process, it takes a little work and foresight and planning on the individual's part. However, the return on the investment of time is significant and it is important when extra motivation is needed when the motivational process is applied.

1. An unsatisfied tension, which stimulates drives within the individual. These drives generate search behavior, to find particular goals that if attained, satisfy the needs and lead to the reduction of tension.
2. In order to relieve this tension, they engage in activity. The greater the tension, the more activity will be needed to bring about relief.
3. Therefore, when we see people working hard at some activity, we can conclude that they are driven by a desire to achieve some goal that they perceive as having value to them.

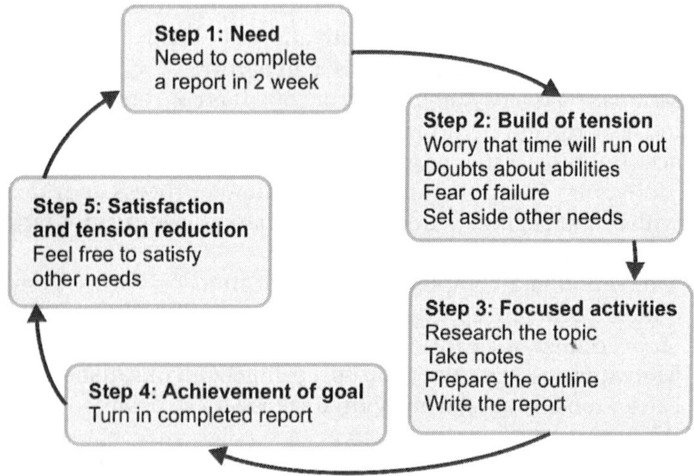

Fig. 3.1: Steps involved in motivation process

COMPONENTS OF MOTIVATION

The three major components to motivation are activation, persistence and intensity. Activation involves the decision to initiate a behavior, such as enrolling in a psychology class. Persistence is the continued effort toward a goal even though obstacles may exist, such as taking more psychology courses in order to earn a degree although it requires a significant investment of time, energy and resources. Finally, intensity can be seen in the concentration and vigor that goes into pursuing a goal. For example, one student might study without much effort, while another student will study regularly, participate in discussions and take advantage of research opportunities outside the class.

Extrinsic vs Intrinsic Motivation

Different types of motivation are frequently described as being either extrinsic or intrinsic. Extrinsic motivations are those that arise from outside of the individual and often involve rewards such as trophies, money, social recognition or praise. Intrinsic motivations are those that arise from within the individual, such as doing a complicated crossword puzzle purely for the personal gratification for solving a problem.

MOTIVE

Meaning

1. Motive is a force that determines the activity of an individual. It energizes and directs the behavior along different channels.
2. When a motive is at work, it creates tension and these tensions arouse the individual towards an activity that will relieve the tension.
3. A motive is a force that initiates, sustains and directs the activity of an organism. A stimulus is an internal or external object, which exiles the receptor or activates a sense organ.

Definitions

1. A need give rise to one or more motives. A motive is rather a specific process, which has been learned. It is directed toward a goal. —*Carroll*
2. A motive is an inclination or impulsion to an action plus some degree of orientation or direction. —*Fisher*
3. A motive may be defined as a readiness or disposition to respond in some ways and not others to a variety of situations. —*Rosen, Fox and Gregory*

Classification

Physiological Motives

Temperature regulation: An organism is active in maintaining a comfortable state of warmth and cold. This motivated activity is the result of the impulses sent to the brain by the skin receptors meant for the sensation of warmth and cold.

Pain: The sense receptors for pain are distributed in all the organs of the body like skin, internal organs, blood vessels, etc. They are in the form of free nerve ending in these organs. Whenever they are stimulated by some sort of injury to the body, there is pain sensation. The organism puts in all possible efforts, consciously or at reflex level to avoid such pain.

Sleep: Need for sleep is one more physiological motive. Though it contains all the activities of the organism, unlike other motives and makes him/her assume an inactive position that can be observed. However, the inactive position is the goal and the motive of sleep, actually it drives the individual toward all the possible efforts to go to sleep.

Hunger: When the individual feels emptiness in the stomach, then the person is hungry. When the person is hungry, two kinds of changes occur. One is the change in the external behavior and other is the change in the internal conditions. The motive of hunger gives rise to the hunger pangs. The actual sensation of a person gets him/her in a type of acting sensation.

Thirst: When deprived of water over some period, the organism becomes excessively restless and needs to intake some water. This drive for water comes from dryness of the mouth and thirst. However, the feeling of thirst is basically related to the degree of dehydration of the body tissues. Thirst is also a physiological need, which promotes activity. This need is very active when it is not immediately satisfied.

Sex drive: Sex is a very powerful drive, which influences the actions of the individual to a very great extent. According to general convention, this drive remains dormant during childhood. Freudian theory shows evidence for sexual behavior right from infancy. With the onset of puberty the sex glands known as gonads start functioning and as a result, the sex drive is simulated.

Maternal drive: What has been said about the sex instinct, applies equally well to maternal behavior. Prolactin, a hormone from the anterior pituitary gland plays an important role in motivating maternal behavior. Human maternal motivation has several aspects. Child rearing practices and attitudes toward children differ from culture to culture and from subculture to subculture.

General Motives

Activity: Men as well as animals are found to be spontaneously active. They enjoy it and spend considerable time in moving about. This innate motive for activity is visible even in a child's behavior. Activity also accompanies other physiological drives. When these drives are stronger, activity increases. Activity is closely related to sensor stimulations. More the stimulations in the environment, more active the organism is.

Exploratory drive: People like to explore new environments. We visit new places; mountaineers even risk their lives in exploratory expeditions. When animals are put in the maze, they are found to explore them without any specific aim to satisfy a physiological drive like hunger. This drives of exploration is stronger when the organism finds itself in a new situation.

Curiosity: This is a motive, which is close to exploration. Exploration is a drive that aids the satisfaction of curiosity. Animals as well as men including children are curious about the several things around them. A small child's curiosity tempts to even break a new toy given to him/her.

Manipulation: This is one more motive, which is a related aspect of the two previously discussed. It is not so easy to differentiate clearly among the drive of exploration, curiosity and manipulation. All three seems to be different aspects of a single motivated activity. Curiosity leads to manipulation and manipulation, in turn, is a counterpart of exploration.

Affectional motive: Love is an important motive of human life. We love our parents, our brothers and sisters, children, friends, etc. The significant people in the environment become love objects through positive contact with him/her. There are enough reasons to believe that it is also an unlearned motive that emerges with maturation.

Fear: It is very powerful motive. Tonic immobility (TI) motivates to escape from fear-producing situation. Fear may also interfere with the satisfaction of other motives. Most of the fears are learned. But there are enough reasons to believe that some fears are unlearned.

Social Motives

Affiliation: The need for affiliation is well-expressed through the affiliation with clubs and other institutions. Marriage is partly a means to satisfy many other needs including the need for affiliation. The motive of affiliation is usually seen in all human cultures. This motive perhaps has its roots in the childhood experiences, when the helpless infant has to associate with others for the basic need satisfaction.

Social approval: People seek social approval for all the things they do. Similarly, they try out their best to avoid from doing anything that may evoke social disapproval. They often show a compulsive tendency to confirm the norms set by the social group. This may be the result of constant parental directions in childhood as to what is right and what is wrong for the child to do.

Status: All people are commonly motivated to achieve status among their fellow men. This motive varies in strength from person to person. Some people show the minimum need for the status in the form of desire, to be thought well of and leave a respectable position in their professional field or in community.

Need for power and prestige: The need for prestige is expressed in the form of striving to feel better than other persons with whom they compare themselves. In daily life, there are many ways through which prestige is sought and achieved. Symbols such as dress, money and other belongings are regarded as ways of feeling superior in comparison to others. The need of power is almost similar though it differs slightly in its expression.

Security: An urge for feeling of security is also an important motive especially in complex modern societies. This feeling involves the ability to hold on to what one has and continue with the assurance to keep it upon the other hand. Insecurity is a haunting feeling that makes one to lose what he/she has now.

Achievements: It is a powerful motive in some societies. This is the motive to accomplish something, to succeed in one's undertaking and to avoid failure. The importance of this varies from culture to culture and from subculture to subculture. The strength of achievement motives depends partly on the past success of an individual.

Unconscious Motives

1. Not all the motives are conscious. A number of motives are operating without awareness. In one's own behavior, they come across instances of acts, the explanation of which cannot be found. All such instances of behavior can be explained with reference to unconscious motives.
2. Origin of unconscious motives can be found in the unconscious mind. The term unconscious should not be taken to mean that it is a part of mind, separated from conscious mind.
3. The repression itself is a function of the unconscious. Hence, constant repression enlarges the domain of the unconscious.

Since the material is related to the motives, it is dynamic in nature and does not remain quiet in unconscious.

4. The material of the unconscious is extremely difficult to top because a considerable part of it is originated in infantile preverbal ideas, which have never become conscious. —*Freud*

Instinctive Behavior

1. An inherited or innate psychophysical disposition, which determines its possessor to perceive and to pay attention to objects of certain class, to experience an emotional excitement of a particular quality upon perceiving such an object and to act in regard to it in a particular manner or at least to experience an impulse to such action. Instincts are innate tendencies, which have a cognitive aspect, emotive aspect to feel certain emotion toward these objects, to act toward them in a particular way. —*McDougall*
2. The human instincts include sucking, crying, locomotion, curiosity, sociality, shyness, cleanliness, pressing downward on the feet, imitation, pugnacity, fear of dark places, acquisitiveness, love and jealousy.

Hierarchy of Motives

1. Hierarchy of motives helps us to understand the potency of different motives in man's behavior.
2. Motives at the lowest rung are those originating from homeostatic mechanism. Thus, all the motives are important for survival including the safety motives, which are included in this class. Affiliation motives are placed still higher. These motives include the need for social acceptance and belongingness. —*White*
3. The need for self-actualization is a complicated concept, which needs some further explanations. —*Maslow*

THEORIES OF MOTIVATION

Drive Reduction Theory

1. One of the earlier theories of motivation was the drive reduction theory. It was proposed by Clark Hull.

2. This theory proposes that, "Organisms experiences the arousal of a drive when an important need is not satisfied and they engage in behavior to reduce the arousal and satisfy the need."
3. Primary drives are those that motivate the organism to fulfill some basic needs necessary for its survival such as hunger, thirst or sex.
4. An important component of the drive reduction theory is homeostasis. The term homeostasis refers to a state of balance or equilibrium necessary in many physiological systems.
5. Primary drives are biological drives necessary for personal and species survival. Acquired drives develop through learning.
6. The drive is the force that motivates an organism to action. An action, which the organism finally performs, depends on the strength of the organism's habit.
7. A habit is a response to some stimulus. The strength of the habit depends on the connection between the stimulus and the response that influences what kind of behavior will drive the energy.

Optimum Level of Arousal Theory

1. The optimum level of arousal theory states that drives do not necessarily motivate an organism to seek the lowest level or arousal. Instead, they provide motivation to seek an optimum level of arousal.
2. Robert Yerkes and JD Dodson (1908) conducted an experiment to examine the effects of different arousal levels on learning. They varied arousal levels in mice by changing the intensity of electric shocks and by observing how well the animals performed in simple and complex mazes.
3. The Yerkes-Dodson law states that, performance on a learning task is related to arousal; the best performance results from intermediate levels of arousal. Performance is also related to the difficulty of the task.
4. Yerkes-Dodson found that the mice performed simple tasks better when the stimulation was more intense. For complex tasks, low to intermediate arousal was the best.

Cognitive Theory

1. A cognitive theory (the word comes from the Latin, which means knowing) emphasizes some sort of understanding or

anticipation of events through perception or thought or judgment as in the estimation of probabilities or in making a choice, on the basis of relative value.
2. Any organism with memory is capable of recognizing some similarities between the present and the past and hence is able to form some sort of experience with regard to the consequences of its behavior.
3. According to cognitive theory, motivated goal-seeking behavior comes to be regulated by these conditions, which are based on the past, modified by circumstances of the present and includes expectations about the future.
4. Cognitive dissonance theory: Festinger (1957) proposed a theory in which certain kinds of unbalanced cognitions are described as dissonant and the subject is under stress to remove this dissonance.

Expectancy Theory

1. Expectancy theory emphasizes the importance of rewards and goals as well as how person's expectations of consequences can influence the behavior. This theory stresses 'pull' rather than 'push'.
2. According to expectancy theory, the hunger drive is only a part of the reason. A hungry rat is motivated to find its way through a maze. It is also motivated because of previous learning experiences in which it has come to expect a bit of food at the end.
3. Motivation is composed of two major features—the valence or attractiveness of the goal and the expectancy or the likelihood of its behavior will lead to the goal.
4. A simple way of explaining the expectancy theory is to say that; motivation = valence × expectancy. The actions, which a hungry person takes to satisfy the hunger, depend very much on valence and expectancy.
5. Economic theories assume that the individual can assign value or utility to possible incentives and then makes decision according to the risk involved.

Psychoanalytic Theory of Modification

1. Freud believed that, all behavior stemmed from two opposing groups of instincts. The life instincts (Eros) that enhance life

and growth, and the death instincts (Thanatos) that pushes toward destruction.

2. The energy of the life instincts is libido, which involves mainly sex and related activities. The death instinct can be directed inward in the form of aggression toward others. Freud pointed out several forms of behavior:
   a. In dreams, people often express wishes and impulses of which they are unaware.
   b. Unconscious mannerisms and slip of speech may reveal hidden motives.
   c. Symptoms of illness (particularly symptoms of mental illness) often can be shown to serve the unconscious needs of the person.

Maslow's Hierarchy of Needs

1. The behavior of an individual at a particular moment is usually determined by the strongest need. These needs have a certain priority.
2. The lower level needs (e.g. physiological needs) have the highest strength until they are reasonably met. When the lower level needs are met, man goes to satisfy the higher needs.
3. The hierarchy of needs is organized step-by-step to the satisfaction of other needs such as physiological needs, safety and security needs, social needs, esteem needs and self-actualization needs. A satisfied need is no longer a motivator of behavior.

Herzberg's Two-factor Theory

1. According to Herzberg, there are ten factors called maintenance factors and six factors called motivational factors of satisfactory.
2. The absence of maintenance factors causes dissatisfaction in the employees, but their presence may not produce motivation in the employees.
3. The presence of motivational factors is necessary to produce motivation and job satisfaction in the individual, but their absence may not produce strong dissatisfaction.
4. The maintenance factors are policy and management, supervision, good interpersonal relationship with supervisor, good international peer review (IPR) with peers and subordinates, fair salary, job security, personal life, good working conditions and status.

5. The motivational factors are achievement, recognition, work itself, advancement and responsibility.
6. The Herzberg model has given several insights. One of the insights is job enrichment. The idea behind job enrichment is to keep maintenance factors constant or higher, while increasing motivational factors by attaching more responsibility satisfying working conditions and power to the job. Relationship between Herzberg and Maslow models is shown in the Figure 3.2.

McClelland's Needs Theory

1. McClelland identified three types of basic motivating needs. They are need for power, need for affiliation and need for achievement.
2. Power motive is the need to manipulate others or to drive for superiority over others. Such individuals are generally seeking positions for leadership.
3. The affiliation motive is concerned with maintaining pleasant social relationships, sense of intimacy, understanding and to enjoy in consoling and to help others who are in trouble.
4. Achievement-motivated people can be the backbone of most organizations, because they progress faster. They are highly task oriented and work to their optimum capacity.

Carrot and Stick Approach of Motivation

1. Carrot and stick approach of motivation comes from the old story that the best way to make a donkey move is to put a carrot in front of the donkey and beat the donkey with a stick from behind.

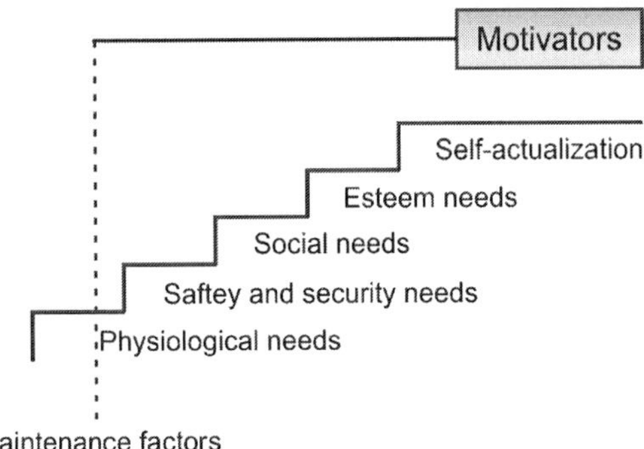

Fig. 3.2: Relationship between Herzberg and Maslow models

2. The carrot is the reward for moving and the stick is the punishment for not moving.
3. To motivate people for better production in an organization, some carrots (rewards) are used such as money, promotion and other incentives.
4. Some sticks (punishments) are used to push the people for desired behavior or to retrain from undesired behavior.

FRUSTRATION

When the pursuit of a goal is thwarted or blocked in any situation, the result is frustration. That is, frustration is the consequence of the blockage of motives or when competing, motives work at the same time and the individual is not in a position to make appropriate choice.

Definition

Frustration is defined as the blocking of a desire or need. It also refers to the failure to satisfy a basic need because of some conditions, either in the individual or external obstacles.

Meaning

1. Frustration is a condition of extreme tension; it is commonly interpreted as a strong emotional tension, caused by the blocking of impulses.
2. The individual is said to be frustrated because he/she does not know how to rid himself/herself of the tension. These tensions make the frustrated person highly uncomfortable.
3. Frustration involves an 'insurmountable' obstacle and the inability to overcome it and a sense of defeat as well as feeling of stress or strain.

Sources

Environmental forces: The frustration may be caused by environmental situations or conditions, which cannot control. Such environmental conditions include a contagious disease, the death of a friend or a beloved relative, unusual rains and storms or floods.

Personal inadequacies: It may be in the form of poor ability or skill in the individual. On the other hand, the person's level of inspiration may be high. This may come in the way of reaching the goals. It may also be due to any physical handicap in the individual.

Conflict of motives: Sometimes frustration results because of interference of one motive with other motives. For example, in the society, sexual motivation is often in conflict with the society's standards of approved sexual behavior.

CONFLICT

Definition

Conflict is a state when two or more incompatible motivations or behavioral impulses compete for expression. In other words, the individual is faced with more than two incompatible demands, opportunities, goals or needs.

Mental conflict is an inner state of mind characterized by tension as a result of the presence of mutually exclusive or opposing tendencies, impulses or desires.

Types

Approach-approach conflict: In this type of conflict, a person is faced with two appealing/attractive goals or choices and he/she is forced to choose one of them. For example, a young computer engineer is offered jobs in two popular multinational companies. The young man is in a dilemma choosing between the two.

Avoidance-avoidance conflict: In this type of conflict, an individual has to make a choice between two unattractive goals. Here the individual is repelled by two undesirable alternatives at the same time. For example, a person has a long history of painful backache for which he/she is advised to undergo surgery. Here the person is faced with the prospect of living with painful backache or undergoing dreadful surgery. This conflict is partly described in the proverb caught between the devil and deep blue sea.

Approach-avoidance conflict: Here the goal has both attractive and repulsive aspects. The choice has pleasant and unpleasant consequences. A prospective young professional bride has an offer to marry a non-resident Indian in America. Here going to America is appealing and at the same time, leaving the parents in India is distressing.

Resolution of conflicts: Conflict often produces stress; stress includes a number of unpleasant responses. Every individual is equipped with capacity to overcome obstacles in order to avoid conflict, which is a source of frustration.

MOTIVATIONAL QUALITIES OF NURSE LEADER

Knowledge and skill, effective communication of ideas, confidence, commitment, energy, insight into the needs of others and an ability to take the necessary actions to achieve goals important to others are the motivational qualities of a nurse leader.

Knowledge and skill: It comes from preparation in the responsibilities of healthcare delivery and organizational duty. The leader has the ability to evaluate the likelihood of success in accomplishing goals and is able to support or suggest changes.

Effective communication of ideas: It involves the ability to convey ideas clearly and in such a way that they can be heard positively.

Confidence: It comes from an internal sense of security that one is competent to make a statement or take action and that there is a reasonable chance of success in accomplishing something of value. The motivational leader is secure enough to have a lower need to control and as a result is able to encourage autonomy, participation and empowerment of staff in decision-making.

Commitment: It is the internalization of an idea and a resulting drive to accomplish specific goals. The mere setting of goals does not indicate leadership that motivates. It is the ability of the leader to translate the importance of the goal (or purpose) to others and to elicit actions from others, which support reaching a goal.

Energy: It is also needed to empower and fire the imagination of others, and constantly invent and move ahead toward future events as well as current needs. Different styles of energy can be motivational. The 'high-energy leader' who is effective in one situation may be viewed as 'pushy and aggressive' in another situation.

Insight into the needs of others: It is the acute awareness of the reason behind the events and an ability to anticipate results of actions. When a leader can put goals into a form that has real or personal value to each person, then motivation will exist.

Additional key qualities: The additional key qualities of a motivational leader are—abilities to listen, reserve judgment, give direction and positive feedback, recognize individual value through respect for others and use humor.

Professional practice and shared governance depends on the clinical leader to produce an environment that fosters autonomy in decision-making and provides the skills, resources and information needed for others to make this transition.

SEVEN RULES OF MOTIVATION

1. Set a major goal, but follow a path: The path has mini goals that go in many directions. When people learn to succeed at mini goals, they will be motivated to challenge grand goals.
2. Finish what you start: A half-finished project is of no use to anyone. Quitting is a habit. Develop the habit of finishing self-motivated projects.
3. Socialize with others of similar interest: Mutual support is motivating. We will develop the attitudes of our best friends. If they are losers, we will be a loser. If they are winners, we will be a winner. To be a cowboy we must associate with cowboys.
4. Learn how to learn: Dependency on others for knowledge supports the habit of procrastination. Man has the ability to learn without instructors. In fact, when we learn the art of self-education we will find, if not create, opportunity to find success beyond our wildest dreams.
5. Harmonize natural talents with interest that motivates: Natural talent creates motivation, motivation creates persistence and persistence gets the job done.
6. Increase knowledge of subjects that inspires: The more we know about a subject, the more we want to learn about it. A self-propelled upward spiral develops.
7. Take risk: Failure and bouncing back are elements of motivation. Failure is a learning tool. No one has ever succeeded at anything worthwhile without a string of failures.

A TO Z STEPS IN MOTIVATION

A : Achieve the dreams. Avoid negative people, things and places. Eleanor Roosevelt once said, "The future belongs to those who believe in the beauty of their dreams."

B : Believe in yourself and in what you can accomplish.

C : Consider things from every angle and aspect. Motivation comes from determination. To be able to understand life, you should feel the sun from both sides.

D : Do not give up and give in. Thomas Edison failed once, twice, more than three times before he came up with his invention and perfected the incandescent light bulb. Make motivation as the steering wheel.

E : Enjoy! Work as if money is not needed, dance as if nobody is watching, love as if you never cried and learn as if you will live forever. Motivational momentum takes place when people are happy.

F : Family and friends are life's greatest 'F' treasures. Do not lose sight of them.

G : Give more than what is enough. Where does motivation and self-improvement take place: At work? At home? At school? Always give 110 percent.

H : Hang on to the dreams. They may dangle for a moment, but these little stars will be the driving force. Define the target and keep trying, until you hit it.

I : Ignore those who try to destroy you. Do not let other people get the best of you. Stay away from toxic people, the kind of friends who hates to hear about your success. Stay away from negativity.

J : Just be yourself. The key to success is to be yourself and the key to failure is to try to please everyone.

K : Keep trying; no matter how hard life may seem. When a person is motivated, eventually sees a harsh life finally clearing out, paving the way to self-improvement.

L : Learn to love yourself. Now, is it not that easy?

M : Make things happen. Motivation is when the dreams are put into work clothes.

N : Never lie, cheat or steal. Always play a fair game.

O : Open the eyes. People should learn the horse attitude and horse sense. They see things in two ways—how they want things to be and how they should be.

P : Practice makes perfect. Practice is about motivation. It lets us learn 'repertoire' and ways on how can we recover from our mistakes.

Q : Quitters never win and winners never quit. So, choose the fate—are you going to be a quitter or a winner?

R : Ready yourself. Motivation is also about preparation. We must hear the little voice within us telling us to get started before others will get on their feet and try to push us around. Remember, it was not raining when Noah built the ark.

S : Stop procrastinating. Do not put off the work until tomorrow what you can do today; we never know what tomorrow will bring.

T : Take control of life. Discipline and self-control lives synonymously with motivation. Both are key factors in self-improvement.

U : Understand others. Know how to talk; should also learn how to listen. Learn to understand first and to be understood the second. We have two ears and one mouth. Use them proportionately.

V : Visualize it. Motivation without vision is like a boat on a dry land. You need to have a crystal clear path.

W : Want it more than anything. Dreaming means believing. And to believe is something that is rooted out from the roots of motivation and self-improvement.

X : X factor is what will make you different from the others. When you are motivated, you tend to put on 'extras' on your life like extra time for family, extra help at work, extra care for friends and so on.

Y : You are unique. No one in this world looks, acts or talks like you. Value your life and existence, because you only get to spend it once.

Z : Zeal, motivation provides strong courage and inspiration to achieve the desired goal.

APPLICATION OF MOTIVATIONAL THEORY IN NURSING EDUCATION

Motivation theory proposes reasons for behavior. One classic approach is Abraham Maslow's 'Toward a Psychology of Being' in 1946. Maslow explains in his later text, 'Motivation and Personality' (in 1954), that individuals move through a hierarchy of motivating needs from physiological safety to social esteem and finally, self-actualization. He suggests that individuals meet each category of needs in that order. Nursing students can identify situations where these needs are met in their practice of nursing.

'Role Play' Application of Theory

1. Teach the students the hierarchy of needs. Ask students to identify an experience to match each level of need. One example is to address the experience of safety in walking across a large hospital parking lot late at night.
2. Tell the students to list needs of patients in the same way. An example is the physiological need to address bleeding or pain from an injury.
3. Present a scenario of hospital duties that includes a nurse acting to address a need. One example is meeting the need for safety in the intake and medical history process.
4. Identify the roles played in the scenario such as patient, parent and nurse. Assign the roles to students. Ask the role players to act out the scenario. In the discussion of the role played, review the hierarchy of needs. Discuss these needs in the areas of physiological safety, social esteem and self-actualization.
5. Instruct the other students to assess the nurse's behaviors that met the identified need. Give examples such as meeting a safety need by asking about allergies to medicines.
6. Discuss what needs the nurse may have experienced such as a need for esteem by being seen as competent.

CONCLUSION

Motivation influences many aspects of life and helps to explain different causes of behavior. It aids survival, accounts for variations in any individual's behavior and guides the actions. Motivation operates in a cycle.

Homeostasis involves maintaining various bodily processes within a narrow range of acceptability. Deviations from that norm lead to automatic corrective actions.

Motivation is the drive forces, which begins, sustains and directs human activities. Motivation is the 'why' of human behavior. Motivation is made up of need, drive, response and goal. All human beings are motivated by something. Very little human behavior is completely random or instinctive. Most human behavior is goal directed. People do things for some reason to get certain results. Motivation drives the human beings to reach their goals and organization goals through every challenge and constraint they face in their workplace; considering it as an advantage to go ahead in the direction they have put for themselves. The need of achievement always results in a desire to put extra effort to have something done better and have the desire for success.

SUGGESTED READING

1. Edward Ellsworth Jones. Ingratiation: A Social Psychological Analysis. New York: Appleton-Century-Crofts; 1964.
2. Edward L Walker, Roger W Heyns. An Anatomy for Conformity. Englewood Cliffs: NJ Prentice Hall; 1962.
3. Harter, Susan. A new self-report scale of intrinsic versus extrinsic orientation in the classroom: Motivational and informational components. Developmental Psychology. 1981;17(3):300-12.
4. Irving Lester Janis. Psychological Stress: Psychoanalytic and Behavioral Studies of Surgical Patients. New York: Wiley; 1958.
5. Jane Thomas. Guide to Managerial Persuasion and Influence. Upper Saddle River, New Jersey: Prentice Hall; 2004.
6. Jones, Marshall R (Eds). Nebraska Symposium on Motivation. Lincoln: University of Nebraska Press; 1956-1962.
7. Jung Carl G. The Integration of the Personality. New York: 1932, 1936, 1939.
8. Leonard Thompson Troland. The Fundamentals of Human Motivation. New York: D Van Nostrand Company Inc; 1928.
9. Martin EP Seligman. Learned Optimism: How to Change Your Mind and Your Life. New York: Alfred A Knopf Inc; 1991.
10. Robert C Gardner, Wallace E Lambert. Attitudes and Motivation in Second-Language Learning. Rowley, MA: Newbury House Publishers; 1972.
11. Whyte Cassandra B. An additional look at orientation programs nationally (reprint of 1986 article in same journal). National Orientation Directors Association Journal. 2007;15(1):71-7.
12. Whyte, Cassandra B. Effective counseling methods for high-risk college freshmen. Measurement and evaluation in counseling. 1979;6(4):198-200.
13. Whyte CB. In: Lauridsen K (Ed). An Integrated Counseling and Learning Assistance Center. New Directions Sourcebook. Jossey-Bass Inc; 1980.

REVIEW QUESTIONS

1. Define motivation. Explain the nature and the meaning of motivation.
2. Discuss motivational process.

3. Describe the components of motivation.
4. Define motive. Explain the various types or classification of motives.
5. Discuss and describe the theories of motivation.
6. Explain frustration. List down the sources of frustration.
7. Explain the types of conflict in detail.
8. Discuss the motivational qualities of a nurse leader.
9. Explain the need and importance of motivation in nursing.

CHAPTER 4

Emotion

LEARNING OBJECTIVES

1. Definitions of emotion.
2. Expression and perception.
3. Emotions in sickness.

INTRODUCTION

Emotions occupy an important place in our life. Life has become enjoyable because of the emotions like love, affection, personal happiness and the like. But all emotions do not have pleasantly toned effect, those just mentioned. Emotions like fear, anger and jealousy bring about a good deal of disturbance. Our emotions have a great impact on others, when we express them in ways that can be perceived by others. When we perceive the emotional responses of other people, we respond in appropriate ways, perhaps with an emotional expression of our own.

MEANING

1. An emotion is a strong feeling. It is a conscious stirred-up state of any organism.
2. Emotion experienced as certain feelings, pleasant or unpleasant, accompanied by marked physiological changes, involving both visceral and peripheral areas.
3. The subjective experience of an emotion is the cognitive component. Here the conscious experience could be pleasant or unpleasant.

4. The bodily arousal is the physical component; this is reflected by the activation of the autonomic nervous system, which regulates the activity of glands, smooth muscles and blood vessels.
5. Emotion is the mode of experience that accompanies the working of an instinctive impulse.

DEFINITIONS

1. Emotion is a distinct psychological state, which involves subjective experience, physical arousal and behavioral response. In other words, it has a cognitive component, physical component and a behavioral component.
2. Emotion is an affective experience that accompany generalized inner adjustment, mental and physiological stirred-up states in the individual and that shows itself in his/her overt behavior.
3. Emotion is a complex affective experience that involves and diffuses physiological changes and can be expressed overtly in characteristics of a behavior pattern.

PHYSIOLOGY OF EMOTION

Physiological reactions and changes that are associated with emotions have their roots in one's body chemistry. They are controlled by the endocrine glands, the autonomous nervous system and the brain.

Emotion and Autonomic Nervous System

1. Our autonomic nervous system plays a significant role in controlling and regulating the emotional behaviors.
2. The autonomic nervous system consists of sympathetic and parasympathetic system.
3. The sympathetic system activation leads to dilated pupils, dryness of mouth, goose pimples of the skin, sweaty palms, dilation of the lung passages, increased heart rate, increased blood supply to the muscles, increased activity of the adrenal glands and inhibited digestion.
4. The parasympathetic system activation leads to constriction of the pupils, salivation, dryness of palm, absence of goose pimples, constriction of lung passages, decreased heart rate, increased blood supply to internal organs, decreased adrenal gland activity and stimulation of digestion.

Emotion and the Brain

1. The brain controls the autonomic responses that accompany emotions. The seat of emotion in the areas of brain is the hypothalamus, amygdala and the adjacent structures in the limbic system.
2. Emotions appear to be triggered by activity in the centers of the brain, medicated by neurotransmitters. Dopamine has a major role in pleasant emotions.
3. Reticular formation: This mass of cells discharges impulses diffusely and some of them ascend to the cerebral cortex, where they have an alerting function. When the reticular formation is activated, the relaxed or passive organism becomes aroused or alert.
4. Hypothalamus: The limbic system consists of a series of interrelated brain structures, which include the hypothalamus and the septal area, both important in emotions. Impulses from the hypothalamus also activate the viscera and muscles, as when the adrenal gland is stimulated to secrete adrenaline.
5. The hypothalamus, in every way, tries to coordinate the activities of the internal organs associated with the emotional behavior. Impulses that come from the hypothalamus increase both smooth muscle (involuntary) and skeletal muscle (voluntary) activities.
6. The connection between the emotional behavior and stimulation of the various parts of the brain has brought the electric stimulation of the brain, as a method for treating violent behavior in human being, particularly epileptics whose brain malfunction causes unusual aggressive behavior.

CHANGES IN EMOTION

External Changes

1. Emotions are complex experiences; they are psychical as well as physiological and physical. In psychical experiences, the individual feels them as pleasant or unpleasant state of mind.
2. Emotion is a conscious and intellectual perception of a situation, intense and important enough to provoke a person emotionally.
3. The body or organism gets stirred up. Changes occur in breathing, circulation of blood, heart rate and other physiological functions.
4. There are many external changes in the body—changes in our voice, gestures, postures, facial expressions, etc.

5. The changes in facial expressions serve as indices to the nature of emotions. The face of a person experiencing joy is radiated with a smile. The angry man's red face betrays his anger.
6. There is a feeling tone accompanying these physical and physiological changes. All this results in some overt responses or behavior such as laughing, crying and shouting, hitting, crouching and cringing.
7. Bodily postures and gestures too can be used as clues to identify emotions. In sorrow, a person tends to slump his face downward and in joy, he holds head high and chest out.

Internal Changes

1. There is a greater intensity of heart action, which results in palpitation.
2. Blood pressure (BP) increases during emotional excitement.
3. There is a shift of blood from the viscera to the surface of the body causing flushing of face, e.g. anger.
4. There are many changes in the gastrointestinal (GI) tract. For example, churning movements slow down or stop in the stomach and the flow of saliva and other gastric juices necessary for digestion, is reduced by 85% to 90%.
5. There is a greater secretion of glycogen into the blood, sweat glands become more active.

Physiological Changes

Psychologists believed that emotions can be measured quantitatively by observing different physiological responses of the individual, equal indicators of emotions. They also believed that they themselves are of different emotional states. The major physiological changes that occur during emotions are respiratory changes, GI changes, etc.

Respiratory Changes

Respiratory changes are the most apparent and obvious change during emotions. During emotions, respiration increases; also occurs when the person is happy or excited. But the production and secretion of saliva decreases as the process of respiration increases.

Changes in Blood Pressure and Heart Rate

Variations in BP occur during emotions; usually increases during an emotional state. Heartbeat also increases during emotions. Increased BP and heightened heart rate for prolonged periods may lead to coronary heart disease.

Glandular Responses

During strong emotional states such as anger or fear, excessive amounts of hormones like adrenaline and noradrenaline are secreted into the bloodstream. Due to this secretion; liver secretes excessive amounts of glucose directly into the bloodstream that causes the blood to clot rapidly in case of injury or damage. Blood pressure and sugar level rises, pulse becomes fast, air passage of the lungs enlarges and causes more air into the lungs, pupil enlarge, sweat appears all over the body, particularly on hands and temperature of the skin rises. Noradrenaline helps to constrict the blood vessels, thus making it available to other parts of the body in case of injury. Pituitary and thyroid glands are also responsive to emotional states. All the glandular responses help to cope physically with the emotional as well as emergency situations.

Gastrointestinal Changes

Stomach and intestines are also very responsive to emotional states. They either start working at a very high rate or stop entirely. During strong emotional arousal, its working speed decreases and flow of blood is more toward the brain and the skeletal muscles, rather than these organs.

Neural Reactions

Besides affecting visceral organs of the body, emotions also bring changes in the neural/nerve activity. Autonomic division of the peripheral nervous system (PNS) is more effective in this regard in which sympathetic and parasympathetic nervous systems work successively.

Galvanic Skin Response

When perspiration appears during emotions, two important changes occur in skin's electrical stimulation: rapid generation of electromotive energy and the electrical resistance of skin changes. These changes can be measured through a measurement of 'galvanic skin response (GSR)'; formerly called 'psychogalvanic response (PGR)'.

Emotional Intensity and State of Arousal

Most of the times, we are aware of our emotional states such as angry, excited or afraid, in all these states, the physiological conditions are the same, e.g. heartbeat increases, face blushes or becomes pale. That is why we are unable, at times, to differentiate between different emotions and the associated arousal.

Other Common Bodily Changes

1. Dryness of throat and mouth.
2. Muscle tension.
3. Weakness or fainting.
4. Trembling.
5. Sinking feeling in heart or stomach.

CHARACTERISTICS OF EMOTION

1. Emotions are universal—prevalent in every living organism at all stages of development, from infancy to old age.
2. Emotions rise abruptly, but subside slowly. An emotion once aroused, tends to persist and leave behind emotional hangover.
3. Emotions are personal and thus differ from individual to individual.
4. An emotion can give birth to a number of other similar emotions.
5. The emotional experiences are associated with one or the other instincts or biological drives.

TYPES OF EMOTION

Pleasure

1. Pleasure is a reaction to the satisfaction of a motive or the attainment of a goal, i.e. satisfaction of motive state results in the emotion of pleasure.

2. We derive a great deal of pleasure from daydreams in which we think about attaining certain goals.
3. The emotion of pleasure manifest in smiling, laughing, hugging and kissing or in contentment is evoked by situations, which give physical comfort to the infant or a young child.

Fear

1. In general, fear is triggered by situations that are perceived as physically threatening, damaging to one's sense of well-being.
2. Fear is produced in children by sudden happenings, when the child is not prepared for what is coming. In infancy, strange and intense stimuli like noise produce fear.
3. An adolescent boy or girl is afraid of social humiliation and ridicule. In adulthood, we are afraid of situation, which threatens our needs to obtain recognitions, prestige and economic security.
4. Several factors are important in determining what are the specific sources of fear will be for an individual.

Anxiety

1. Anxiety is a vague fear experienced unknowingly, just what the matter is. One cause of anxiety can be unconscious memory of a fear stimulus.
2. When we learn a response to a particular situation, we have learned a response to all situations that are similar to the earlier one.
3. A child who learns to fear a strict father may later feel uneasy or anxious in the presence of other men.

Anger and Hostility

1. Anger and hostility are reactions to the frustration of motives, insults and threats.
2. Frustrating a motive by imposing restraints and behavior is likely to provoke anger in a person of any age. For infants, a simple restraint (which frustrates exploratory motive) is common cause of anger.
3. Social frustrations are also common cause of anger in adults. We seldom observe and outright display it. Most frequent are the feelings of anger that we call 'annoyance'.

4. Ways of expressing anger changes with age. Among preschool children, anger is likely to take the form of temper, tantrums and fighting.
5. An adult feels angry when his prestige is at stake, the desires are being thwarted and plans are being foiled.

Depression and Grief

1. When depressed, people often feel inadequate and worthless because of their failure to reach important goals. The depressed person loses the joy of living.
2. For most of us, depression does not last long because the situation in the environment changes and we are able to reach at least some of our goals. But for some people, perhaps because of an innate predisposition, depression can be prolonged and severe enough to make suicide.
3. Grief or sorrow and depressions are closely related, but there are differences between them. We usually call the emotion as grief, when it is triggered by a specific loss, such as the death of a family member or friend.

Classification of Emotion by Robert Plutchik

Humans express a wide variety of emotions. Robert Plutchik, who was a professor emeritus at the Albert Einstein College of Medicine, did research on emotions and designed a color wheel that depicts the intensity level of emotions. Eight primary emotions, in three strengths, for a total of 24 emotions, form this wheel. These are: joy, trust, fear, surprise, sadness, disgust, anger and anticipation. Eight other and secondary emotions are: love, submission, awe, disapproval, remorse, contempt, aggressiveness and optimism.

Serenity

Serenity and its increasingly intense companions such as joy and ecstasy, demonstrate increasingly positive feelings. Serenity is calmness; and joy shows happiness or gaiety, while ecstasy flows forth as pure delight or bliss.

Acceptance

Acceptance, trust and admiration show increasing feelings of respect. Acceptance means approval; trust means a firm belief in someone or something and admiration signifies esteem.

Apprehension

Apprehension, fear and terror signify emotional discomfort. Apprehension means a sense of uneasiness and fear represents aversion, but terror means phobia.

Distraction

Distraction, surprise and amazement are related to unexpected. Distraction shows a lack of focus. Surprise means unexpected, usually in reference to a gift or event. Amazement is astonishment or sudden wonder.

Pensive

Pensiveness, sadness and grief represent intensified feelings of sorrow. Pensiveness shows sad thoughtfulness. Sadness means unhappiness, but grief generally relates to sorrow over death.

Boredom

Boredom, disgust and loathing show aversion. Boredom represents a lack of interest; and disgust is repugnance. Loathing means extreme hatred.

Annoyance

Annoyance, anger and rage demonstrate levels of ire. Annoyance shows mild irritation and anger may be spoken or non-verbal, but demonstrates hostility. Rage vents as intense fury.

Interest

Interest, anticipation and vigilance show increasing concern. Interest is beginning attention. Anticipation marks a pleasurable expectation. Vigilance signifies watchfulness.

Love and Submission

Plutchik introduced the secondary emotions with love, although most people would consider it a primary emotion. Love demonstrates strong affection, but submission is a feeling of service.

Awe and Disapproval

Awe represents wonder combined with slight fear; and disapproval means censure.

Remorse and Contempt

Remorse means deep sorrow or disappointment; and contempt is disdain.

Aggressiveness and Optimism

Aggressiveness signifies the powerful outward expression of strong emotion such as that shown by bullies. Optimism shows a positive belief in the best possible outcomes.

EMOTION AND HEALTH

1. Emotions play an important role in human life. We wish to influence other persons actions, we can do so by raising the appropriate emotions. They give us energy to carry out the activity.
2. Modern discoveries in medicine have shown to us that uncontrolled emotionality plays a vital role in the causation of many physical disorders.
3. Persistent emotional disturbances caused by anger, fear and worries, have been found to be one of the causative factors of psychosomatic disorders.
4. The continuous worries, fears and anxieties cause perpetual tensions. As a result, one's mental health is bound to be affected.
5. A relatively new field of investigation known as psychosomatic disease has thrown some light upon it. It has shown how an emotional strain can cause bodily harm.
6. Illness like asthma, chronic headache, certain skin diseases, nervous pains, etc. are believed to have a psychosomatic origin. Their symptoms may be physiological, but origins are psychological.
7. Other illnesses in which emotions play a vital role are bronchial asthma, high BP, insomnia, chronic constipation and others.
8. Good, pleasant emotions contribute to good health. But intense and unpleasant emotions disturb us sometimes to a great extent, if they persist. They may cause certain illnesses or may worsen the conditions of one already ill.
9. The responsibility of a nurse is not only to practice the nursing skills and provide physical comfort but also to reduce the intensity of emotional disturbances, as much as it is possible.

THEORIES OF EMOTION

Theories of emotion can be categorized in terms of the context within which the explanation is developed. The standard contexts are evolutionary, social and internal. Evolutionary theories attempt to provide a historical analysis of the emotions, usually with a special interest in explaining why humans today have the emotions that they do. Social theories explain emotions as the products of cultures and societies. The internal approach attempts to provide a description of the emotion process itself. Theories of emotion are organized around these three categories and it will discuss the basic ideas that are associated with each one of them. Some specific theories, as well as the main features of emotion will also be explained.

James-Lange Theory

1. William James, an American psychologist and Lange, a Danish physiologist have independently brought forward a theory of emotions that explains the relationship between the components of emotions (Fig. 4.1) in just the opposite direction of the one given above.
2. According to this theory, an emotional experience has primarily a physiological basis. The psychical part is the resultant phenomenon.
3. Studies of patients with spinal cord damage have supported the James-Lange theory. These patients have no feedback from their muscles or viscera, before the injury and many of them reported that their feelings of emotion changed considerably, after the injury.
4. The James-Lange theory of emotions is subject to certain criticisms. The bodily changes in themselves are not seen to be the

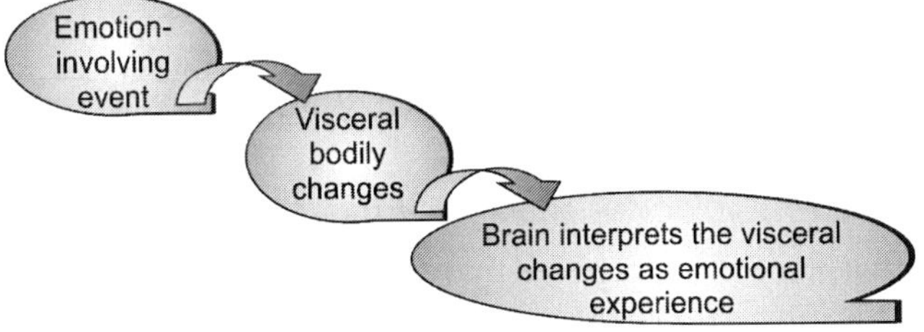

Fig. 4.1: Sequence of events in James-Lange theory of emotions

essential basis of emotions in experimental situations. Such changes brought about by drugs do not cause an experience of emotions.

5. Recently, some scientists have proposed the 'facial feedback hypothesis', which suggests that feedback from the facial muscles and the viscera contribute to the experience of emotion.

Cannon-Bard Theory

1. Walter B Cannon objected to the James-Lange theory for several reasons. Cannon argued that people, whose viscera were surgically separated from the CNS, still reported some kind of emotional experience.
2. This theory emphasizes the role played by hypothalamus in emotional behavior. It says that both the feeling aspect and the bodily changes are set simultaneously by the hypothalamus.
3. Cannon-Bard theory of emotions suggested that emotions originate in the activity of lower brain areas, rather than in the viscera; these circuits then activate both the cortex and viscera. Activity in the brain is critically important for certain emotions.

Cognitive Theories

1. The American psychologists Stanley Schachter and Jerome Singer, while adopting an eclectic approach to both the earlier theories of emotion, introduced a new theory named cognitive theory of emotion.
2. This theory suggested that whenever people are emotionally aroused, they decide, which emotion they are feeling, by cognitively evaluating and appraising situational cues.
3. Network model of emotions is a recent view of the relationship between emotions and cognitions. This theory suggests that manifestations are linked in the brain to memories, for the experience in which those emotions were aroused.

Cognitive Physiological Theory of Emotion

1. Schachter (1959) proposed that emotional states are the function of the interaction of cognitive factors and a state of physiological arousal.

2. Feedback to the brain from physiological activity gives rise to an undifferentiated state of affect. But the felt emotion is determined by the 'label' (cognition), the subject assigns to the aroused state. The assignment of a label is a cognitive process.
3. To interpret the feelings, the subject uses information from past experiences and the perception of what is going around.
4. Experienced and inexperienced users of alcohol and other drugs, label their bodily sensations differently in terms of emotional tone. The initial users have to learn to label the physiological sensations as enjoyable. Hence, emotion is an internal physiological arousal in interaction with cognitive process.

Activation Theory

1. The term activation theory of emotion was actually coined in 1951 by Donald B Lindsley. In general, activation theory refers to the view that emotion represents a state of lightened arousal, rather than a qualitative unique type of psychological, physiological or behavioral process.
2. Arousal is considered to lie on a wide continuum, ranging from a very low level such as deep sleep to such extremely agitated states as rage or extreme anger.
3. According to Lindsley (1951), emotion provoking stimuli activate the reticular activating system in the brainstem, which in turn sends impulses, both upward (toward the cortex) and downward (the musculature). For the occurrence of a significant emotional behavior, the reticular formation must be properly activated.

Somatic Theory

1. Many psychologists held that consciousness was more directly associated with the muscles, than with the brain.
2. Jacobson trained the subjects to relax completely. In this condition, their minds were blank. If the subject thought of moving the arm, electrical potentials showed up in the muscles. Similarly, tension in the region of the eyes accompanied visual images. These experiments clearly show that consciousness is intimately associated with muscular activity.

STRESS AND ADAPTATION

Stress is a term that is difficult to define; it is used loosely and means different things to different people. Some use it to describe an upset feeling or response; others use it to describe the source or stimulus for their feeling upset. Study in the field of stress and adaptation has been pursued by researcher in different disciplines, according to their individual conceptual views.

Definitions

1. Hans Selye (1976) defined stress, as the state manifested by a specific syndrome, which consists of all the non-specifically-induced changes within a biologic system.
2. George Engel (1960) defines stress, as referring to all processes, whether originating in the external environment or within the person, which impose a demand or requirement upon the organism, the resolution or handling of which necessitates work or activity of the mental apparatus, before any other system is involved or activated.
3. Stress is a state produced by a change in the environment that is perceived as challenging, threatening or damaging to the individual's dynamic equilibrium. There is an actual or perceived imbalance in the individual's capability to meet the demands of the new situation.

Nature of Stress

1. Stress is mediated by two factors, the individual's ability to cope and the social support he/she receives.
2. The change or stimulus that evokes this state is the stressor. The nature of the stressor is variable.
3. Stress is any situation in which a non-specific demand requires an individual to respond or take action. It involves physiological and psychological responses.
4. Stress can lead to negative or counterproductive feelings or threaten emotional well-being.

Sources of Stress

Physiologic Stressors

1. The primary physiologic stressors are chemical agent, infectious agent, physical agent, faulty immune mechanisms, genetic disorders, nutritional imbalance and hypoxia.
2. All the stressors have both general effect and a specific effect.

Psychosocial Stressors

1. Accidents and the survivors.
2. The experience of others in our social networks.
3. Horrors of history.
4. Intrapsychic, unconscious conflicts and anxieties.
5. The fear of aggression, mutilation and destruction.
6. The events of history brought into our living room.
7. The changes of the narrower world in which we live.
8. Phase-specific psychosocial crisis.
9. Other normative life crisis—role entries and exits, inadequate socialization, underload and overload.
10. The inherent conflicts in all social relations.
11. The gap between culturally-included goals and socially-structured means.

Factors Influencing Stressors

The nature of the stressor involves the following factors such as intensity, scope, duration, number and nature of other stressors. Each factor influences the response to a stressor. A person may perceive the intensity or magnitude of a stressor as minimal, moderate or severe. The greater the magnitude of stressor, the greater is the stress response. The response to any stressor depends on physiological functioning, personality and behavioral characteristics.

Models of Stress

Response-based Model

1. The response-based model is concerned with specifying the particular response or pattern of responses that may indicate a stressor.

2. Selye's model of stress is a response-based model that defined stress as a non-specific response of the body to any demand made on it.
3. Stress is demonstrated by a specific physiological reaction the general adaptation syndrome (GAS). Thus, the response of a person to stress is purely physiological and is never modified to allow cognitive influences.
4. The response-based model does not allow individual differences in response patterns. This lack of flexibility may produce some differences and must be identified in the assessment phase.

Adaptation Model

1. The adaptation model proposes that, four factors determine whether a situation is stressful or not. The ability to cope with stress, the first factor, usually depends on the person's experience with similar stressor, support systems and overall perception of the stressor.
2. The second factor deals with the practices and norms of the person's peer group. If the peer group is considered, it is normal to talk about a particular stressor; the client may respond by complaining about it or discussing it.
3. The third factor is the impact of the social environment in assisting an individual to adapt to a stressor.
4. The last factor involves the resources that can be used to deal with the stressor.
5. The adaptation model is based on the understanding that people experience anxiety and increased stress, when they are unprepared to cope with stressful situations.
6. Using this model and appropriate interventions, nurses can help clients and families to promote health, in all human dimensions.

Stimulus-based Model

The stimulus-based model focuses on disturbing disruptive characteristics within the environment. The classic research that identified stress as a stimulus has resulted in the development of the social readjustment scale, which measures the effects of major life events on illness. The assumptions of the stimulus-based model are:

1. The life change events are normal and they require the same type and duration of adjustments.

2. People are passive recipients of stress and their perceptions of the event are irrelevant.
3. All people have a common threshold of stimulus and illness results, at any point after the threshold.
4. As with the response-based model, the stimulus-based model does not allow for individual differences in perception and response to stressors.

Transaction-based Model

1. The transaction-based model views the person and environment in a dynamic, reciprocal and interactive relationship.
2. This model, developed by Lazarus and Folkman, views the stressor as an individual perceptual response, rooted in psychological and cognitive process.
3. Stress originates from the relationship of the person and the environment. This model focuses on stress-related process such as cognitive appraisal and coping.

RESPONSE TO STRESS

The classical research by Selye has identified the two physiological responses to stress; the local adaptation syndrome (LAS) and the general adaptation syndrome (GAS). The LAS is a response of a body tissue, organ or part to the stress of trauma, illness or other physiological change. The GAS is a defense response of the whole body to stress.

Local Adaptation Syndrome

The body produces many localized responses to stress. This includes blood clotting, wound healing, accommodation of the eye to light and response to pressure.

Characteristics

1. The body produces many localized responses to stress. These include entire body systems.
2. The response is adaptive, which means that a stressor is necessary to stimulate it.
3. The response is short-term, which means that it does not persist indefinitely.

4. The response is restorative, which means that the LAS assist in restoring homeostasis to the body region or part.

Reflex pain response: The reflex pain response is a localized response of the CNS to pain. It is an adaptive response and protects tissue from further damage.

Inflammation response: The inflammatory response is stimulated by trauma or infection. This response localizes the inflammation, thus preventing its spread and promoting healing. The inflammatory response may produce localized pain, swelling, heat, redness and changes in functioning.

General Adaptive Syndrome

The general adaptive syndrome is a physiological response of the whole body to stress. It involves several body systems, primarily the autonomic nervous system and the endocrine system.

Alarm Reaction

1. The alarm reaction involves the mobilization of the defense mechanisms of the body and mind, to cope with the stress.
2. Hormone levels rise to increase blood volume and thereby prepare the person to act. Other hormones are released to increase blood glucose levels, to make energy available for adaptation.
3. This extensive hormonal activity prepares the person for the fight-or-flight response.
4. During the alarm reaction, the person is faced with a specific stressor. The person's physiological response is extensive, involving major systems of the body and it may last from a minute to many hours.

Resistance Stage

1. In the resistance stage, the body stabilizes and hormone levels, heart rate, blood pressure and cardiac output return to normal.
2. The person is attempting to adapt to the stressor. If the stress can be resolved, the body repairs damage that may have occurred.
3. If the stressor is present, as in continued blood loss, debilitating disease or long-term severe mental illness and adaptation fails, the person enters the third phase of GAS exhaustion.

Exhaustion Stage

1. The exhaustion stage occurs when the body can no longer resist stress and when the energy necessary to maintain adaptation is depleted.
2. The body is unable to defend itself against the impact of the stressor, physiological regulation diminishes and if the stress continues, death may result.

Types of Stimuli

Focal Stimuli

The provoking focal stimuli command the attention of the person. Stimuli become focal because of size, intensity, position, novelty quality, movement and internal predisposing factors such as set and attitude.

Contextual Stimuli

The contextual stimuli category includes those stimuli that surround the focal stimulus. They include all other environmental stimuli present—physical surroundings, other people present and so on.

Residual Stimuli

Residual stimuli are the recalled remnants of past experiences that influence the meanings attached to other stimuli. It includes attitudes, values, beliefs and other factors that influence an individual's behavior in a given situation.

ADAPTATION TO STRESS

Adaptation is a constant, ongoing process that occurs along the time continuum, beginning with birth and ending with death. Also existing along with lifetime continuum is the dimensions of health and illnesses. Adaptation is a continuous process of seeking harmony in an environment. The desired end goals of adaptation for any system are growth and reproduction. A major nursing objective is to support and promote the efforts of the individual to achieve a healthy adaptation.

Concept of Adaptation

1. Adaptation is a term used to describe the work expended by the body, in attempting to maintain homeostasis and toward the off effect of the stressor.
2. The current usage of the term includes the multiplicity of genetic, physiologic, psychic and social phenomena through which adjustment (homeostatic balance) is achieved in response to changes within the environment.
3. According to Helsen's concept of adaptation, constant and varied stimuli impinge on each individual at all times.
4. The basic premise of the adaptation level theory is that an individual's attitudes, values, ways of structuring experiences, judgments of physical, esthetic and symbolic objects, intellectual and emotional behavior, learning and interpersonal relations—all represent modes of adaptation to environmental and organism forces.

Modes of Adaptation

In the Roy adaptation theory, humans are conceptualized as having four modes of adaptation.

Basic Physiologic Needs

As human respond to environmental changes, they will need to keep balance in exercise, nutrition, elimination, fluid and electrolytes, oxygen, circulation and regulation (temperature, sense, endocrine system).

Self-concept

Self-concept includes all the ideas, feelings, beliefs and attitudes that persons have about them. To maintain psychological adaptation, defense mechanisms may be used to protect the ego, when the self-concept is threatened.

Role Mastery

In this mode of adaptation, humans are viewed as regulating their performance of duties, according to their varying positions in society.

Interdependent

Environmental changes may threaten conflict in a person's interactions with other persons.

ADAPTATION CONCEPT IN NURSING

In the conceptual framework of adaptation, nursing intervention becomes the means through which the nurse's knowledge and skills are interposed in supporting and promoting the patient's adaptive potential to the highest level of effectiveness.

Assessment

First level: Recognizing patient's level of wellness behavior in each adaptive mode.
Second level: Identifying positive and negative behaviors related to problem areas.

Planning

Selecting appropriate intervention from basic seven adaptations:

1. Reducing or limiting stress.
2. Preventing additional stress.
3. Supporting adaptations.
4. Limiting and supporting adaptations.
5. Altering, limiting and supporting adaptations.
6. Interrupting, altering, limiting and supporting adaptations.
7. Supplementing, interrupting, altering, limiting and supporting adaptations.

Intervention

Saxton and Hyland point out seven objectives to nursing intervention, related to stress and adaptation.

1. Reduce or limit the extent and intensity of the present stress.
2. Prevent additional stress.
3. Support the individual's adaptations to assist in sustaining and maintaining the defensive responses.
4. Limit and support the individual's adaptations to confine and restrict the compensatory responses.
5. Interrupt, alter, limit and support the individual's adaptations to modify and adjust the symptoms or response.

6. Interrupt, alter, limit and support the individual's adaptations, to discontinue or stop the responses that have become stresses.
7. Supplement, interrupt, alter, limit and support the individual's adaptations to complement or replace the responses that are failing to control stress.

Evaluation

Reassessing patient's level of wellness behavior in each adaptive mode to determine satisfactory resolution of problem area or need for reassessment and replanning.

NURSING IMPLICATIONS ON STRESS REDUCTION

Copying behavior should be remembered that the individual is in constant interaction with his/her environment, both internal and external. This implies that change is constant and necessary for optimal psychosocial and physiological growth. The development of a nursing database that supplies the essential information for making decisions about patient care is a necessity.

Strategies of Stress Reduction

Modification of the Situation

Techniques to reach these goals may include changing jobs, if the workplace is the source of excessive stress. Through health appraisals, nurses may identify patient stressors. The stress control requires self-care and motivation and therefore, the patient must actively and willingly participate in appraising, identifying and managing the sources of stress.

Modification of the Meaning of the Problem

It may require taking a longer range view of situation or putting it into perspective. Compulsive behavior, deadlines and clock watching may need to be re-evaluated.

Control or Management of the Symptoms of Stress

The individual needs to be able to anticipate the development of stress and to know how to typically react.

Stress Reduction Methods

Self-regulation of Stress

Sutterley (1982) has described six categories of approaches to self-regulation of stress. Proper nutrition, adequate rest and regular exercise improve one's well-being and help develop resistance to stressors. Regular exercise assists in weight control, decrease a sense of fatigue and monotony and increase the exercise tolerance for patients with angina pectoris and peripheral arterial disease.

Biofeedback

The purpose of biofeedback is to gain some degree of mental control over the autonomic nervous system and possibly decrease blood pressure, control heart rate and prevent migraine headaches, hyperactive stomach, etc. Some form of electronic instrumentation is used to monitor a biological function such as measuring skin conductance with the galvanic skin responder.

Relaxation Response

Benson (1975) has described what he calls the 'relaxation response', which is a calming state opposite to the arousal state or stress. Four elements are necessary to produce the relaxation response: a quite environment, a comfortable position, a passive attitude and a mental device or object, such as a word, sound or phrase occupy the mind and keep out thoughts.

Social Supports

The importance of social support as a mediating resource in stress has already been identified. To reinforce the information, the function of social networks includes the maintenance of positive social identity, the provision of emotional support, the provision of material aid and tangible services, access to information and access to new social contacts and new social roles.

ROLE OF NURSE IN EMOTIONAL CONTROL

A number of patients show emotional reactions like anxiety, worry, fear, irritability, anger and resentment. Such negative feelings need to be replaced by hope, courage and cooperation. A nurse should listen sympathetically, develop cooperative relationship with the patients and help them to reduce the tensions.

Emotions are controlled as follows:

1. The causes, reactions and consequences of emotions are studied.
2. Emergency situations are avoided because they cause strong emotional reactions. Adequate planning is useful in preventing emergencies.
3. Mental conflicts and emotional tensions are avoided by adopting a sound philosophy of life.
4. Hobbies and sound social relationships are developed, so as to direct one's attention away from emotion-provoking situations.
5. Unreasonable and uncontrolled external expression of emotions is avoided, since it increases the intensity of emotions further.
6. A sense of humor is developed. It helps overlook irritations and petty annoyances.

CONCLUSION

In hospitals and clinics, there are clients of different ways of behavior. Sometimes nurses face some situations whereby they will be stimulated to change their behavior. There are situations whereby nurses will be ordered to give patient medication at a certain time; some patient will be refusing to take it due to some reasons like religious beliefs. Some nurses will come to an extent of being angry. Some nurses will use the defense mechanism called denial. They normally deny whatever is happening by doing as if nothing is happening. They normally control their anger by talking to the patient with low and slowly explaining them, the importance of the medication. Nurses face different emotions each and every day. Patients show unhappiness, confusion, anger and sadness. So nurses should be able to manage their own emotions, so that they can be able to remain calm during unstable conditions. Nurses have to suppress any negative feelings toward patients in order to demonstrate a non-judgmental manner with patients.

Basically, emotions are socially very important because, through it, people can work together or bind to each other and they make life worth living or sometimes ending. So it is considered important for each and everyone to know and understand more about emotions. For nurses, it is a must to acquire knowledge and understand more about emotions, since they are dealing with people of different characters, who can just arouse their feelings in any other way. Hence by understanding it, they may know how to cope with situation they encounter in their working places. Least, but not last, emotions are like wild horses, so people have to consider it before they take a step forward.

SUGGESTED READING

1. Arnel B Salgado. Psychology for Nurses: Emotions, 1st edition. Malaysia: McGraw-Hill companies; 2009.
2. Burnard P. Counselling: A Guide to Practice in Nursing. Oxford: Butterworth-Heinemann; 1994.
3. Carrothers RM, Gregory SW, Gallagher TJ. Measuring emotional intelligence of medical school applicants. Academic Medicine. 2002;75(5):456-63.
4. Caruso DR, Mayer JD, Salovey P. Relation of ability measure of emotional intelligence to personality. Journal of Personality Assessment. 2002;79(2):306-20.
5. Dennis Coon. Introduction to Psychology: Emotional Intelligence, 9th edition. United States of America; 2003.
6. Dennis Coon. Introduction to Psychology: Emotions, 10th edition. United States of America; 2004.
7. Edward P Sarafino. Health Psychology: Ways of Expressing Emotions, 4th edition. San Francisco: John Wiley & Sons Inc; 2002.
8. Henry L, Roediger III. Psychology, 3rd edition. Canada: Little Brown & Company; 1984.
9. Lester M Sodorow. Psychology, 4th edition. United States of America: McGraw-Hill Companies; 1998.
10. Philip GZ, Richard JG. Psychology and Life, 14th edition. New York: Harper Collins College Publishers; 1996.
11. Raty H, Snellman L. Does gender make any difference? Common-sense conceptions of intelligence. Social Behavior and Personality. 1992;20(1):23-34.
12. Rita LA, Richard CA. Introduction to Psychology, 12th edition. United States of America; 1996.
13. Rogers C. Regarding learning and its facilitation. In: Freedom to Learn, Merrill, Columbus; 1969. pp. 157-64.
14. Samuel EW, Ellen GW, Denise Boyd. Mastering the World of Psychology, 2nd edition. United States of America; 2006.
15. Wayne Weiten, Margaret AL. Psychology Applied to Modern Life, 6th edition. Canada; 1990.

REVIEW QUESTIONS

1. Define emotion. Explain the meaning of emotion.
2. Discuss in detail about physiology of emotion.
3. Describe the internal and external changes of emotion.
4. Enumerate the characteristics and types of emotion.
5. Describe the relation between health and emotion.
6. Explain the theories of emotion in detail.
7. Discuss stress and adaptation.
8. Explain the nursing implications on stress reduction.
9. Role of nurse in emotional control.

CHAPTER 5 Personality

LEARNING OBJECTIVES

1. Definitions.
2. Constituents of personality.
3. Personality in sickness and nursing.

INTRODUCTION

Etymologically the word personality has been derived from the Latin word *persona*. *Persona* means mask used by actors on the stage. Personality in the modern usage of the term means the real individual. Personality covers the whole nature of an individual and hence it is very difficult to define it. The personality system is a complex product of biological endowment, cultural shaping, cognitive style and spiritual groups. When psychologist talk of personality they mean a dynamic concept describing the growth and development of person, as a whole, which is composed of habits, interests, attitudes, will, character, etc. Watson (1930) the father of behaviorism, taking clues from his behavioral studies, tried to conclude that personality is the sum of activities that can be discovered by actual observations over a long enough period of time to give reliable information.

CONCEPTS

1. Personality is a combination of all the behavioral, emotional, temperamental and mental attributes that shape the unique character of a person.

2. Personality includes both physical and mental characteristics of the person, which determine his/her general and specific qualities. The distinct identity of the person is only determined by his/her personality.
3. The impact of personality can always be seen on the behavior, thoughts, conducts, actions and activities of the person.
4. Personality is also described as the unique pattern of traits, which characteristics the individual. Traits are characteristics of an individual like good natured, calm, anxious, shy and irritable.
5. Personality includes the behavior patterns, a person shows across situation or the psychological characteristics of the person that lead to those behavior patterns.
6. Personality includes the cognitive, affective and psychomotor behavior and covers all the conscious, subconscious and unconscious also.
7. Personality is not static, but dynamic in nature. Personality of an individual keeps adjusting itself to the environment on a continuous basis. A fine balance is maintained between the environmental and the inner forces.
8. Personality is the individual characteristic (and relatively during) organization (or integration) of ways of behaving (or trait, motives, interests, abilities, attitudes) and modes of adjustment to others and to his/her total environment.

DEFINITIONS

1. Personality is the dynamic organization within the individual of those psychophysical systems that determine his unique adjustments to the environment. —*Gordon Allport*
2. Personality may be defined as the most characteristic integration of an individual's structure, modes of behavior, interests, attitudes, capacities, abilities and aptitudes. —*MN Munn*
3. The more or less stable and enduring organization of a person's character, temperament, intellect and physique that determines his/her unique adjustment to the environment is defined as personality. —*Eysenck*
4. Personality is that which permits a prediction of what a person will do in a given situation. —*Cattell*
5. Personality is a person's unique pattern of traits. —*Guilford*

6. Personality is the most adequate conceptualization of a person's behavior in all its detail. —*McClelland*
7. Personality is a study concerned with the interaction of the biological organism with the social interaction. —*Gardner Murphy*
8. Personality is the sum total of all the biological innate dispositions, impulses, tendencies acquired by experience. —*Morton Prince*
9. Each individual's characteristically recurring patterns of behavior are known as personality. —*Kolb*
10. Personality refers to the aggregate of the physical and mental qualities of the individual's as these interact and function in characteristic fashion with his environment. —*Taylor*
11. Personality consists of the distinctive patterns of behavior including thoughts and emotions that characterize each individual's adaptation to the situations of his/her life. —*Walter Mischel*
12. Personality is the sum of activities that can be discovered by actual observations over a long enough period of time to give reliable information. —*Watson*
13. Personality refers to deeply ingrained patterns of behavior, which include the way one relates to, perceives and thinks about the environment and oneself. —*American Psychiatric Association (APA)*
14. Personality is defined as enduring patterns of perceiving, relating to and thinking about environment and oneself. —*Diagnostic and Statistical Manual of Mental Disorders-IV (APA)*
15. Personality refers to the organized consistent and general pattern of behavior of a person, which helps us to understand his /her behavior as individual. —*Indira Gandhi National Open University (IGNOU)*
16. Personality is a united multiplex, which means a unity composed of elements. He further stated that personality is continuous in an individual's life, a perpetual and a consistent whole, which represent his/her entire life pattern. —*Stern*

COMPONENTS

Physical appearance: It refers the physique of an individual. Some people place much emphasis on looks and judge mental alertness from personal appearances, it cannot be denied that to some extent, success and failure is determined by personal appearance, which includes not only weight, height, complexion but also voice, dress, other characteristics of personal nature.

Character: It refers to the ethical or moral aspect of a personality, which one possesses. The character of an individual is judged by the level of consistency exhibited in the person behavior.

Temperament: It refers to the deep-rooted emotional trends present in an individual. It is a result of secretion of endocrine glands as well as habit formation. Temperament plays an important role in one's ability to adjust to their environment.

Interest: It refers to a felt need. It is connected to three aspects, the need to know, feel and perform.

Ability: It refers to a special natural power to do something well, physical or mental.

Sociability: It refers to an ability of the individual to socialize them-self in a social environment and how others perceive their presence in the group. This trait is present in varying degree in different people. The young child is inclined to be extremely selfish and self-centered, but gradually they learn to share their things and experiences with others. They play with other children and share their toys with them. This give and take cooperation in childhood lays the foundation of social solidarity at the adult level.

Emotionality: It refers to the ability of an individual to show mature emotional behavior in suitable situations. Emotionality has a powerful role to play in personality. The emotional stability and maturity is required for healthy personality.

Moral character: This trait refers to social approval as to whether to have a balanced personality pursuing well-defined goals that benefit to the individual society.

Intelligence: It is capacity of an individual to learn and solve problems and adjust to relatively new and changing conditions. These are individual differences, but it is desired from well-balanced personality in which intelligence is supplemented by healthy social being.

VARIABLES

There are three basic factors or variable, which have to be considered in describing the analyzation of the personality:

1. The internal aspects of the individual or organism: The basic drives, covert feelings, the physiological systems, glands and inherently determined physical features of a person.
2. The social and material stimuli or situations exterior to the individual. These modify and direct the person impulses and needs. They include the influence of family and other groups to which one belongs, the influence of customs, traditions and cultures.
3. The reaction of behavior or conduct, which results from the interaction of the individual and the stimuli.

From these three basic variables, it will be clear that personality is a dynamic thing. It grows in a social setup through social experiences. These variables do not stand apart from each other; they are related to each other, they are interconnected and as well as a result of this integration give raise to a characteristic behavior pattern or quality called personality.

FACTORS INFLUENCING PERSONALITY

Physiological Factor

Physiological factors include the physique of the individual size, strength, looks and constitution. They also include the physical deficiencies and nature of glandular functioning. The physiological conditions of the body influenced by drugs, diseases, diets, toxins and bacterial infections, may also shape the behavior and personality. The changes are shown below:

1. Physical appearance is the first thing that attracts the attention when they meet a person and the judgment of toward them is inevitably colored by it. An attractive physical appearance helps to create self-confidence, poise, self-reliance and other similar personality traits in the individual. A well-built person generally enjoys a forceful and impressive personality. They may develop a tendency to bully or to dominate or to protect. The smaller person may feel to be titled in the presence of large and tall people. They may try to compensate for this by doing hardworking.

2. Physical attractiveness, strength and general health may determine certain reactions and traits. But it must be remembered that these things in themselves are not the major factors that determine one's personality.
3. Physical handicaps such as orthopedic defects, a bad squint in the eye, snub nose or deafness may cause shyness, reserve and unsociableness in persons.
4. The endocrine glands produce hormones, which have the power to raise or depress the activity of the various organs. They influence emotional behavior and hence color their personality. They bring about changes in physical appearance, motor functioning, intelligence and emotional stability. The parathyroid gland regulates calcium metabolism. Excitability of nervous system is directly dependent on the amount of calcium in the blood. Deficient working of this gland leads to the development of an irritable, quick reactive, distracted, nervous and a tense person. Similarly other glands namely the pituitary, the adrenal and the gonads have their tremendous impact on various personality traits.
5. Syphilis infections of the brain or general paralysis may change a truthful, meticulous person into one who is dishonest and unreliable. Encephalitis, lethargic or sleeping sickness may cause serious behavior problems in a child who has been a joy with parents and teachers.
6. Nervous system: Entire behavior is effectively managed and controlled by the coordination and functioning of the nervous system. The sense impressions, which are received through sense organs, do not bear any significance unless they are given meaning by the nervous system.
7. Hereditary: At conception, when the egg cell of the female is fertilized by the sperm cells of the male, each new human being receives a genetic inheritance that provides potentialities for development and behavioral traits throughout a lifetime. The principle raw materials of personality—physique, intelligence and temperament are the result of heredity.

Environmental or Social Factor

The social aspects of an individual's environment affect personality significantly. Cruze says, an individual's personality is influenced more by the reactions of other people to him and his reactions to other people than by any other factor in the environment. Of these social factors, the most important are the relationship in the home and the family, the influence of the school and the playground, the social codes and social roles, which the individual has to play in the family environment and in the community are given below:

1. Family: The reaction of the family environment toward an individual and the role of parents are very important in the molding of personality. Parents serve as a model that the child imitates and their influence is considerable on the child. Parents influence the development of a child's personality in a wide variety of ways. Children learn the moral values, code of conduct, social norms and methods of interacting with others from parents.
2. School: The children spend much of their time in the schools and hence it can play a very significant part in the formation of the personality of the child. A nurturing school atmosphere provides for all round development of the child.
3. Teacher: A teacher is the most important person in the school who can help in modifying the children's personalities. Teacher is the most powerful source of stimulation for the child.
4. Peer group: Peer group refers to other children of the same age who study with or play with the child. Peer group is much more influential than sibling or parents. The peer group serves as an important reference group in shaping personality traits and characteristics of the growing child. As peer group grows up peers become progressively more influential in molding the child's self-concept.
5. Culture: Culture influences personality because every culture has a set of ethical and moral values, beliefs and norms, which considerably shapes behavior. Cross-cultural studies have pointed out the importance of cultural environment in shaping the personality.

Psychological Factors

Psychological factors include motives, acquired interests, attitudes, will and character, intellectual capacities such as intelligence, reasoning, attention and perception, and imagination. These factors determine their reaction in various situations and thus, affect personality growth and direction

TYPES

Hippocrates Classification

Hippocrates (400 BC) was great physician, known as *Father of Medicine*. Based on the individuals temperaments, human being are classified into four characteristic groups (Table 5.1).

Table 5.1: Hippocrates classification

Sl No	*Type of fluids in the body*	*Personality type*	*Temperamental characteristics*
1.	Blood	Sanguine	Optimistic, happy, hopeful, accommodating and light hearted
2.	Phlegm	Phlegmatic	Cold, calm, slow and indifferent
3.	Black bile	Melancholic	Sad, depressed, pessimistic, dejected, deplorable and self-involved
4.	Yellow bile	Choleric	Irritable, passionate, strong, active, imaginative

Kretschmer's Classification

Kretschmer classificated all human being into certain personality types according to their physical structure (Table 5.2).

Table 5.2: Kretschmer's classification

Sl No	*Physical structure*	*Personality type*	*Characteristics*
1.	Fatty body	Pyknic	Sociable, jolly, easy going and good natured
2.	Balanced body	Athletic	Energetic, optimistic and even adjustable
3.	Lean and thin	Leptosomatic	Unsociable, reserved, shy, sensitive and pessimistic

Sheldon's Classification

Human being was classified by their physical body structures and attached certain temperamental characteristics to them (Table 5.3).

Jung's Classification

Carl G Jung (Table 5.4) classify the personality based on complex network of ideas bound together by a common emotion or a set of feeling.

Table 5.3: Sheldon's classification

Sl No	*Name*	*Description*	*Characteristics*
1.	Endomorphic	Person having highly developed viscera, but weak somatic structure (fat, soft, round—like pyknic type)	Easy going, sociable, affectionate and fond of eating
2.	Mesomorphic	Balanced development of viscera and somatic structure (muscular, strong—like athletic type)	Craving for muscular activity, self-assertive, loves risk and adventure, energetic, assertive and bold tempered
3.	Ectomorphic	Weak somatic structure as well as undeveloped viscera (thin, long fragile—like Kretschmer's leptosomatic)	Pessimistic, unsociable, reserved brainy, artistic and introvert

Table 5.4: Jung's classification

Sl No	*Features*	*Extrovert*	*Introvert*
1.	Interest	The extroverts are interested in the world around them	The introverts are interested in themselves, their self-feeling, emotions and are unable to adjust easily to social situation
2.	Social interaction	Involves in social participation, are sociable, not easily upset by difficulties	Socially they are aloof and withdrawn
3.	Adjustment	They are successful in adjusting to the realities of their environment, are socially active and more interested in leaving a good impression on others	They prefer to work alone and avoid social contacts, are inclined to worry and get easily embarrassed
4.	Influencing factor	Their behavior is influenced more by physical stimulation than by their inner thoughts and ideas	Introverts are the persons who seek the manifestation of their life through inner activities by going inward or dragging up things from within themselves
5.	Area of occupation	Politicians, social worker, lawyers, insurance agents, salesmen, etc. fall in this category	Philosophers, scientists, writers, etc.

Hans Eysenck's Classification

The distinct types in Hans Eysenck (1967) theory of personality are introversion, extroversion, neuroticism and psychoticism (Table 5.5).

Table 5.5: Hans Eysenck's classification

Sl No	*Types of personality*	*Characteristics*
1.	Type A personality	The characteristics of type A personality are competitive, drive, restlessness, hostility, sense of urgency, impatience, hard driving, live under constant pressure; seeks recognition and advancement, multiple activities with deadlines to meet and cope up more constructively with stressors might be useful
2.	Type B personality	Calmer, more philosophical, easy going, non-competitive, little dull, longer life, struggle to control situation, but when they fail to do so, they stop coping

Gordon Allport's Classification

Gordon Allport counted 18,000 traits terms (1937), designated as distinctive and personal forms of behavior and divided into three parts (Table 5.6).

Table 5.6: Gordon Allport's classification

Sl No	*Traits*	*Characteristics*
1.	Cardinal traits	Are traits, which are so dominant that nearly all of the individual's actions can be traced back to them. Each term describes a trait so broad and so deep in its impact that it overshadows the influence of other traits in the same individual. Allport believed that most people have no true cardinal traits.
2.	Central traits	Are traits, which are major characteristics of a person such as trust, worthiness, honesty or conscientiousness.
3.	Secondary traits	Are less important characteristics that are not central to our understanding of an individual's personality such as particular attitudes, performance and style of behavior.

THEORIES

There are six paradigms that have been chosen to represent personality theories (Hergenhahn, 1944). Each paradigm is named after its central theme. All paradigms provide useful information about personality and contribute to understanding personality are given below:

1. *Psychoanalyticl paradigm:* For example, personality theories of Sigmund Freud and Carl Jung. This paradigm focuses on the analysis of the psyche.
2. *Sociocultural paradigm:* For example, personality theories of Alfred Adler, Karen Horney and Erik Erikson. This paradigm emphasizes the importance of sociocultural factors influencing personality.
3. *Trait paradigm:* For example, personality theories of Gordon Allport and Raymond B Cattell. This paradigm emphasizes the importance of various traits that a person possesses.
4. *Learning paradigm:* For example, personality theories of Skinner BF, John Dollard and Neal Miller, Albert Bandura and Walter Barash. This paradigm emphasizes the importance of learning in personality development.

Freud's Psychoanalytical Theory

Sigmund Freud (1939), *Father of Psychoanalytical Theory,* is created as the first to identify development by stages (Table 5.7). He believed that the first 5 years of a child's life to be the most important, as he believed that an individual's basic character had been formed by the age of five.

Table 5.7: Freud's psychoanalytical theory

Sl No	*Theories*	*Description*
1.	Structure of personality	Id, ego and superego
2.	Dynamics of personality	Conscious, preconscious, semiconscious and unconscious
3.	Topography	Cathexis and anticathexis
4.	Stages of personality development	Oral stage, anal stage, phallic stage, latency stage and genital stage

Freud's Psycoanalytical Theory: Personality Conceptualization

The concepts of Freud's personality theory includes structure of personality, dynamics of personality, stages of personality development and topography are given in Tables 5.8 to 5.11 respectively.

Table 5.8: Structure of personality

Sl No	Types	Description
1.	Id	The Id contains all our biological based drives—the urge to eat, drink and eliminate; especially to be sexually stimulated. The Id operates according to the pleasure principle. It aims to achieve immediate gratification. Its driven behaviors are impulsive and may be irrational.
2.	Ego	It is based on rational self or reality principle, it develop between ages of 4 and 6 months. It acts as a mediator to maintain harmony among the external world. It experiences the reality of the external world, adapts to it and responds to it.
3.	Superego	It is based on perfection principle. It develops between 3 and 6 years, internalizes the values and morals set forth by primary caregivers. The superego is important in the socialization of the individual as it assist the ego in the control of Id impulses. When the superego becomes rigid and punitive, problems with low self-confidence and low self-esteem arise.

Table 5.9: Dynamics of personality

Sl No	Theories	Description
1.	Conscious	Consciousness refers to the perception, thoughts and feelings existing in a person's immediate awareness. The conscious includes all memories that remain within an individual's awareness. It is thought to be under the control of the ego, the rational and logical structure of the personality.
2.	Preconscious	Preconscious includes all memories that may have been forgotten or not in present awareness, but that with attention can be recalled into consciousness. Preconscious content on the other hand, is not immediately accessible to awareness.
3.	Unconscious	The unconscious includes all memories that one is unable to bring to conscious awareness. Unconscious material consists of unpleasant or non-essential memories that have been repressed and can be retrieved only through therapy, hypnosis and with certain substances that alter the awareness and have the capacity to restructure repressed memories.

Table 5.10: Stages of personality development

Sl No	*Theories*	*Description*
1.	Oral stage (infancy) 1–18 months	During this stage baby's mouth is the focal point of pleasure; children suck, bite and chew anything that fits into their mouth. Infant obtains gratification by taking in, begins to develop self-concepts from the response of others. Interest in oral gratification from sucking, eating, mouthing, biting.
2.	Anal stage (early childhood) 18 months to 3 years	Gratification from expelling and withholding feces; coming to terms with society's controls relating to toilet training. In early part of this period, the child freely gratifies his love of self with the pleasurable sensation involved in evacuating the bladder and bowels naturally and without restriction. Freud believed that if great success is placed on the child in relation to remaining clean during this period, he may grow up compulsively clean. Other adult attitudes thought to be rigid toilet training include stubbornness hoarding, collecting excessive concern with bowel function and sadistic or masochistic tendencies.
3.	Phallic stage (later childhood) 3–6 years	Interest in the genitals; coming to terms with oedipal conflict, leading to identification with same-sex parent. The focus of pleasurable sensation has shifted from the mouth and the excretory organs to the genitalia. Freud proposed that the development of the oedipus complex occurred.
4.	Latency stage 6–12 years	Sexual concerns largely unimportant. During the elementary school year, the focus changes from egocentrism to one of more interest in group activities, learning and socialization with peers. Sexuality is not absent during this period, but remains obscure and imperceptible to others. The preference is homosexual; children of this age show a distinct preference for same sex relationships, even rejecting members of opposite sex.
5.	Genital stage 12–18 year	Re-emergence of sexual interests and establishment of mature sexual relationships. During puberty and adolescence final stage of personality development is characterized by a reactivation of libidinal energy and focusing of this energy on the genital area. The adolescent is simultaneously drawn toward his parents and driven away from them. This ambivalence is manifested by much conflict between behaving in a dependent, immature, child like way and in an independent, mature adult manner.

Table 5.11: Topography of the mind

Sl No	Theories	Description
1.	Psychic energy	It is the force or impetus required for mental functioning. The psychic energy originates in the Id and instinctually fulfills basic physiological needs is called 'libido'. As the child matures, it is diverted from the Id to the ego and then from the ego to the superego.
2.	Cathexis	It is the process by which the Id invests energy into an object in an attempt to achieve gratification.
3.	Anticathexis	It is the use of psychic energy by the ego and the superego to control Id impulses.

Stages of Personality Development/ Psychosexual Development

Sigmund Freud (1856–1939) described formation of personality through five stages of psychosexual development.

Erikson's Psychosocial Theory

Erik H Erikson born in 1902, build on Freud's theories by identifying eight development stages that encompasses the entire lifespan, referred as eight ages of man (Table 5.12).

Learning Theories of Personality

Social Learning Theory—Bandura and Walters

1. Albert Bandura and Richard Walters in 1963 gave altogether a new approach to personality in the shape of a social learning theory.

Table 5.12: Erikson's psychosocial theory

Sl No	Stages	Description
1.	Trust vs Mistrust (birth to 18 months)	The major development task during this stage is to develop a basic trust with the mothering figure and be able to generalize it to others. The trust depends not on absolute quantities of food or demonstrations of love, but rather on the quality of maternal relationship, when needs, met, trust develops. Distrust can develop if the infant's world is filled with insecurity due to unmet needs, caused by lack of caring on the part of parents and significant others.

Contd...

Contd...

Sl No	*Stages*	*Description*
2.	Autonomy vs Shame (18 months to 3 years) Early childhood	The major developmental task during this stage is to gain some self-control and independence within the environment. Achievement of the task results in a sense of self-control and ability to delay gratification. Autonomy is achieved when parents encourage and provide opportunities for independent activities. Non-achievement results in a lack of self-confidence, lack of pride in the ability to perform, a sense of being controlled by others and a range against the self.
3.	Initiative vs Guilt (4–5 years) Middle childhood	The major development task during this stage is developing a sense of purpose and ability to initiate and direct own activities. Achievement of the task results in ability to exercise restraint and self-control of inappropriate social behavior, enjoys learning and personal achievement, achieve, initiative when creativity is encouraged and performance is recognized and positively reinforced. If this initiative and curiosity are discouraged, the child may be prevented from setting future goals by a sense of guilt and shame for holding such ambitions.
4.	Industry vs Inferiority (6–11 years) Late childhood	The major developmental task during this stage is to achieve a sense of self-confidence by learning, competing, performing successfully and receiving recognition from significant others, peers and acquaintances. Achievement of the task results in a sense of satisfaction and pleasure in the interaction and involvement with others; master's reliable work habits and develops attitudes of trust-worthiness; feels pride in achievement. This industry is achieved when encouraged for activities and responsibilities given in home, school and community. Non-achievement results in difficulty in interpersonal relationships owing to feeling of personal inadequacy; neither cooperate and compromise with others in group's activities nor problem solver or complete task successfully.
5.	Identity vs Role confusion (12–20 years) Adolescence	The major developmental task during this stage is to integrate the tasks mastered in the previous stages into a secure sense of self. Childhood comes to an end during this stage and youth begins. Puberty brings on a physiological revolution with each adolescents must learn to cope. Achievement of this task results in a sense of confidence, emotional stability and a view of self as unique individual. Identity is achieved when adolescent are allowed to experience independence by making decisions that influence their values. Non-achievement results in sense of self-consciousness, doubt and confusion about one's role in life.

Contd...

Contd...

Sl No	Stages	Description
6.	Intimacy vs Isolation (20–30 years) Young adolescence	The major development task during this stage is to form as intense, lasting, relationship or a commitment to another person. Intimacy is achieved by the task results in the capacity for mutual love and respect between two people and the ability of an individual to pledge a total commitment to another, personal sacrifices are made for another; capacity for giving of oneself to another. This is learned when one has been the recipient of this type of giving within the family unit. Non-achievements results in withdrawal, social isolation, aloneness unable to form lasting intimate relationships, often seeking intimacy through numerous superficial sexual contacts.
7.	Generativity vs Stagnation (30–65 years) Adulthood	The major development task during this stage is to achieve the life goals established for oneself, while also considering the welfare of future generations. Achievement of the task results in a sense of gratification from personal and professional achievements and form meaningful contributions. Non-achievement results in lack of concern for the welfare of others and total preoccupation with the self becomes withdrawn, isolated and highly self-indulgent with no capacity for giving of self to others.
8.	Ego integrity vs Despair (65 years to death) old age	The major developmental task during this stage is to review one's life and derive meaning from both positive and negative events, while achieving a positive sense of self-worth. Achievement of the task results in a sense of self-worth and self-acceptance as one reviews life goals; derives a sense of dignity from his/her life experiences and does not fear death. Non-achievement results in a sense of self-contempt and disgust with how life has progressed; feels worthless and hopeless to change; feels anger, depression and loneliness; fears death.

2. The theory emphasizes that what one represents through their personality is very much acquired through a process of continuous structuring and restructuring of their experience through social learning.
3. Observational learning from social situations may involve both real and symbolic models. Children, for example, may learn social etiquette by watching their parents and elders as well as by direct instructions.

Learning Theory of Personality—Dollard and Miller

1. John Dollard and Neal Miller (1950), in The Institute of Human Relations at Yale University provided their own theory of

personality. In this theory, they tried to substitute Freud's concept of a pleasure principle with the principle of reinforcement, concept of ego with the concept of learned drive and learned skills, concept of conflict with competing reinforces, etc.

2. It emphasizes that what they consider as a personality is learned. The child at birth is equipped with two types of basic factors; reflexes and innate hierarchies of response and a set of primary drives, which are internal stimuli of great strength and are linked with known psychological processes.
3. Dollard and Miller's theory of personality stressed the acquisition of personality in the same way as learning of most of the responses and behavior through the process of motivation and reward.

Self-theory—Carl Rogers

1. Carl Ransom Rogers, an American psychologist, in 1947 brought out a new theory of personality named self-theory, quiet distinct from the earlier theories of personality.
2. He stressed the importance of an individual's self for determining the process of his growth and development and unique adjustment to his environment. There are two basic systems underlying his personality theory—the organism and the self.
3. Rogers considers them as system operating in one's phenomenological field (a world of subjective experience, the personal and separate reality of each individual). The organism is an individual's entire frame of reference. This represents the totality of experience—both conscious and unconscious available with him.
4. The second system, the self is accepted, awareness part of experience. The self as a system of one's phenomenal field can perhaps best be understood in terms of our concepts of I, me or myself. Human beings have inherited a tendency to develop their self in the process of interpersonal and social experiences, which they have in the environment.
5. Rogers does not propose a set of specific stages in the development of personality as proposed by Freud in his history, rather his advocate's continuity of growth in terms of the continuous evolution of the concept of self.
6. Once a concept of self is formed, the individual strives to maintain it. In order to do this, he regulates his behavior. What is consistent at conscious level while what threatens the image of self may be totally ignored or buried deep in his conscious?

7. The most unfortunate results in the environment of one's personality lie in the cases where an individual develops some false self-images. This false image is often so strong that obvious reality can be stoutly denied.

Trait Approach Theory

Trait Approach—Allport GB

Allport GB (1897–1967) was the first personality theorist who adapted trait approach in providing a theory of personality. According to him, an individual develops a unique set of organized tendencies or traits, generally, these traits are organized around a few cardinal (primary) trait. Allport's theory asserts that no two individuals are alike. Allport regarded traits as responsible for these individual differences. According to Allport, trait is a predisposition to act in the same way in a wide range of situations. Allport deeply committed to study of individual traits. He started calling them as personal dispositions. Common traits were simply called traits. Allport proposed that there are three types of personal dispositions are shown in Table 5.13.

Table 5.13: Allport's three types of personal dispositions

Sl No	*Types*	*Description*
1.	Cardinal disposition	A cardinal disposition is so dominant that all actions of the person are guided by it. Very few people possess cardinal dispositions.
2.	Central disposition	These are not a dominant as cardinal dispositions, but they influence the person's behavior in a very prominent way. Therefore, they are called the building blocks of personality.
3.	Secondary disposition	These are not very consistent and are thus less relevant in reflecting the personality of the individual.

Trait Theory—Raymond Cattell

The most recent advanced theory of personality based on trait approach has been developed by Raymond B Cattell, a British born American researcher. He defined trait as a structure of the personality inferred from behavior in different situation and describes four types of traits as shown in Table 5.14.

According to Cattell, personality is that, which permits us to predict what a person will do in a given situation. In line with his mathematical analysis of personality, prediction of behavior can be made by means of a specification equation:

R = f (S, P)

According to this formula the response (R) of the person is a function (f) of the stimulus (S) at a given moment of time and of the existing personality structure (P). This equation conveys Cattell's strong belief that human behavior is determined and can be predicted.

Table 5.14: Cattell's four types of traits

Sl No	*Types*	*Description*
1.	Common traits	The traits found widely distributed in general population like honesty, aggression and cooperation
2.	Unique traits	Unique to a person as temperamental traits, emotional reaction
3.	Surface traits	Able to recognize by our manifestations of behavior like curiosity, dependability, tactfulness
4.	Source traits	Underlying structures of source that determine one's behavior such as dominance, submission, emotionality, etc.

Trait-type Theory of Personality—Hans Eysenck

Hans Eysenck approach tries to synthesis the type and trait approaches. Eysenck gave it more specification by grouping traits into definite types (Table 5.15). The essence of personality can be arranged hierarchically. In this scheme certain super traits and types such as extroversion exert a powerful influence over behavior. According to Eysenck's focus has been on a small member of personality types, defined by two major dimensions:

1. Introversion-extroversion.
2. Stability-instability (neuroticism).

Based on his categorization of personality types, Eysenck constructed an inventory called 'Eysenck Personality Questionnaire (EPQ)'. It covers item from each of the personality types identified by them throughout his writing, Eysenck consistently emphasized the role of genetic factors and neurophysiologic factors, role of the cerebral cortex, autonomous nervous system, limbic system and reticular activating system in explaining individual differences in behavior.

Table 5.15: Hans Eysenck's trait-type theory of personality

Sl No	*Types*	*Stable*	*Unstable*
1.	Introvert	Calm	Moody
		Reliable	Anxious
		Controlled	Rigid
		Peaceful	Pessimistic
		Careful	Reserved
2.	Extrovert	Leader	Restless
		Easygoing	Aggressive
		Talkative	Impulsive
		Outgoing	Optimistic
		Sociable	Active

PSYCHOMETRIC ASSESSMENT OF PERSONALITY

Personality testing is done for various reasons. A personal psychologist may want to identify people for a salesman's job. A clinical psychologist often uses personality tests to evaluate psychological disorders. They want to describe it and know what type of personality or the personality traits possessed by us their self, or others. It needs the knowledge and skill for the assessment or measurement of personality.

Subjective Methods of Personality Assessment

Personality assessment is that approach where methods employed provide an opportunity to the individuals to speak about themselves. The methods followed under this approach are called subjective methods (Table 5.16).

Objective Methods of Personality Assessment

Objective data are collected by experts using specific tools or devices based upon certain methodologies. These methods, which are used to collect objective data regarding varied personality aspects of an individual, are called objective methods of assessing the personality of an individual. These methods are also known as observational methods as these are based upon the observation of experts rather than the answers given by individuals in the case of subjective methods. The observation methods are rating scales, verbal behavior, situation tests and sociometric method.

Table 5.16: Subjective methods of personality

Sl No	*Types*	*Description*
1.	Autobiography	The subject (individual) is asked to write his autobiography either on a structured pattern or an unstructured pattern. Generally, only those subjects should be asked of guidance. Such autobiographical material provides data on the personal qualities of an individual, for instance, goals, aspirations, hopes, wishes, disappointments, frustrations, etc.
2.	Case history method	The case history method takes into consideration are the time factor and the changes in the personality of an individual during this time. Following steps should be followed in the case history method: a. Identification data. b. Family background. c. Health history. d. Educational achievement. e. Emotional and social behavior. f. Interpretation of the data. g. Evaluation treatment. The above information helps in making predictions about the personality of an individual. This method has a limited application for educational institutions, but it is more useful in clinics for the treatment of patients.
3.	Case study method	This method is concerned with the intensive study of an individual with the aim of having a holistic view of that individual. The cases of the problems of an individual are found on the basis of the collected information and remedial treatment is suggested for better adjustment in the society, school or home environment. Following steps should be taken into consideration while following the case study method: a. Selection of the subject or the case. b. Reason for the selection of the case/subject. c. Tools for recording data like cumulative records, tests, medical reports, etc. d. General information about the subject. e. Health records. f. Family background. g. Educational data. h. Social relations. i. Hobbies, interests, attitudes, etc. j. Interpretation of data. k. Remedial treatment to the case/subject under study.

Contd...

Contd...

Sl No	*Types*	*Description*
		The following points should to taken into consideration for selecting a case for case study: a. Preferably, problem children that are those who are truants, delinquents, low achievers, shy, quite and retiring, etc. should be selected for the case study. The teacher is free to select any student for case study depending upon the situation. b. Selection of the case by the teacher should be made from his/her class. c. Time and facilities should be taken into consideration for the case study in question.
4.	Questionnaires -	A questionnaire is a valuable tool for collecting information directly given by a person. Such information may consists of personal knowledge, likes and dislikes (values and preferences), attitudes and beliefs, experiences (biography) and present status of things or events. This information can be both qualitative (verbal, description, comments or views) and quantitative (numbers or scores as in the case of rating scale or opinion scores elicited by attitude scales). Any assembly of questions cannot be called questionnaire. It must reflect an objective, a design and a framework. It is a way of obtaining data about persons by asking them rather than watching them behave or by sampling a portion of their behavior. A good questionnaire embodies a beginning, middle and an end. There is an introductory section comparing a note on the purpose of the questionnaire, an appeal and a direction for responding to the various questions and a basic data part of which is to filled in accurately by the respondents.
5.	Interviews	An interview is face-to-face talking with a purpose. It is a systematic method by which one person enters more or less imaginatively into the inner life of another who is generally a comparative stranger to them. An interview can be formal or informal. For good interview, there is a need for establishing a rapport between the interviewee and the interviewer.

Observation Methods

The observation method can be used to observe intellectual functioning, emotional development, interests and hobbies, and to study habits, etc.

Four psychological process involved in collecting data in the observation method, i.e. attention, sensation, perception and conception.

Attention: It implies a mental set or a state of alertness, which an individual assumes in order to perceive selected events and conditions of things.

Sensation: It means the awareness of the internal and external environment through one's senses. It is the immediate results of a stimulus to the sense organs.

Perception: It is the art of linking what is sensed with some past experience to give meaning to sensation.

Conception: It is the quality of mental activity associated with observing by which one removes blocks to perception through the creation of imaginative concepts. It is an intellectual representation of some aspects of reality, which is derived from the perception of a phenomenon.

Steps of observation method: Following are the four elements of the observational method:

1. Deciding major phenomenon to be observed.
   a. Defining the phenomenon to be observed.
   b. Modalities for the observation of the phenomenon: structured, semistructured or unstructured.
   c. Person conducting the observation.
   d. System involved in recording various features of the phenomenon: videotape, tape recorder or any other devices.
2. Recording.
3. Organizing.
4. Interpreting the observations.

Precautions: The following are the precautions to be taken in observation method:

1. Training of the observer is a must.
2. Subjective of the observer should be involved to be minimum possible extent.
3. The observer should have knowledge of personality aspects.
4. A member of observations should be taken for the purpose of making the observation more reliable.

Phenomena amenable to observations: These are as follows.

Characteristics and conditions of individuals: Like people's attributes and states such as physical appearance, physiological symptoms that can be observed directly through the senses or with the aid of observational apparatus such as radiography.

Verbal communication behaviors: Like observing the content and structure of people's conversations, e.g. nurses giving information to parents, nurses conversation with grieving relatives.

Non-verbal communication behaviors: Include facial expressions, touch, posture, gestures and other body movements.

Activities: Like patient's eating habits and trends and aggressive actions among children in the hospital playroom.

Skill attainment and performance: Like behavior assessment through skill development by patients and nurses.

Environmental characteristics: Noise levels in different areas of a hospital, cleanliness in homes in a community, safety, hazards of children's classroom, shelters of homeless, etc.

Situational Test Methods

In situation tests, certain artificial situations resembling real-life situations are created before the students. The reaction of the students are recorded and interpreted. The interpretations on the recorded responses under certain situations reveal the personality of the individual. These tests provide opportunities to observe the behavior in life situations. Traits like leadership, initiative, cooperation, persistence, risk-taking capacity, honesty, flexibility, imagination, etc. can be assessed. Reliability and validity of these tests have not been ascertained as given below.

Group discussion: It is a general part of the selection procedure for admission. Group discussion is a situational test. A group is given a problem on a certain theme. No one is assigned the duty of a group leader. Everyone in the group is free to express ideas on the problem. In this situation, qualities like initiative, imagination, accommodation, suggestibility, flexibility, etc. can be assessed.

Situations created to assess honesty: A teacher may create the following situations in the class to assess the honesty traits of his/her student:

1. The teacher holds a class test.
2. Evaluates the written performance, but does not show marks on the answer books.
3. Distributes the answer book to the student expressing their inability to mark the answer books due to certain reasons. Teacher asks his/her students to handover the answer books the next day.

4. The answer book is collected again.
5. Those students are located whose awards are found higher due to additions. Thus, some students may reveal their dishonesty traits or honesty trait.

Imaginary situations: It can be created and responses of students to these imaginary situations may reveal personality aspects of the individuals. For example, suppose one of us comes across an individual who inquire about a certain place and approach the road to reach that place.

Situational test by May and Hartshorne: May and Hartshorne mention a number of situational tests in their book studies in deceit. One example related to honesty from this book is mentioned. The teacher had a box containing coins. Coins from the box were distributed to some of the students in a class. The coin left in the box was counted and then the box was placed in a corner. Students were asked to place back the coins given to them. The coins were again counted. Some students kept the coins with themselves.

Sociometric Methods

The sociometric method involves studying relationship among the members of a group, which helps in assessing the personality traits of the members of the group. Moreno devised this method. Social preferences with specific references to a specific criterion are recorded. For example, social preferences of students are recorded on the following questions:

1. With whom would you like to sit in the class?
2. With whom would you like to go on the educational tour?

The sociometric data so obtained can be expressed graphically. Such graphical expression is called 'sociogram'. A sociogram reveals information regarding subgroups, cliques, stars, isolated, neglected and rejected. Appropriate steps can be taken on the basis of the sociometric data to improve the personality of the individuals.

Rating Scale

A rating scale is an instrument designed to facilitate appraisals of a number of traits or characteristics by references to a common quantitative scale of values. The rating scale is used to know from others where an individual stands in terms of some personality traits.

Three points are taken into consideration in this method:

1. The specific traits or traits to be rated are specified.

2. The scale range is also decided, i.e. 3-point scale, 5-point scale, 7-point scale or 11-point scale.
3. Those persons are decided who required to use the scale to quantify the trait regarding a specific person whose personality is to be measured, e.g. one may decide that these specific persons will submit their observations on the scale for a particular trait (s) regarding a person.

Precautions while using a rating scale: The rating scale method can be made more effective if the following precautions are taken:

1. The raters should be impartial.
2. A number of rater should give their rating and these should be taken into consideration for framing the final assessment on the traits.
3. Generally, the halo effect is there in the rating of the raters for different traits. It should be checked. It is a tendency for transfer to occur so that a rater many rate the same individual high or low for many different traits. One impression may color the rest.
4. Avoid being too lenient or too strict in standard.
5. Avoid the tendency to either remain at the neutral points or the extreme points in the rating scale.

Purposes of rating scale: According to Freemen (1965), the purposes of rating scales are as follows:

1. Rating scales are chiefly useful for finding out what impression an individual has made of persons with whom he has come in contact with respect to some specified traits or attitudes.
2. It is a device that rates social values, occupational efficiency, group status and the like in certain specified areas.
3. It reflects the impression, the subject has made upon the persons who do the rating.
4. For the evaluation of an individual, rating scales are submitted to teachers, counselors, employers, colleagues, parents and others who have had sufficient contact with the person in question.
5. Rating scales may be devised for a variety of traits such as tact, generosity, leadership, cooperativeness, resourcefulness, punctuality, industriousness, honesty, personal attractiveness, etc.

Points for the construction and use of rating scale: These are as follows:

1. Each trait should be clearly defined.
2. The degree of the trait should be defined. Each trait should be rated on a scale, most frequently of five or seven intervals.

3. The mean or the median of the rating by different judges should be taken for having a reliable rating.
4. Guidance counselors, employers and personal officers find them helpful if the judges are carefully selected and if the rating are properly made.
5. Overt traits are more reliably rated than covert traits. For example, overt traits like emotional expression, social acceptability, manifest fear and anxiety, aggressive or impulsive acts are related with greater reliability than the covert traits like a person's inner life and feeling about one's self.
6. Degree of certainty of rating should be stated, e.g. very strong, strong and moderate.
7. Extroverted persons are more reliably judged than introverted ones.

Types of rating scale: The following are the types of rating scale:

1. Scoring rating scale.
2. Ranking rating scale.

Projective Tests

Projective test technique has been developed by Swiss psychologist, Hermann Rorschach. Projective methods involve an unstructured stimulus or situation. In this process, the individual projects his/her unconscious a desires, fears, motives, drives, needs, etc. Subjective and objective methods do not clear the study of unconscious mind of an individual. Projective methods deal with the conscious as well as the unconscious mind. The unconscious mind is 9/10th of the mind and inner urges, wishes, emotions, etc. are not visible to the outsiders and the individual himself/herself.

Definition

Projective test is an instrument that is considered sensitive to covert or unconscious aspect of behavior. It permits or encourages a wide variety of subject's responses. It is highly multidimensional it invokes rich and profuse response data with a minimum of subject's awareness, concerning the purpose of the test. —*Lindsey*

Characteristics

According to Rastogi (1983), following are the characteristic features of a projective test:

1. Brief instructions are given to the subjects who are necessary for them to respond.
2. The test material is kept ambiguous, projects their characteristic ideas, attitudes, strivings, fears, conflicts, aggressiveness, hostility, etc.
3. The purpose of the test is hidden from the subject.
4. The projective tests reflect the influence of psychoanalytical school.
5. The test reveals emotional and social characteristics, maladjustments, attitudes and motives. Certain intellectual aspects of individual behavior are also revealed.

Rorschach Inkblot Test

Description: This test developed by Hermann Rorschach has ten cards with vague inkblot on them. Five of the cards are chromatic stimuli, while rest of the five is achromatic stimuli, subjects are asked to tell what they see on these cards. Each response has elaborate scoring system and well-developed interpretation. Rorschach inkblot test reveals structural aspects of personality such as individual stability, value system, ego strength, etc.

Procedures: The procedure of Rorschach inkblot test as follows:

1. The card is presented one at a time in a specific order. When the subject takes their seat, the examiner gives the first card with necessary instruction. Examiner is asked to say what he/she sees in it, what it looks like, etc.
2. The subject is allowed as much time as he/she wants of a given card and it is permitted to give as many responses to it as his/her wishes. Examiner is also allowed to turn the card around and look at it from any angle to find things in it.
3. Besides keeping a record of the response of the subject concerning these inkblots on different pieces of paper, the examiner notes the time taken for each response, position in which cards are being held, emotional expression and other incidental behavior of the subject during the test period, etc.
4. After all the cards have been presented; the second phase of enquiry follows. It is intended to seek clarification or addition to original responses.
   a. Verbal projective test: Present subjects with an ambiguous verbal stimuli rather than a pictorial one. There are two types of verbal methods:

i. Association technique: An example of an association technique is word association method, which represents subjects with a series of words, to which the individual respond with the first thing comes to mind. The word list often combines both neutral and emotionally tinged words, which are included for the purpose of detecting impaired thoughts processes or internal conflicts, anxiety or any problems in relationships.

ii. Sentence completion test: This test includes a list of incomplete sentences generally open at the end and is asked to complete them in any desired manner. This approach is frequently used as a method of measuring attitudes or some aspect of personality.

b. Expressive method: These techniques encourage self-expression, through the construction of some product out of raw materials. The major expressive methods are play techniques, drawing, and painting and role playing. It is believed that people express their feelings, needs, motives and emotions by working with or manipulating various materials.

Scoring of responses: Responses to the test are scored in terms of location, determinants, content and popularity or originality taken for responses.

Location: The response of the subject in the context of the whole inkblot or a part of it is recorded. The subject may observe the whole ink for giving a response or a part of it. The subject may give large details or small details.

Determining quality: Scoring is done with specific responses of the subject in the form of shape, shades and movements (human movement, inanimate movement or animal movement) perceived by the subject.

Contents: The subject may respond on the inkblot on the basis of human figures, human details, parts of human figure, animal figure, details of animal figure, inanimate objects, plants, maps, clouds, blood, nature (light), sexual objects and other symbols. The responses are recorded keeping in view the above contents of the inkblot.

Popularity or originality: Some responses are given frequently by normal subjects. These are called 'popular responses'. Some responses may be extremely different, which can be considered original responses.

Analysis: The recorded responses are analyzed in the light of location, determining quality, contents and popularity or originality.

Interpretation: It is done on the basis of the analyzed data. Interpretation of the responses is a different job. Generally, subjectivity comes in the way and reduces the validity of the test as such. There is need for further experimentation on the test to make valid.

A few examples of responses of the subject to Rorschach inkblot test and the corresponding interpretation are given in Table 5.17.

Table 5.17: Response and interpretation of Rorschach inkblot test

Sl No	*Response*	*Interpretation*
1.	The response is associated with the whole inkblot (location)	The subject has the ability to solve the problems in a comprehensive manner; they possess high mental ability
2.	The response is linked with large details (location)	The subject has a practical approach toward problems of life
3.	The response is linked with small details (location)	Subject expresses emotional conflicts
4.	The response involved too many colors (determining quality)	The subjects are impulsive
5.	Predominance of human figure movement (determining quality)	The subject has vivid imagination
6.	The response frequently involved animal figures (determining quality)	Subject has stereotyped thinking and perhaps he/she is of low intelligence

Thematic Apperception Test

Apperception test consisting of perception of a certain picture in a thematic manner (revealing imaginative themes) is called thematic apperception test (TAT). This test was developed by Murray and Morgan in 1935.

Description: This standard test contains 30 pictures, 10 pictures for men alone, 10 for women alone and 10 mixed ones for both men and women. All the pictures are more or less vague. Each picture shows a dramatic or emotional scene that might have a number of explanations.

Administration of the test: These are as follows:

1. The picture is shown to the subject one by one and he is asked to develop a story about each picture. The subject is asked to explain the picture and to give an imaginary reconstruction of

what went before, and what followed. Although a good deal of emotion is portrayed in each picture, yet it is not clear just what the excitement is all about.

2. Thus, a man may be shown pointing excitedly toward something, but there is no clue as to what he is pointing at. The subject therefore, reads into the pictures some fantasies or interpretations of his own.
3. In giving meaning to the pictures, a person is certain to reveal something about him/her.
4. The raw material for a pupil's story comes from his/her own experiences and is colored by his own personality needs. His stories are scored for evidence of basic, unsatisfied urges and for environmental pressures.
5. The nature of the outcome is also examined, since it is the product of the needs and the pressures. Environmental and psychological aspects can be analyzed.

Thematic apperception test type pictures: The test type pictures are as follows:

1. Achievement motivation.
2. Need for affiliation.
3. Parent-child relationships.
4. Inner fantasies.
5. Level of aspiration.
6. Social and family relationships.
7. Functioning of sex urge.
8. Emotional conflicts.
9. Attitudes to work, minority groups or authority.
10. Outlook toward future.
11. Frustration.
12. Creativity.
13. Fear of success.

Modification of TAT: These are as follows:

1. The number of pictures can be reduced depending upon the nature of the subjects and the experience of the expert.
2. Some other pictures can be combined with the original ones.
3. The test can be determined to act as a group test. Pictures can be projected and the group of individuals can be required to write stories after necessary instructions. Stories are evaluated individually to assess the personality of concerned students.

4. Bellak modified TAT for using it for children of 3 to 11 years. This test is known as children's apperception test (CAT). The test consists of 10 pictures depicting situations of family relationships, toilet training, feeding habits, etc.

Children's Apperception Test

Children's apperception test was developed by Leopold Bellak D. The TAT test is used among adults and adolescents, but not suitable for children between 3 and 10 years.

Description: It consists of 10 cards. The cards have pictures of animals instead of human character, since it was thought that children could identify themselves with animal figures more readily than with persons. These animals are shown in various life situations. For both sexes, all the 10 cards are needed. Whatever story the child makes, he projected himself. The pictures are designed to produce fantasies relating to the child's own experience, reactions.

Administration of the test: All the 10 cards are presented one by one and the subject is asked to makeup stories on them. The child should have confidence and he should take story making a pleasant game to play with.

Interpretation: The following 11 variables of interpretation of the stories are centered:

1. Hero: The personality traits of the hero as revealed by the story.
2. Theme of the story: What particular theme has he selected for the story building?
3. The end of the story: Happy ending or unhappy, wishful, realistic or unrealistic.
4. Attitude toward parental figures: Hatred, respectful, devoted, grateful, dependent, aggressive and fearful, etc.
5. Family role: With whom in the family the child identifies himself/herself?
6. Other outside figures introduced: Objects of the elements introduced in the story, but not shown in the picture.
7. Omitted or ignored figures: Which figures are omitted or ignored should be not as they may depict the wish of the subject that the figures were not there.
8. Nature of the anxieties: Harassment, lose of love, afraid of being left alone, etc. should also be noted.

9. Punishment for crime: The relationship between a crime committed in the story and severity of punishment given for it.
10. Defense and confidence: The types of defenses, flight, aggression, passivity, regression, etc. The child takes nature of compliance or dependence, involvement in pleasure and achievement of sex desire, etc.

Word Association Test

A word is presented to a subject and he/she is asked to answer as quickly as possible with the first word that comes in his/her mind. The interpretation depends upon two factors, responses and the reaction time. In this technique there are a number of selected words. The subject is told that:

1. The examiner will utter a series of words, one at a time.
2. After each word the subject is to reply as quickly as possible with the first word that comes to his/her mind.
3. There is no right or wrong responses.

The examiner than records the reply to each word spoken by him/her, the reaction time and any unusual speech or behavior manifestations accompanying a given response. The contents of the response along with other recorded things give clues for evaluating the human personality and thus help a psychologist in his/her work.

Sentence Completion Test

Sentence completion tests include a list of incomplete sentences, generally open at the end, which require completion by the subject in one or more words. The subject is asked to go through the list and answer as quickly as possible (without giving a second thought to his/her answer). For example, we can have the following sentences:

1. I am worried over ________
2. My hope is ________
3. I feel proud when ________
4. My hero is ________

The sentence completion tests are regarded as superior to word association because the subject may respond with more than one word. Also there it is possible to have a greater flexibility and variety of responses and more area of personality and experiences may be tapped.

In addition to the projective techniques mentioned above, there are some others, which may prove useful in many situations. These are play techniques; drawing and painting tests, etc. both of these techniques are very useful in the case of small children. In the former, the examiner observes the spontaneous behavior of the children, while playing or constructing something with the help of given material and in the later, the natural free hand drawing and painting of the children are the matter of the study. Both of these techniques provide a good opportunity for the careful analysis of a child's personality.

Minnesota Multiphasic Personality Inventory

One of the most commonly used personality test is the Minnesota Multiphasic Personality Inventory (MMPI). It was developed during 1930s. This test asks for answers of true or false, or cannot say to 567 statements (one for men and another for women) about different personality traits such as attitudes, emotional reactions, physical and psychological symptoms, and past experiences. The answers are quantitatively measured and personality assessment is done based on the norm scores. Dr NH Murthy of NIMHANS, Bangalore, Karnataka, has reduced it to 100 items called 'multiphasic questionnaire'.

Millon Clinical Multiaxial Inventory

Items on this test correspond more closely than those on the MMPI to the categories of psychological disorders currently used by psychologists. This makes the test especially useful to clinical psychologist, who must find identity individuals problems before recommending specific forms of therapy for them.

NURSE AND PERSONALITY

1. The nurse needs know the basic structure of personality for providing effective care in the community and hospital set-up.
2. The nurse interacts with different individual everyday so evaluation of character and personality is essential in planning the care.
3. The nurse should have basic understanding about the uses of defense mechanisms, it is important in making determinations about maladaptive behaviors, in planning care clients to

assist in creative change, if desired or in helping clients accept themselves as unique individuals.

4. The nurse is not only to acquire skills and correct knowledge; she should have and develop a pleasing and string personality, if she wants to be a successful nurse.
5. Possessing professional qualities are the essential characteristics of a nurse such as integrity, dignity, mental alertness, poise, self-confidence and dependency. Nurse ought to have such personal qualities as sympathetic, understanding, friendliness of spirit, gracious manners, kindness and adaptability.
6. The nurse interacts with patients, doctors, coworkers and other important members of the society. So the nurse should develop certain behavior patterns and practice well-adjustable personality.
7. The patient appreciate a nurse who brings physical comfort to them with her skills and is prepared to understand their emotional reaction and difficulties that have been caused by illness.
8. Personality is the total quality of an individual's behavior as it is shown in his habits of thinking in their attitudes, interests and their members of acting and personal philosophy, which facilitates quality patient care.
9. Personality is dynamic, growing thing, different in each person. Individuals are different from each other even at birth in physical appearance, motility or temperament, the needs to understand the individual differences, while planning the care or education.
10. Many individuals with mental health problems are still struggling to achieve tasks from a number of developmental stages. Nurses can plan care to assist these individual in fulfilling these tasks and moving to a higher developmental level.
11. Assisting teaching and advising the parents, teachers and family's responsibility in developing and achieving developmental task in personality.
12. It incorporates sociocultural concepts into the development of personality.

Personality Disorders

The terms and description of personality disorders are given in Table 5.18.

Table 5.18: Terms and description of personality

Sl No	*Terms*	*Description*
1.	Personality disorder	Deviate from the characteristic trait that goes beyond normal
2.	Meaning	Personality disorders are usually recognized in early adolescence
3.	Definition	An abnormal personality is one in which there are deeply ingrained maladaptive patterns of behavior recognizable by the time of adolescence or earlier and continuing through most of adult life (ICD-9)*
4.	Classification–DSM-IV[†]	Cluster-A: Schizoid, paranoid, schizotypal Cluster-B: Histrionic, antisocial and borderline, narcissistic Cluster-C: Avoidant, dependent, obsessive compulsive, aggressive and passive
5.	Etiology	Hereditary—chromosomal abnormality or genetic predisposition Biological factors—brain dysfunction and changes in neurotransmitters Developmental factors—emotional, physical and sexual abuse Sociocultural factors—involuntary isolation, long-term psychiatric diseases Precipitating stressors—instability in the family or divorce Psychological stressors—high anxiety
6.	Group psychotherapy	Widely used in antisocial personality
7.	Individual psychotherapy	Effective in antisocial, dependent and inhibited personality disorder
8.	Behavior therapy	It is useful in anger control and social skills training of some valve
9.	Cognitive behavior therapy	Effective in antisocial personality disorder

*ICD-9 = International statistical classification of diseases and related health problems; [†]DSM-N = Diagnostic and statistical manual of mental disorders.

CONCLUSION

Personality is something that enables a person to stand out distinct from others. It is the total quality of an individual's behavior. It includes person's physical, mental, emotional and temperamental make up and how it shows itself in behavior. Personality is a dynamic thing that grows in a social setup. It is different in each person. The growth is affected by one's physique, glandular functioning and physical appearance and physiological conditions of the body brought about by drugs, disease and toxins, the growth is also influenced by one's environmental and social factors as the relationships in the home and the school, social codes and roles, which one has to play, the cinema, the agencies of social communication and the radio. Maternal factors influence the growth of our motives, acquired interests, our attitudes, will or character and our intellectual capacities. Personality can assessed or evaluated by means of interview, observation of behavior, rating scales, questionnaire and case study method. A successful nurse needs to develop a pleasing and strong personality; such qualities as dignity, mental alertness, self-confidence, dependability, sympathetic understanding, a strong desire to help, a high standard of values and the ability to develop healthy interpersonal relationships, are generally associated with the personality of a successful nurse.

SUGGESTED READING

1. Eysenck HJ. Dimensions of Personality. London: Kegan Paul; 1947.
2. Eysenck HJ. The Structure of Human Personality, 3rd edition. New York: Methuen and Co; 1971.
3. Hall CS, Lindzey, Garner. Theories of Personality, 2nd edition. John Wiley and Sons Inc; 1970.
4. Kuppuswamy B. Advanced Educational Psychology. Delhi: University publication.
5. Mangal SK. Advanced Educational Psychology, 2nd edition. New Delhi: Prentice Hall; 2002.
6. Stiagner R. Psychology of Personality. New York: McGraw-Hill Book Co.
7. Travers, Robert MW. Educational Psychology. New York: Macmillan; 1973.
8. Williams, Jessie. Psychology for Student Nurses. New York: Methuen and Co Ltd.
9. Young, Kimball. Personality and Problems of Adjustment. London: Kegan Paul, Trench, Trubner and Co Ltd.

REVIEW QUESTIONS

1. Define personality. Explain the components of personality.
2. Describe the various factors influencing personality.
3. Enumerate different types of personality and explain.

4. Explain various theories of personality.
5. Discuss in detail about psychometric assessment of personality.
6. Short answers:
   a. Projective test.
   b. TAT test.
   c. MMPI.
   d. Observation method.
7. Describe the role of nurse in personality.

CHAPTER 6

Psychological Aspects of Nursing

LEARNING OBJECTIVES

Psychological needs of:
1. Child and adolescents.
2. Adult.
3. Aged.
4. Attendants.
5. Chronically ill individual.
6. Behavior and sickness.

CHILD (PRESCHOOLER)

The preschool years span 3 to 6. Although physical growth slows, this is a time characterized by reinforcement of the cognitive and social skill begins during the toddler years. The preschooler establishes control of body systems as indicated by the ability to toilet, dress and self-feed, and is able to tolerate longer periods of separation from caregivers and interact cooperatively with adult and other children.

Characteristics

Period of slow and steady growth: Where the preschooler is the period of rapid and intensive growth, the stage of childhood is characterized as the period of slow, steady and uniform growth occurs.

Independence: In fact, at this stage child feels more at home with the world and takes satisfaction by doing work with own efforts. By acquiring experiences and developing physically and socially, the child tries to adjust himself/herself in his/her environment

Emotional stability and control: The preschoolers exercise control over emotions and express them in appropriate and socially approved ways. The emotional behavior is not guided by instinctive causes, but has an appropriate rationale behind it.

Developing social tendency: Child likes to play with group and share his/her toys with others. Feeling of mutual cooperation, team spirit and group loyalties are developed among children of their age.

Realistic attitude: Child at this stage begins to accept and appreciate the hard realities in place of imaginative idealist. He/she begins to take close interest in the world of realities and tries to adapt in real environment.

Formation of sentiments and complexes: The child at this stage is not in the habit of hiding the feelings and checking his/her emotions. Therefore, no complexes are formed at this stage is, whereas childhood stage. At this stage, preschooler's emotional behavior gets itself structured into sentiments. Various sentiments like religious, moral, patriotic and esthetic sentiments begin to develop at this stage.

Physical Development

Biological growth: Children in preschooler grow relatively slowly; they become taller and thinner without gaining much weight.

Weight and height: The preschooler gains approximately 1.8 kg per year. At 3 years of age, the child weighs an average of 14.4 kg and at 5 years, the average weight is 18.3 kg.

Body proportions: The typical preschooler looks more like adult than the toddler because of skeletal maturation. The head and neck continue to decrease in proportion to the size of the rest of the body. The lower extremities grow faster than the head, trunk and arms.

Cardiovascular system: By age of 4, heart size is four times than birth size and is now similar to that of the adult heart. Murmurs may be discovered during the late preschooler period.

Blood values: During the preschooler years, fat replaces the red marrow of the long bones. The total leukocyte count is slightly higher—5,000 to 13,000 from 4 to 6 years of age.

Respiratory system: With growth, the length of structures in the respiratory tract has increased and the incidence of the infection decreases.

Gastrointestinal system: The process of digestion is mature at this time, but the gastrointestinal system is vulnerable to stress, which may be manifested by mild to moderate dysfunction.

Genitourinary system: The urinary system is nearly mature by the age of 5. The urine output in the age group is 600 to 750 mL for a period of 24 hours. Daytime bladder control is achieved by the end of the preschooler period, but nightmare control still variable.

Immune system: Adult level of immunoglobulin A (IgA) are reached during the preschool years. In addition, children develop antibodies to the agents they are exposed to and to the normal flora in their body.

Nervous system: By 5 years of age, the nervous system comprises one-twentieth of the total body weight. Cerebral dominance is achieved, as demonstrated by the acquisition of handedness.

Motor development: As children use their muscles, muscle fibers increase in strength and size. Coordination and the ability to voluntary control movements are increases significantly, allowing them to refine their skills.

Emotional Development

1. The preschooler watches adults and attempt to imitate their behavior. Imagination and creativity allow them to fantasize, trying out roles and behaviors.
2. Preschool children look forward to become like their fathers and mothers. They learn adult roles from their parents, who serve as role models for behavior.
3. A feeling of conflict may also arise from thoughts; the child realizes actions were not appropriate. Feeling of guilt may also arise from thoughts in the child that are different from expected behaviors.
4. The goal of caregivers during this period is to assist children to learn about the world and other people. With this help, preschooler gradually modifies their egocentricity.

Sexual Development

1. Sexual generally, energy at this stage remains dominant, but merges with great forces at the end of the stage.
2. The sexual behavior of the children at this stage is characterized by the development of an attitude of antagonism and indifference toward opposite sex.

3. While this stage, the boys and girls play together, they wish to play with the members of their own sex.
4. Due to their varied interests, they gradually develop a general attitude of antagonism toward the sexes, naturally draws apart. Even when brought together in family gathering, boys and girls of this age are barely civil to one another.
5. Sex antagonism is more pronounced in boys than in the case of girls, the attitude of antagonism, generally takes the form of indifference.

Cognitive Development

1. During Piaget's preoperational stage, between the ages of 2 and 6 years, the child develops the ability to perform mental operations governed by personal perceptions and linkage to events previously experienced.
2. At this stage, the child acquires new experiences and tries to adopt in his/her environment. The child prepares himself/herself to solve the problems.
3. The preschooler gains power of reasoning, thinking, observation, concentration, perception, imagination, etc.
4. The child develops the concept of length, time and distance and learns to express himself/herself in various ways.
5. The preschooler uses a personal system for organizing objects and events in his/her mind and reasons from one particular to another, often by unrelated events, when in reality the particulars are not linked at all.

Moral Development

1. The child's moral development is at the most basic level, and right and wrong are determined from the rules parents have established.
2. Preschoolers conform to rules strictly for the purpose of self-interest, i.e. to avoid punishment and to have favors returned.
3. According to Kohlberg, moral growth occurs in specific sequences of developmental stages such as preconventional or premoral stage.

Spiritual Development

1. Preschool children continue in Fowler's stage of intuitive-projective faith.

2. The preschooler has a concrete conception of God, who has physical characteristics and can understand simple religious stories.
3. The preschool children accept the religion of their parents because for them, parents are omnipotent and powerful.
4. Preschool children are old enough to go to Sunday school. Any discussion of religion should be shared experience between parents and their children.

Language and Speech Development

1. Preschool children use language in a symbolic way. They not only imitate sounds at this stage but also use words to represent things.
2. Language is used by preschoolers to communicate their feelings and ideas.
3. They consistently ask questions and learn about the outside world by seeking the meaning of what they experience through sensory stimulates.
4. Preschool children use progressively longer and more complex sentences and their vocabulary grows rapidly.
5. An analysis of child's questions shows a need for information, for relief from anxiety and for attention.
6. Preschoolers delight in trying out a variety of words. They are unconcerned about the consequences of language and are prone to pick up words that parents may prefer they do not have their vocabulary.

Play Activities

1. Play facilitates the development of an optional self-identity by establishment of an imaginary friend, which helps a child to work through a particular time.
2. Activities that promote small muscle development encourage a child's creativity and fine motor skills.
3. Preschool children play actively; they climb, run, hammer, open doors with a bang and slam them shut.
4. The repetitive play of preschool children is an imitation of the life about them. Many play themes stem from a confusion in children's minds about experiences they have had a real life.
5. The children need to be encouraged to express their own creativity rather than fitting them within a mold of adult expectation.

They should be allowed and encouraged to play with toys of their choice independent of gender, role and designation.

Nurse's Role in Health Promotion

Nutrition: Preschooler needs to eat only one-half as much as adult. The daily requirements range from 1,300 to 1,700 calories, including 30 g proteins. The preschoolers enjoy five meals a day to keep up with energy demand. Food should be selected from the basic four food groups, with a limit of 16 ounces of milk daily.

Accident prevention: During the preschool years, the child begins to explore outside the home and into the neighborhood. It is also important to remember that the preschool-aged child is less reckless, will listen more to rules and is aware of potential dangers such as hot objects, sharp instruments or dangerous heights.

Hygiene: Many preschoolers enjoy their bath time, but the parental assistance may be needed for hair washing and cleaning fingernails and ears.

Dental health: The number one dental problem during this time is dental caries, which may cause the premature loss of teeth and a consequent alteration of dental arch, compromising development of the permanent teeth. The preschool child should visit a dentist at least 6 months.

Rest and sleep: The preschooler sleeps a total of 12 hours a day. Preschoolers may have difficulty sleeping in a dark, a proper parental support and guidance is essential during this time.

SCHOOLCHILD

The phase of development from 6 to 12 years, the school-age years, is crucial for establishing positive self-esteems, a sense of belonging and feeling of competence. The schoolchildren gain new ideas from adults outside the family: teacher, parents of their friends, police, television performers, newspaper writers and authors of textbooks with those of their parents.

Schoolchildren learn to think of themselves as person in their own right, may resent limits that parents continue to improve on their behavior. Parents need help in understanding the normal growth and development of their child when conflicts arise. Today, child can experience the world beyond the classroom with the help of the internet, electronic mail, educational videotapes and cable television.

Physical Growth and Development

Biological growth: Weight and height during the school years show a sex related difference. Boys tend to gain slightly more weight through 12 years.

The yearly height gain is similar in boys and girls, although boys tend to be taller.

Cardiovascular system: The heart assumes a more vertical position in the chest because of left ventricular development and downward placement of the diaphragm. Heart murmurs peak, during 6 to 9 years of age.

Immune system: The immune system continues to develop; response to infection is specific and localized. Normal adult levels of the immunoglobulins reached during the school years. The increased amount of lymphatic tissue in the nasopharynx continues to cause blockage of the eustachian tube.

As the child reaches puberty and the amount of lymphatic tissue decreases, ear infection decreases in direct proportion.

Nervous system: By 10 years of age, the nervous system is essentially mature. The maturity is evident in the sensory and motor functions as well as in the cognitive process.

Sensory development: By the time the child reaches age of 6, central visual acuity is established. At age 7, visual acuity should be 20/20, which is the adult level. The accommodative and refractive powers of the eye also reach stability.

The sense of taste and smell fully mature prior to the school years, allows for greater discrimination.

Skeletomuscular development: Skeletal growth is particularly noticeable in the long bones of the extremities. Growing pain occurs because the long bone grows faster than the attached muscles.

Muscle strength and size also increase at a gradual rate during school-age years and six basic gross motor skills such as balancing, catching, throwing, running, jumping and climbing continue to be refined.

At the same time, improved balance and coordination enable the school-aged child to explore new physical activities such as bike riding and roller blading.

Boys have a greater number of muscle cells than girls, so it is common to find they do well gross motor activities such as throwing and running.

Motor development: The motor development progress in a cephalocaudal and proximal to distal direction, with reinforcement of both gross motor and fine motor skills occurring as the central nervous system matures.

The developmental theory of Erik Erikson identified the major task of the school age period as identity versus inferiority.

During this time, energy is channeled into activities such as school projects, sports and hobbies. The school-age child also develops the ability to work with others on school projects and athletic terms in preparation for becoming a citizen of the world.

Schoolchildren must grow out of the dependency on their family and must find satisfaction in the company of peer groups and adults outside the home environment.

During the school years, the child develops wholesome attitudes toward a set of persons and learns the appropriate masculine or feminine social role.

Psychosexual Development

1. Freud believed that, starting at age of 6 and throughout school age, the child enters a calm period in the development of their sexuality called latency.
2. Freud theorized the school-aged child identified with the same-sex parent by modeling the behaviors and emotional of this parent and learned about sex-role behavior and identify by observing caregiver instructions, the media and friendship with children of the same gender.
3. School-aged children become much less ecocentric and direct their energies beyond themselves. During the early latency period, children associate with same-sex peers and tend to ignore members of the same age and tend to draw apart from them.
4. Boys and girls should be informed about the reproductive cycle and their respective roles as they approach puberty.

Spiritual Development

1. In school years, Fowler identified schoolchildren as being in the mythic-literal faith stage.
2. During these years, children are learning many specifics about their culture that will develop into a religious philosophy to be used in their interpretation of the world.
3. As children reach pubescence, they begin to be less mythical in their thinking and their beliefs are more controlled by reason.
4. As the child enters preadolescence, he/she realizes self-centered prayers are not always answered and there is no magic involved in religious beliefs. Blind faith that previously existed in the younger child is replaced by reason.

Cognitive Development

1. Piaget suggested that around 6 years of age, children start to move from the egocentric view of the preschool age to the more open and flexible thought of the school-aged child.
2. By 7 to 11 years, during concrete operational stage, characterized by considerable growth in thinking, imagination and language, which allows school-aged children to expand and understand their world.
3. School-aged children are increasingly able to classify objects in a more complex manner than they could during the preschool years.
4. The schoolchildren mental ability permits them to carry on converse and reverse process. They can solve problems because they can manipulate symbols.
5. During the school-age periods, children think not only of the present but also the past and future. Since, children can recall events that happened in the past, they become aware that exist over a period.

Moral Development

1. The school-aged child is at the conventional level of moral development, when the conscience develops an internal set of 'rules' that must be followed in order to 'be good'.
2. During third stage of moral development, the child's morality is based on avoiding the disapproval of others and maintaining a positive relationship with friends, family and teachers.

3. Children at this level can also demonstrate rigid behavior in an effort to obey the law. These children can take into account circumstances surrounding and incident rather than just looking at the result.

Language and Speech Development

1. During this period of development, children show tremendous growth in their ability to use words.
2. They extend their vocabulary by 20,000 to 30,000 words.
3. Their sentence structure and use of grammar continue to improve and the use of adjectives and pronouns increases.
4. Speech proceeds from egocentric to social. The unique culture of the children is reflected in language acquisition and speech patterns.

Play Activities

1. Play activities vary with age, number of play activities decreases, whereas the amount of time spent in one particular activity increases.
2. Likes games with rules because of increased mental abilities.
3. Likes games of athletic competition because of increased motor ability.
4. Play serves as a learning tool for children and their play changes with developmental needs.
5. Play becomes more formal, more organized, more competitive and a degreeless physical activity.
6. Parents can assist the schoolchildren with learning the rules of organized sports. Although, parents may not be attending sports events and others activities in which their children participate.

Mental Abilities

Readiness for learning, especially in perceptual organization: names of months in year, knows right from left, can tell time and can follow several directions at once.

The schoolchild acquires use of reason and understanding of rules needs consistency.

Trial-and-error problem solving becomes more conceptual rather than action oriented. Reasoning ability allows greater understanding and use of language.

Role of Nurses in Health Promotion

Nutrition: Children aged 7 to 10 years require 80 cal/kg of body weight. After age in years through adolescence, boys require more protein and iron. Careful meal and physical activity are crucial for the physical and emotional health of the school-aged child.

Accident prevention: Factors contributing to the high incidence of accidents for this group are their increased independence, desire to have peer approach and increased involvement in physically challenging activities.

Most accidents are related to motor vehicles, but firearm injuries continue to increase in incidence. The second most frequent cause of accidental death is drowning. Accidents also occur when children are skating, skateboarding or riding a bicycle or minibike.

Elimination: Schoolchildren are old enough to attend school all day, they have learned to control and independently care for their own elimination patterns. Usually, stools are well formed and school-aged children have one to two stools per day. The amount of urine passed is depended on intake, temperature, time of the day and child's emotional state.

Hygiene: Children older than 6 or 7 years of age are capable of caring out their own personal hygiene practices daily and by the time, they are 8 or 9 can be held responsible for independently bathing, grooming, dressing and properly discarding their soiled clothing.

As children become more aware of changes in their bodies or they reach late school age, they begin to take more interest in and are more reliable in their own grooming and cleanliness.

Dental health: Dental caries resulting from poor nutrition is still a significant problem in the school age population. Raw sugars and candies are common contributors to the development of dental caries.

Dental checkups are recommended every 6 months; the school system should incorporate a dental health educational program into the curriculum.

Sleep and rest: The 6-year-old child may need 11 to 12 hours of sleep, whereas the 12-year-old child generally, needs only 10 hours.

Sleep is essential during the school age years to foster physical growth and academic performance and failure to receive adequate rest can lead to irritability and lack of attention span at school.

Nightmares and night terrors are less common, during the school age years.

Sex education: It is important that school-aged children be educated about pubertal changes and responsible sexual practices.

Sex education should be incorporated into health education throughout the school years in a manner that is appropriate to age and development.

Common Problems Associated with Schoolchildren

School Phobia

School phobia is fear of attending school. It is a type of 'social phobia' similar to agoraphobia (fear of going outside the home).

Children who resist attending school this way may develop physical signs of illness such as vomiting, diarrhea, headache or abdominal pain on school days.

The causes of resistance to school, the child may be over dependent on the parents or may be reluctant to leave home because he/she feels that younger siblings will usurp the parent affection, while he/she is at school.

Handling school phobia requires coordination among the school, school nurse and healthcare providers who diagnoses the problem.

The nurse is the ideal person to coordinate such efforts and to help the parents allow the child some independence not only in going to school but also in other activities.

Stealing

During early school age, most children go through a period in which they steal loose change from their mother's purse or father's dress.

This usually happens at around 7 years of age, when they are learning how to make change and discovering the importance of money.

Youngsters, who continue to steal, may require counseling, because they should have progressed beyond this normal development step by this age.

Recreational Drug Use

Recreational drug use was once considered a college or high school problem is now a problem of school age. Illegal drugs are available to children as early as elementary school and certainly by the time, they reach the 7th or 8th grades.

Alcohol is available in so many homes and often can be purchased in small stores without proof of age; it is a commonly abused drug of this age group. Cocaine is becoming increasingly easy for children to obtain.

Parents should suspect of recreational drug use if their child regularly appears irritable, inattentive or drowsy. School health personnel should be aware of the increase in this practice among students and look for warning signs.

Children need to be counseled against this, because the recreational drug use leads to cardiovascular irregularities, uncontrollable aggressiveness and possible cancer in later life. Both nurses and parents should be role models of excellent health behaviors when earning for school age children.

Obesity

Many of the teenagers, particularly boys, become overweight. Some have been overweight since infancy. Their prepubertal neutral weight gain makes them obese.

Obese children begin to develop many of the same health problems as obsess adults such as hypertension and elevated total cholesterol level with possible atherosclerosis.

A weight reduction program for school-aged children that emphasis long-term life changes such as intake about 1,200 calories low in fat and designed to reduce weight, active exercise program and counseling program.

ADOLESCENT

Adolescent is the time period between 13 years and 18 to 20 years, which serves as a transition period between childhood and adulthood. It is a time of explosion, excitement and discovery and sometimes confusion and despair. Adolescent consist of early, middle and late stages. Each is distinguishing by several aspects of adolescent lives and constitutes the ages 12 to 14, 15 to 17 and 18 to 21 years.

Physical Growth and Development

Weight and height: Most of the girls are 1 to 2 inches taller to boys reaching adolescence and generally, stop growing within 3 years from menarche. Thus, those girls who start menstruating at 10 years of age may reach their adult height by age of 13.

Musculoskeletal development: Significant changes occur in skeletal size, muscle mass, skin and adipose tissue. Full bone length is first reached in the extremities and moves inwards.

The skeletal system grows faster than the muscles and muscle mass increases more rapidly than the height.

Teeth: Adolescent gains their molars (wisdom teeth) between 18 and 21 years of age. The jaw reaches about size only toward the end of adolescence.

Adolescent, whose third molars erupt before the lengthening of the jaw is complete, may experience pain and may need these molars extracted because they do not fit their jaw line.

Central nervous system: Brain growth continues during adolescence. The cells that support and nourish the nerves proliferate even though the number of neurons does not increase.

Continuing growth of myelin sheath allows faster neural processing and it is reflected in the adolescent's increasing ability to think abstractly and hypothesize.

Cardiorespiratory development: The heart almost doubles in weight and increase in the size by about one-half during adolescence.

The lung increases in length and diameter during adolescence and the respiratory rate averages 16 to 20 breaths per minute.

Males have greater capacity, volume and rate because of their shoulder width and chest size.

The slower of respiratory system growth relatives to the growth of other body system may be another cause of the inadequate oxygenation and fatigue, sometimes experienced by adolescents.

Gastrointestinal system: Rapid maturation of the gastrointestinal system occurs during adolescence and by the 21st birthday, all 32 teeth have erupted.

Gastric acidity and capacity increase up to 1,500 mL to accommodate and facilitate digestion of the increased food intake that occurs in response to rapid growth.

Genitourinary system development: Secretion of neurohormonal releasing factors by the hypothalamus stimulates the anterior pituitary gland to release follicle-stimulating hormone (FSH) and luteinizing hormone (LH).

In females, FSH stimulates ovarian follicle growth and estrogen production. Estrogen causes breast changes, including enlargement and darkening of the reproductive organs such as vagina, uterus, ovaries, and growth and darkening of pubic and axillary hair.

In males, FSH is responsible for sperm production and maturation of the seminiferous tubules. LH promotes testicular maturation and testosterone production. Testosterone causes the musculoskeletal system development of the male reproductive system.

Sexual Development

1. Adolescence is the physiologic period between the beginning of puberty and cessation of bodily growth.
2. Puberty is the stage of life at which secondary sex changes begin. Girls began dramatic development and maturation of reproductive organs at approximately age of 10 to 13 years, for boys 12 to 14 years.
3. Androgenic hormones are responsible for muscular development, physical growth and increase in sebaceous gland secretions that cause typical acne in both boys and girls.
4. In girls, pubertal changes typically occurs such as growth spurt, increase in the transverse diameter of the pelvis, breast development, growth of pubic hair, onset of menstruation, growth of axillary hair and vaginal secretions.
5. The average age at which menarche (the first menstrual period) occurs is 12.5 years. It may occur as early as age of 9 or as late as age of 17, however, still be within a normal age range.
6. A menstrual cycle can be defined as periodic uterine bleeding in response to cyclic hormonal changes. It is the process, which allows for conception and implantation of a new life.
7. Education regarding menstruation is an important aspect of comprehensive sexuality education.

Psychosexual Development

1. According to Freud, the physical changes of puberty reawaken the sexual and aggressive energies felt toward parents, during latency or late childhood.

2. Freud argued, many psychological issues adolescents face are attributable to physiological changes.

Psychosocial Development

1. According to Erikson, the development task of youngsters in early and midadolescence is to form a sense of identity. If the young person's do not achieve a sense of identity, they develop a sense of role confusion.
2. Body image: Adolescents, who developed a strong sense of industry during their school age, have learned to solve problems. They are best equipped to adjust to their new body image.
3. Value system: Adolescents need to be able to talk to peers to develop the values. They dress identically with other members of the group.
4. An important part of adolescents is self-understanding. It is the value they place on their definition of who they are, which involves self-competency and self-worth.
5. According to Erikson, the youth who is not sure of his/her identity, stays away from interpersonal intimacy or throw himself/herself into acts of intimacy, which may involved in intimate relations.

Cognitive Development

1. The final stage of cognitive development is the state of formal operations, begins at age 12 or 13 years and grows in depth over the adolescent years.
2. This step involves the ability to think in abstract terms and use the scientific method to arrive at conclusions. Problem solving in any situation depends on the ability to think abstractly and logically.
3. They can create a hypothesis and think through the probable consequences. Thinking abstractly is what allows adolescent to project themselves into the minds of others and imagine how others view them or their actions.
4. Another significant change is cognitive development. Adolescents generally, become more sophisticated in their ability to understand words and their related concepts.
5. Another important aspect of adolescent's cognitive development is their broadening ability to assume another perspective.

Moral Development

1. Kohlberg's conventional level of moral reasoning has been shown to emerge during adolescence and to persist as the predominant stage of moral functioning thought of adulthood.
2. Adolescent male would likely reflect judgment-based reasoning of fourth stage thinking, whereas female adolescents would more likely reflect the relationship based on the third stage.
3. Abstract thinking—new level of social communication and understanding can comprehend satire and double meanings. They can say one thing and mean another.

Spiritual Development

1. Almost all adolescent's question the existence of God and any religious practices they are taught.
2. This questioning is a part of forming a sense of identity and establishing a system value, at a time in life when they draw away from their families.
3. Religious and scientific views are often compared as teens decide what is true. More emphasis is placed on internal aspects of religious commitment rather than on attending church.
4. Adolescents become more oriented toward spiritual and ideological matters and less oriented toward practice, rituals and strictly observing religious customs.
5. The late adolescent tends to re-examine and re-evaluate the beliefs and values of childhood and become more personalize, and less bound to the traditional, religious practices when expressed to younger.

Health Promotion During Adolescence

Nutrition

1. The nutritional objective is to provide nutritional support for demand of rapid growth and higher energy expenditure.
2. Support development of appropriate eating habits through variety of foods, regular pattern and good quality snacks.
3. Nutrition education may be made through association with teenagers concerns about physical appearance, finger control, complexion, physical fitness, athletic ability.

Safety Measures

1. Accidents, most common those involving motor vehicles, are the leading cause of death among adolescents.
2. Drowning is one of the chief accident and athletic injuries tend to occur during adolescence because of the vigorous level of competition that occur.
3. Appropriate education regarding sexual maturity, reproduction, sexual behavior, driver education, hazards associated with smoking, alcohol and drug abuse.

Elimination

1. The elimination patterns for adolescents are similar to adults. They should void an average of 700 to 1,400 mL per day and have stool every day.
2. Constipation in adolescents may be due to a physiological disorder, eating disorder or improper nutritional patterns.

Hygiene

1. Skin care is especially important during this age because of the increased activity of the sebaceous gland. Which contributes to acne, increased sweat gland activity requires careful cleansing as well as the use of deodorant and body powders.
2. For female, menstrual hygiene is especially important and may require extra attention.
3. It is important to remind parents and other adult as well as the adolescent that these physical changes may require more attention to hygiene are normal.

Dental Hygiene

1. Adolescents are generally, very conscious about tooth brushing because of fear of developing bad breath.
2. During adolescence malocclusion, gingivitis and dental trauma may occur. Malocclusion occurs due to dental crowding or mandibular/facial bone growth changes.
3. The dental teaching should include brushing the teeth at twice a day using a soft-bristle brush and fluoride toothpaste, flossing daily, eating a well-balanced diet and regular dental visits.

Rest and Sleep

1. Protein synthesis occurs most readily during sleep. Because of this, adolescents need proportionately more sleep than school-age children to support the growth spurt during this time, which demands the formation of so many new cells.
2. Nurses need to educate both parents and adolescents on the importance of adequate rest and sleep and encourage teens to have realistic activity schedules that do not overextend their time.
3. An adolescent's excessive anxiety and fatigue may also result in sleep disturbances, which can continue into adulthood, since adult sleep cycles and habits are formed during adolescence.

Health Problems During Adolescence

Alcohol Abuse

1. Alcoholism and alcohol abuse in adolescence are increasing. Many adolescents who drink use it as a mind altering device, since it allows participation in risk taking activities they might otherwise avoid.
2. There are numerous hazards of alcohol ingestion. Some may be seen in adolescents, including hepatitis, pancreatitis, gastritis, neuritis and cirrhosis, ulcer of gastrointestinal tract, cerebellar degeneration and delirium tremens.
3. Parents and nurses with adolescents who abuse or other mind-altering drugs and their family members need to explain about detrimental effects.

Homosexuality

1. Nurses need to recognize that even though many young people explore their own sexual orientation or homosexual attractions, few who engage in homosexual behavior during adolescence, continue the practice into adulthood.
2. Nurses and caregivers recognize that homosexual experimentation is not same as establishing homosexual orientations acknowledge same bisexual relationships and attractions and phrase questions about sexuality and sexual activity carefully.

Suicide

1. The number of adolescents committing suicide has increased dramatically over the last few decades.
2. Stresses related to psychosocial, psychosexual or psychological issues have been identified as cause for the increasing number of adolescent suicides.
3. Risk factors of adolescents are previous history of suicide, family history of psychiatric disorders, living without home, history of physical or sexual abuse, unable to meet scholastic expectations of parents and teachers.
4. Suicide programs for teens should be directed by school staff, community agency personnel and students themselves by providing information relative to warning signs, fact and programs, which can enhance self-esteem and social competence.

ADULTHOOD

The young and middle adulthood is a period of challenges, rewards and crisis. Challenges may include the demand of work and raising families, although adult can also be rewarded by successes in their carrier endeavors and in their personal lives. Adult development involves orderly changes in characteristics and attitudes. Developmental changes are based on earlier characteristics, which help to shape subsequent behavior and characteristics.

Concepts of Young Adulthood

1. Young adulthood is the period between the late teens and the mid to late 30's.
2. During young adulthood, individuals increasingly separate from their families of origin, establishing carrier goals and decide whether to begin families or remain single.
3. Young adults are active and must adapt to new experiences. The transition into middle age occurs when young persons become aware that changes in reproductive and physical abilities signify the beginning of another stage in life.
4. Middle age is a time of continuing transitions when individuals may reassess their goals in life and add new goals.
5. The adult face such crisis as caring for their aging parents, possibilities of job loss in a changing economic environment and

dealing with their own developmental needs as well as their family members.

Maturity Developmental Task

1. People are said to have reached maturity when they have reached a balance of growth in physiological, psychological and cognitive areas.
2. Mature individual feels comfortable with abilities, knowledge and responses that they have developed over the years.
3. They look at the world with a broad view, based on a blend of insight, emotion and imagination. They take problems that can solve, but recognize and learn to live with unsolvable problems.
4. Mature people are open to suggestion and can accept constructive criticism without a major loss of self-esteem.
5. They weigh other person's input and recommendations in making decisions, but are not overly influenced or intimated by others; above all, mature people develop by learning from their own and others experiences.
6. Other characteristics of maturity are related to interpersonal communication and behavior.
7. Mature person acknowledge accomplishments and shortcoming. The mature adults confront tasks openly, use decision-making techniques to solve problems and are accountable and responsible for their actions.

Theories of Young Adulthood

Levinson's Phases of Young and Middle Adult Development

1. Early adult transition (ages 18–20), when the person separates from the family and desires independence.
2. Entrance into the adult world (ages 21–27), when the person prepares for and tries out career and lifestyles.
3. Transition (ages 28–32), when the person may greatly modify life activities and thinks about future goals.
4. Setting down (ages 33–39), when the person experiences greater stability.
5. The payoff years (ages 40–65), a time for maximal influence, self-direction and appraisal.

Gilligan's (1993) Intellectual and Moral Development

1. Gilligan's theory proposes that intellectual and moral development differ between men and women.
2. Women struggle with the issues of care and responsibility and in turn, their relationships progress toward a maturity of interdependence.
3. As women progress toward adulthood, the moral dilemma changes from how to exercise their right without interfering in the right of others to how to lead a moral life, which includes obligations to themselves and their families not people, in general.

Gordon (1991)

1. As women entered professional areas, they hoped to develop the caring and nurturing roles in their male colleagues.
2. Women have long recognized that, without caring, the perceived quality of life is changed. As a result, women maintained caring in the home and educational frustration in their development.
3. However, women become frustrated in their development because the responsibility of caring was not shared and frequently nurturing become a gender-specific responsibility.

Diekelmann Developmental Tasks

1. They activate independence from parental controls.
2. They begin to develop strong friendship and intimate relationships outside the family.
3. They establish set of personal values.
4. They develop a sense of personal identity.
5. They prepare for life work and develop the capacity for intimacy.

Physiological Development

1. The young adult has completed physical growth by the age of 20. The young adult is usually quite active; experiences severe illnesses commonly less than older adults.
2. A personal life assessment of the young adult includes assessment of general life satisfaction, hobbies and interests.

Cognitive Development

1. Rational thinking habits increase steadily through the young and middle adult. Formal and informal educational experiences, general life experiences and occupational opportunities dramatically increase the individual's conceptual, problem solving and motor skills.
2. Identifying preferred occupational areas is a major task of young adults. When people known their educational preparation, skills, talents and personality characteristics, occupational choices are easier and they are generally, more satisfied with their choices.
3. The young adults are continually evolving and adjusting to changes in the home, workplace and personal lives; their decision-making processes should be flexible.

Psychosocial Development

1. The young adult is usually caught between wanting to prolong the irresponsibility of adolescence and wanting to assume adult commitments.
2. The years from 35 to 43 are a time of vigorous examination of life goals, relationships; alterations are made in personal, social and occupational lives.
3. During young adults, generally, people give more attention to occupational and social pursuits. During this period, individuals attempt to improve their socioeconomic status.
4. During young adult, they take major decisions concerning career, marriage and parenthood.

Health Promotion During Young Adulthood

1. Young adult lifestyles may put them at risk for illnesses or disabilities, during their middle or older adult years. Young adults may also be genetically susceptible to certain chronic diseases such as diabetes mellitus and familial hypercholesterolemia.
2. Violence is the greater cause of mortality and morbidity in the young adult population. Death and injury can occur from physical assault, motor vehicle or other accidents and suicidal attempts.

3. Intoxicated young adults may be severely injured in motor vehicle accidents that may result in death or permanent disability to other young adults as well.
4. Sexually transmitted diseases have immediate effects such as discharge, discomfort and infection. They may also lead to chronic disorders, which can result from genital herpes, infertility, gonorrhea or even death.

OLDER ADULTHOOD

Geriatrics, the care of aged, aging is a normal process of time-related change that occurs throughout life. It involves all aspects of the human being. It is largely characterized by decline in functional efficiency and decreased capacity to compensate and recover from stress. It does not necessarily occur in an inter-related or synchronous manner, but it does involve physiological, psychological and social changes that interact to influence behavior and adaptation.

Concepts of Old Age

1. Old age is a normal part of human development and is the final phase of the life cycle.
2. Aging is not something that happens to the other person, but is a unique and highly personal experience that affects everyone who lives long enough.
3. Successful adaptation to the aging process probably correlates with the person's previous ability to cope and adopt to change.
4. Other influences include environmental factors, education and sociocultural determinants as well as the health status of the entire body.
5. Gerontology, the study of the aging process and its effects on older persons, become more important with each passing day.

Developmental Theories of Old Age

1. Certain theoretical models of human development help to point out important turning points, during the late years of the cycle.
2. The theories concerning the life cycle incorporate the social, psychological and biological factors of developmental growth and relate them to age to identity milestones and time development.

3. The theories of Buhler, Jung and Erikson, which are considered to be three of the most prominent theories of adult development, have a common theme, the goal of personal resolution in the second half of life.
4. Buhler's theories perceived that the period from 65 is one of awareness of the experience of fulfillment or failure and the remaining years are spend in either a continuance of previous activities or a return to the need satisfying orientations of childhood.
5. Jung suggested that in the second half of life, the individual direct attention inward, so that through an intensive inner exploration he/she may find a meaning and totality in life that makes the acceptance of death possible.
6. Erikson's theory explains that the years between 40 and 50 challenge those values that a person places on physical power in favor of the value placed on wisdom. People who cling to their waning physical powers, becoming more and more depressed, but persons who shift to using their mental abilities as a primary resource, appear to age more successfully.
7. The theorists view the first part of life as growth and expansion and the later part of life as inner withdrawal and contraction.
8. The task of later life involves finding meaning and wholeness in life and considerations about oncoming death.

Types of Aging

Biological Aging

1. Aging occurs with such changes as whitening of the hair, wrinkling of the skin, decline in eye focus and high-register hearing.
2. Biological aging depends on a combination of factors including genetic inheritance, finances and good health.
3. The most serious change for most people is their heightened vulnerability and lessened ability to recuperate from various illnesses.

Psychological Aging

1. Psychological aging refers to a role; the individual assigns to himself/herself as reaches a certain chronological age.
2. The two major threat felt by the older persons are the deterioration of his/her concept of self, which results in loss of

self-esteem and extensive and continual grief over frequently occurring losses.

3. The part of the aged in the youth-oriented society continues to receive attention and the process of gerontological counseling is now recognized as a specialized form of helping.
4. The older person should encourage seeing himself/herself as in a dynamic period of growth rather than in a period of rapid deterioration. The older person, for the most part, wishes to be treated as a person on worth and dignity.

Sociogenic Aging

1. Society imposes role on people as they reach a certain chronological age. Older persons are considered as either non-people or expendable people by many people in our society, merely because they lived longer.
2. Older people have been told by our society that they are supposed to be physically, socially, sexually and intellectually infirmed—slow in comprehending events going on around them and rigid in their ways of thinking and behaving.
3. Society also seems to take the attitude that older people should run away and hide until they die. It is important to note the combination of psychological than biological aging for many people.

Physiological Changes During Old Age

Changes in Homeostasis

1. Homeostasis is the body's ability to maintain a stable internal environment. The complex mechanism of homeostasis regulates fluid and electrolyte balance, blood pressure, temperature and food intake.
2. Man is dependent upon the functional integrity of the cell and the stability of the internal environment. If the homeostatic mechanisms are functioning properly, the body is able to adapt or react with stress.
3. However, with aging, these mechanisms become less efficient and reserve power is lost. This in turn makes the person more vulnerable to disease. Recovery is also affected, since more time is required for the body to return to normal after illness.

Changes in the Nervous System

1. The nervous system is extremely vulnerable to the aging process, as is seen in the progressive loss of cells that occurs with advancing years.
2. There are approximately half as many brain cells in the frontal area at age 80 as at 40, with resulting decrease in brain weight.
3. The steady loss of neurons begins surprisingly early in life and affects both brain and spinal cord. There is also a decrease in the blood flow to the brain.
4. Both physiologic changes in the brain and the reduced blood supply may be related to personality changes, sometimes encountered elderly.

Changes in Special Senses

1. The aging process produces varying degree of impairment in hearing, vision, smell, taste and pain perception as well as diminished sensation of touch and slowing reflexes.
2. A decrease in the sense of smell and in the number of taste buds at times contributes to a loss of appetite.
3. Diminished sensitivity to thirst needs can lead to dehydration and confused behavior as a result of fluid imbalance.
4. Hearing impairment, which usually is first noticed in the higher frequencies, can result in impairment of speech discrimination and loss of the full sense of background noises.
5. Vision is affected by a decrease in visual acuity and accommodation to glare and by a marked diminution of night vision and peripheral field of vision.
6. Perception of some types of pain decreases and referral of pain from one part of the body to another seems to become more common with advancing age.
7. The temperature-regulating mechanisms are less reliable and heat-generating activities are reduced.

Cardiovascular Changes

1. In older people, the heart is able to pump effectively under normal circumstances, but because it lacks much of its physiological reserve, it reaches poorly to sudden stress such as blood loss, excessive parenteral fluids or sudden effort.

2. When normal homeostasis is upset, congestive heart failure, arrhythmias and myocardial ischemia may develop.
3. The signs of arteriosclerosis become clinically recognizable when it has reached the advanced stage in the elderly.

Respiratory Changes

1. Most of the changes that occur in pulmonary function in the aged result from loss of elastic tissue surrounding the alveoli and alveolar ducts and from changes in the anteroposterior of the chest owing to rib and vertebral calcification.
2. There is also changes in the tissues of the lungs and decline in its functional capacity, size and structure as well as weakening of the respiratory muscles.
3. Vital capacity becomes reduced, while there is a concurrent increase in residual volume. Changes in the pulmonary vasculature also occur.

Changes in the Kidney Function

1. Kidney function declines with age because of reduction in the number of glomerulus, and diminished filtration and tubular function.
2. The blood flow to the kidney is reduced as a result of decreased cardiac output and increased peripheral resistance.

Metabolic Changes

1. As the body ages, the basal metabolic rate slows and the quantity of oxygen used by the tissue is reduced.
2. As metabolic processes change, the glucose tolerance curve tends toward that of the diabetic. If normal standards for glucose tolerance tests were applied to the aged, 50 percent of this population would be classified as diabetes.

Musculoskeletal Changes

1. Generally, there is a slow and steady atrophy of muscles that result in muscle wasting, particularly the trunk and extremities.
2. With loss of muscle power, there is a decrease in strength, endurance and agility.
3. Bones gradually lose calcium and porous bone is lighter, because bone become more brittle, falls are especially dangerous in the elderly.

4. Ligaments calcify and ossify and joints become stiffened from erosions of cartilaginous joint surfaces. Changes in the lining of joint cavities can produce degenerative changes.

Skin and Connective Tissue Changes

1. The skin is among the first structures to show the most obvious associated with aging.
2. As the person ages, there is loss of subcutaneous supporting tissue and resultant thinning of the skin. With the loss of subcutaneous fat, the skin assumes the characteristic appearance of aging folds, lines, wrinkles and slackness.
3. The dermis become relatively dehydrated and loses strength and elasticity. The skin in general is prone to excess dryness and itching.
4. As a preventive measure, older people should avoid overexposure to the sun, which tends to accelerate aging of the skin and increases the tendency to skin cancer.

Reproductive Changes

1. Physiologic changes occurring with menopause can affect sexual function and activity in older women. Atrophy of the vaginal canal and diminished vaginal secretions can lead to local irritation, bleeding and pain with sexual activity.
2. In older male, there may be diminished and delayed ability to achieve a full penile erection and a reduction in the frequency associated with psychological changes.

Health Promotion Measures for Elderly

Health Appraisal

1. Varied health assessment techniques can be implemented to help, detect and identify elderly people at risk.
2. Many authorities believe that a comprehensive physical examination, including blood examinations, urinalysis and stool test should be carried out annually.
3. Assessment of health habits is necessary as a basis for health counseling. Positive measures for maintaining health include weight control, exercise and proper nutrition, avoidance of cigarette smoking and protection of accident prevention.

Nutritional Support

1. Dietary inadequacies in the elderly result from factors such as poor nutritional habits, economic constraints and underlying disease condition.
2. Nutrition can have a tremendous impact on health maintenance and disease prevention as well as on the treatment of disease.
3. Older people are vulnerable to low nutrient intake. Dietary studies show that calcium, thiamine, ascorbic acid and other vitamins are the nutrients most commonly lacking in the diets of the aged.
4. The addition of moderate amount of fiber to the diet may alleviate constipation and flatulence. The high incidence of osteoporosis in older women seems to be age related.
5. Other factors contributing to nutritional deficiencies are social isolation, lack of interest in cooking and eating and problems in food shopping.

Exercise

1. Activity is one key to the prevention of premature aging. Many of the health problems of the aged arise from a lack of conditioning and diminished response to stress.
2. Exercise maintains muscular tone throughout the body and is effective in the prevention and rehabilitation following cardiovascular diseases.
3. Exercise training improves functional capabilities, increase vitality and has psychological benefits.

Temperature Regulation

1. Older people cannot tolerate a cold environment and are very susceptible to hyperthermia. The nursing approach is to provide extra blankets may be added for warmth.
2. Efforts are directed to maintain heat and humidity at comfortable levels by fans, air conditioning and humidifiers or dehumidifiers during hot weather.

Hygienic Care

1. With aging, the skin becomes thin and inelastic, predisposing the elderly patient to prevent pressure sores.
2. For elderly people, foot care is essential in order to maintain mobility, physical well-being and independence. A common

foot disorder of this age group includes calluses, bunions, toenail problems, corns and fungal infections.

3. The components of dental care for the aging patients include eating a proper diet, maintaining oral health and denture-bearing structure, being motivated to speak proper care and having adequate dental services available.
4. Problems of constipation and bowel incontinence often can be reduced through systematic habit training. Constipation occurs because of altered mobility, decreased mucus secretion and changes in muscle tone and elasticity of the colon, as well as changes in diet.

Recreation

Recreation is more than just having fun; it is fundamental to physical and mental well-being. No matter how old or disabled one becomes, the desire for the dignity that comes only through purposeful activity is never lost.

Common Health Problems of Elderly

Disease and Aging

1. The aged are particularly vulnerable to diseases because of such factors as their decreased physiological reserve, a less flexible homeostatic mechanism and lessened defensive mechanism of the body.
2. Chronic diseases have been called companions of the aged and most persons over 65 are affected by at least one chronic disease.
3. The major disorders of old age include heart disease, malignancy, cerebrovascular disease, influenza and pneumonia.
4. Disease in the aged does not always present with classic signs and symptoms. The usual clinical manifestations may be absent, attenuated or disguised and atypical signs and symptoms may be present.

Falls in the Elderly

1. A fall may be a frightening experience that can lead to immobilization and possibly to pneumonia and complete loss of the ability to walk.
2. Falls by the elderly result from age-related physiologic decline in postural control and deterioration of the central nervous

system from lightheadedness, postural hypotension, heart block and arrhythmias.

3. Special danger arises from osteoporosis, a condition in which the bones lose calcium and thus become thin and brittle. This condition renders an elderly person susceptible to major fractures.

Depression

1. Depression is the most common emotional disorder in the aged. Depression and grief are common with aged since losses are inevitable.
2. Depression resulting from losses can easily be overlooked and may be mistaken for physical or organic mental illness. The patient may exhibit anger, denial, withdrawal or other maladaptive responses that move him/her further away from reality.
3. Depression in the aged is usually manifested by feelings of apathy, quietness and emptiness, which may be mistaken for senile changes.
4. Treatment in elderly, usually referred to community health resources such as the community mental health services, can be very beneficial.

Chronic Organic Brain Syndrome (Senile Dementia)

1. The term dementia refers to signs and symptoms of intellectual dysfunction owing to differing etiologies and varying pathophysiologic mechanisms that can occur alone and in combination.
2. It is believed to result from diffuse impairment of brain tissue. The most common long-term disorders of cognitive functions (attention, learning, memory) in the elderly are seen in senile dementia (often called Alzheimer's disease).
3. Senile dementia generally refers to a disturbance of mental status or mental deterioration occurring after the age of 65. There are neuropathological changes associated with changes in the patient's cognitive function, which may include loss of neurons, neurofibrillary tangles, granulovascular changes and neurotic (senile) plaques in the brain.
4. Senile dementia is devastating to the human personality and is a source of anguish and frustration to the patient and loved ones.

5. Senile dementia and related disorders are associated with a high motility rate and significantly shortened life expectancy.

Acute Brain Syndrome

1. Acute brain syndrome is a temporary psychiatric state caused by a physiologic or an anatomical insult to brain tissue.
2. The disorder have a relatively sudden onset and potentially reversible. They associate with acute physical illness of physiologic disturbances, cardiac and circulatory problems, neurological conditions, cerebrovascular disorders, dehydration, electrolyte imbalance, alcohol or drug toxicity and wide variety of infections.
3. In management of acute brain syndrome, the basic disease must be treated or the etiologic toxic agent must be removed.
4. Specific treatment is aimed at alleviating or curing the condition that underlies the confusion: antimicrobials for infection, removal of drugs, removal of fecal impaction, correction of heart failure, treatment of stroke.
5. Appropriate medications such as the phenothiazines, which exert much of their calming action on the lower brain centers, may be administered.

BEHAVIOR AND SICKNESS

1. Health in its broadest sense is a dynamic state in which the individual adapts to changes in internal and external environments to maintain a state of well-being. The internal environment includes many factors that influence health, including genetic and psychological variables, intellectual and spiritual dimensions and disease processes.
2. The external environment includes factors outside the person that may influence health including the physical environment, social relationships and economic variables, because both environments continuously change, the person must maintain a state of well-being.
3. Health and illness, therefore, must be defined in terms of individual. Health can include conditions that the client or nurse may have previously considered to be illness. Health is also closely related to an individual's workplace and home life and stressors can be the result of those environments.

Concepts of Health, Illness and Sick Behaviors

1. It is useful for the nurse to be aware of the behavioral components of health, illness and sick-role behavior.
2. Every person develops a system of health beliefs and attitudes and these tend to fall within the framework provided by society or cultural heritage.
3. Health behavior, activities a person engages in when feeling well, to take measures to prevent disease and illness to detect them before symptom occur.
4. Illness behavior, activities a person edges in when feeling ill, that will lead to the defining of the state of health and that will gain help.
5. Sick-role behavior, activities a person engages in believing himself/herself ill. For any individual, the level of health behavior is determined by the significance of symptoms—danger value, visibility, ambiguity, fear of unknown, the expectations of those whom from help is sought, feeling about dependence and fear of loss of control, the expectorations of the illness position, including past experiences with illness.

Illness Behavior

1. Illness is not merely the presence of disease process. Illness is a state in which a person's physical, emotional, intellectual, social, developmental or spiritual functioning is diminished or impaired, compared with that person's previous experiences.
2. Illness behavior involves the ways persons monitor their bodies, definite and interpret their symptoms, take remedial actions and use their healthcare system.
3. The important internal values influencing the way clients behave when they are ill are their perceptions of symptoms and the nature of the illness. A client's illness behavior can also be affected by the nature of the illness.
4. Acute illness involves symptoms of relatively short duration that are usually severe and may affect functioning in any dimension.
5. Chronic illnesses persist, usually longer than 6 months and can affect functioning in any dimension.
6. External variables influencing a client's illness behavior include the visibility of symptoms, social groups, cultural background,

economic variables, accessibility of the healthcare system and social support.

Stages of Illness Behavior

Symptom experience: It is as follows:

1. During the initial stage, a person is aware that something is wrong. A person usually recognizes a physical sensation or a limitation in functioning, but does not suspect a specific diagnosis.
2. The person's perception of symptoms includes awareness of a physical change such as pain, rash or a lump.

Assumptions of the sick role: These are as follows:

1. The assumption of the sick role results in emotional changes such as withdrawal or depression and physical changes.
2. Emotional changes may be simple or complex, depending on the severity of the illness, the degree of disability and anticipated length of the illness.

Medical care contact: It is explained below:

1. If symptoms persist despite home remedies, become severe or require emergency care, the person is motivated to seek professional health services.
2. In this stage, the client seeks expect acknowledgment of the illness, as well as treatment. In addition, the client seeks an explanation of the symptoms, the cause of the symptoms and the course of the illness for future health.
3. Client's illness can be validated at any point on the health illness continuum. A health professional may determine that they do not have an illness or that illnesses are present and may belief threatening.

Dependent client role: It is given below:

1. After accepting the illness and seeking treatment, the client enters the fourth stage of illness behavior.
2. In this stage, the client depends on healthcare professionals for relief of symptoms. The client accepts care, sympathy and protection from the demands and stresses of life.
3. It is socially permissible for clients in the dependent role to be relieved of normal obligations and tasks.

Recovery stage: It is explained below in detail:

1. The final stage of illness behavior is recovery and rehabilitation —can arrive suddenly such as when a fever subsides.
2. The recovery is not prompt; long-term care may be required before the client is able to resume an optimal level of functioning.
3. In the case of chronic illness, the final stage may involve an adjustment to a prolonged reduction in health and functioning.

Impact of Illness on Family

Behavioral and emotional changes: Are given below:

1. People react differently to illness. Individual's behavioral and emotional reactions depend on the nature of the illness, the client's attitude toward it, the reaction of others to it and the variables of illness behavior.
2. Severe illness, particularly one that is life threatening, can lead to more extensive emotional and behavioral change such as anxiety, shock, denial, anger and withdrawal.

Impact of family roles: It is given below:

1. When an illness occurs, the roles of client and family may change. Such a change may be subtle and short term or drastic and long term.
2. An individual and family generally, adjust more easily to subtle, short-term changes. In most cases they know that the role change is only temporary.
3. Long-term changes, however, require an adjustment process similar to the grief process. The client and family often require specific counseling and guidance to assist them in coping with role changes.

Impact on body changes: It is given below:

1. Some illnesses result in changes in physical appearance and clients and families react differently to these changes.
2. When changes in body image occur such as results from a leg amputation, the client generally, adjusts in the following phases: shock, withdrawal, acknowledgement, acceptance and rehabilitation.
3. Withdrawal is an adaptive coping mechanism that can assist the client in making the adjustments.

Impact of self-concepts: It is explained below:

1. Self-concept is individual's mental image of themselves, including how they view their strengths and weakness in all aspects of their personalities.
2. Self-concepts depend in part of body image and roles but also include other aspects of the psychological and spiritual self.
3. Self-concept changes because of illness and may no longer meet the expectations of the family, leading to tension or conflict.

Impact of family dynamics: It is given below:

1. Family dynamics is the process by which the family functions, makes decisions, give support to individual members and copes with everyday changes and challenges.
2. If a parent in a family becomes ill, family activities and decision-making often come to a hault as the other family members wait for the person to recover, or they delay action because they are reluctant to assume the ill person's roles or responsibilities.

Health and Illness Continuum

1. According to Neumann (1990), health on a continuum is the degree of client wellness that exist at any point in time ranging from an optimal wellness condition, with available energy at its maximum to death, which represents total energy depletion.
2. According to health-illness continuum model, health is a dynamic state that continuously alters as a person adapts to changes in the internal and external environments to maintain a state of physical, emotional, intellectual, social, developmental and spiritual well-being.
3. The continuum is thought of a complex, dynamic process that includes physical, psychological and social components. There are adaptive or maladaptive behavioral responses to internal and external stimuli.
4. Health and illness tend to merge, but may represent patterns of adaptive change along the continuum. The direction of change may be reversible, depending on the quality of the individual's adoptive efforts.
5. The individual at the illness end of the continuum is characterized by feeling of uncertainty, helplessness, loss of control, loss of identity and incapacity for problem solving.

6. As the patient is in the sick-role, there is incapacity to meet other social roles, the person has sought diagnosis and get treatment.
7. Less far along the illness end of the continuum, as illness behavior are brought into play, the person may be tried, run-down and irritable with complains of loss of sleep, appetite, dependence, self-absorption, minor illnesses such as colds, infections, headaches and backaches.
8. Between illness and wellness there is the ambiguous area, where no symptoms are present and the person is neither especially well nor especially ill.
9. At the health end of the continuum, as health behaviors are utilized, the persons is not only unaware of disease and without pain, fatigue or somatic complications but also tends to be resistant to infections, industrious, vigorous and physically agile, with a strong sense of identity and autonomy, caring out usual social roles and needing no health care.
10. The goal in preventive health care is to maintain equilibrium between health and illness, with balance in favor of maximum wellness for the individual.

Models of Health and Illness

Health-wellness model: Is described below:

1. It was developed by Dunn (1997); the high-level wellness model is oriented toward maximizing the health potential of an individual.
2. This model requires the individual to maintain a continuum of balance and purposeful direction within the environment.
3. It involves progress toward a higher level of functioning open-ended and expanding challenges to live at the fullest potential.

Agent-host-environmental model: Is described below:

1. The agent-host-environmental model of health and illness is originated in the community health work of level.
2. According to this approach, the health or illness of an individual or group depends on the dynamic relationship of the agent, host and environment.
3. The agent is any internal or external factors that its presence or absence can lead to disease or illness.

4. The host is the person or persons who may be susceptible to a particular illness or diseases.
5. The environment consists of all factors outside of the host. It includes physical environment, social environment and biological environment.

Health belief model: Is described below:
1. Rosenstock's (1794), Becker and Maiman's (1975) health belief model addresses the relationship between a person's belief and behavior.
2. It provides a way of understanding and predicting how clients will behave in relation to their health and how they will *comply* with healthcare therapies.
3. The 1st component in this model involves the individual's perception of susceptibility to an illness.
4. The 2nd component is the individual's perception of the seriousness of the illness. This perception is influenced and modified by demographic and sociopsychological variables, perceived threats of the illnesses and cues to action.
5. The 3rd component—the likelihood that a person will take preventive action—is the person's perception of the benefits of taking action.

Health promotion model: Is described below:
1. The health promotion model was proposed by Pender (1996). It was designed to be a complementary counterpart to models of health protection.
2. Health promotion is directed at increasing a client's level of well-being. The model focuses on three functions.
3. The model also organizes cues into a pattern to explain the likelihood of a client's participation in health-promotion behavior.
4. The focus of this model is to explain the reasons that individuals engage in health activities. It is not designed for use with families or communities.

Biopsychosocial Aspects of Health and Illness

Physical, social, cultural and psychological factors interact dynamically and have an important influence on patient care needs. There are needs common to everyone, no matter their sociocultural background, so called human needs. These needs, when they are not met, create tensions and these tensions may give rise to anxiety that can hamper recovery, if not relieved.

Developmental Needs

Prenatal: This stage determines many characteristics of the person and to some extent, the requirements for use of adaptive resources throughout life.

Neonatal: Developmental tasks are mostly physical; foundations are begun at this time for later personality responses.

Infancy: This is a time of much physical, but foundations are begun at this time for later personality responses.

Childhood: Marked physical growth continues during this time. There is the beginning of role identification and moving out from the family to the peer group and community.

Adolescence: Many physical and emotional changes occur as growth and maturation continues; changing hormonal activity and search for identity are major stresses for the adolescent.

Young adulthood: Physical maturation is completed. There are many psychosocial stresses related to family and community roles during this stage.

Middle adulthood: Developmental tasks are mostly psychosocial, relating to reassessment of goals, physical stamina and hormone output beginning to decline.

Older years: Physical conditioning is generally declining and decreased sensory acuity may be noticeable. Developmental tasks are related to sharing accumulated experiences and evaluating achievements.

Cultural Influences

1. Culture may be thought of as the total way of life of people, the social legacy and the individual acquires from his/her groups.
2. The culture concept is cardinal to an understanding of ourselves and our world.
3. Custom and group habits are referred to as folkways and mores. Folkways are the accustomed and time-honored ways of doing things, the social habits that become routine and that are often performed without thinking.

4. The patient's cultural background helps to determine the way the relationship with the physician or nurse in perceived and facilitates or impedes interaction or communication.

Religious Aspects

1. Religion traditionally has focused on a God beyond the individual and has concerned itself with relating the individual to that God.
2. Religious beliefs are seldom held to oneself, but are part of group processes, so that there is immediate family or group support for the patient.
3. It helps the patient's own attitude or belief that recovery is possible and that there are forces available to facilitate the healing process.
4. It is important if the nurse is to help, to understand not only the spiritual needs of the patient but also the means and methods that organized religion has for meeting those needs.

SUGGESTED READING

1. Jacob A. Psychology for Graduate Nurses, 4th edition. New Delhi: Jaypee Brothers Medical Publishers (P) Ltd; 2007.
2. Khan MA. Psychology for Nurses in India. New Delhi: Academic Publications; 2004.
3. Mangal SK. General Psychology. New Delhi: Sterling Publishers Pvt Ltd; 2006.
4. Perry AG, Potter PA. Clinical Nursing Skills and Techniques, 3rd edition. St Louis: Mosby-Year Book Inc; 1994.
5. Potter PA, Perry AG. Fundamentals of Nursing Concepts, Process and Practice, 3rd edition. St Louis: Mosby-Year Book Inc; 1993.
6. Purtilo R. Health Professional and Patient Interaction, 4th edition. Philadelphia: WB Saunders; 1990.
7. Stuart GW, Sundeen SJ. Principles and Practice of Psychiatric Nursing, 4th edition. St Louis: Mosby-Year Book Inc; 1991.
8. Thompson RF. Introduction to Psychology. New Delhi: Harper and Row; 1975.
9. Timby BK, Lewis LW. Fundamental Skills and Concepts Patient Care, 5th edition. Philadelphia: JB Lippincott Co; 1992.

REVIEW QUESTIONS

1. Define preschooler. Explain the physical and emotional development. Discuss the nurse's role in health promotion.
2. Define schoolchild. Discuss the psychosexual development during school age. Explain the nurse's role in health promotion.
3. Discuss the common problem associated with schoolchildren.
4. Define adolescent. Discuss the sexual, psychosocial, cognitive and moral development during adolescence.
5. Enumerate the health problems during adolescence. Discuss the nurse's role in health promotion of an adolescent.
6. Define adulthood. Explain the maturity developmental task. Explain the psychosocial and cognitive development during adulthood.
7. Define old age. Explain the developmental theories of old age.
8. Discuss the physiological changes during old age. Enumerate health promotion measures for elderly.
9. Explain the common health problems of elderly.
10. Enumerate the details of health and illness continuum. Explain the biopsychosocial aspects of health and illness.

CHAPTER 7 *Individual Differences*

LEARNING OBJECTIVES

1. Significance of individual differences.
2. Heredity and environment.
3. Role of individual differences both in health and sickness.
4. Implications of individual differences in nursing.

INTRODUCTION

No two persons are born alike, but each differs from the other in natural endowments. Individual differences in psychology focus on this second level of study. It is also sometimes called differential psychology, because researchers in this area, study the ways in which individual people differ in their behavior. This is distinguished from other aspects of psychology, although psychology is ostensibly a study of individuals, modern psychologists often study groups or biological underpinnings of cognition that people differ from each other is obvious. How and why they differ is less clear and is the subject of the study of individual differences (IDs). Although to study of individual differences seems to be the study variance, how are people different from each other, it is also to study central tendency, how well can a person be described in terms of an overall average person. Indeed, perhaps the most important question of individual differences is whether people are more similar to themselves over time and across situations than they are to others and whether the variation within a single person across time and situation is less than the variation between other people.

Individuals differ from each other. One individual is never like another in all respects. Each one has his own peculiarities, which presents him as a separate individual from the others.

In psychological terminology, differences between individuals that distinguish or separate them from one another and makes the person one distinct, unique and standout from the rest are termed as individual differences.

MEANING OF INDIVIDUAL DIFFERENCES

Difference between the individual is normally attribute to both hereditary and environment. A related question is that of similarity, for people differ in their similarities to each other. Questions of whether particular groups (e.g. groupings by sex, culture, age or ethnicity) are more similar within than between groups are also questions of individual differences. Individual differences research typically includes personality, motivation, intelligence, ability, intelligence quotient (IQ), interests, values, self-concept, self-efficacy and self-esteem (to name just a few). There are few remaining 'differential psychology' programs in the United States, although, research in this area is very active. Current researchers are found in a variety of applied and experimental programs, including educational psychology, individual psychology, industrial psychology, personality psychology, social psychology and developmental psychology programs, in the neo-Piagetian theories of cognitive development in particular. Earlier studies show us a higher risk with the factors of social and behavioral domains in young children with a single parent. However, the variety of single-parent families regarding gender of the main parent has rarely been taken into reason when understanding the relation between family and child's negative outcomes.

According to 'Dictionary of Education' by Carter B Good, 1959

1. Individual differences stand for the variations or deviations among individuals in regard, to a single characteristic or a number of characteristics.
2. Individual differences stand for those differences, which in their totality distinguish one individual from another.

Similarities Among Individuals

1. Intellectual capacity—all individuals have sense organs, brain, muscles and glands. They have an intellectual capacity to gain through education and experiences.
2. All individuals have the emotions of love, fear and the feelings of pleasure and pain.
3. All individuals feel the need for independence, success, acceptance, etc.
4. All individuals are influenced by the traditions and customs of the society.
5. All individuals have some rights and the society imposes certain obligations upon them.

TYPES OF INDIVIDUAL DIFFERENCES

Types of individual differences and its description are given in Table 7.1.

Table 7.1: Types of individual differences

Sl No	*Types*	*Description*
1.	Physical or physiological differences	Physical differences among individuals are related to the differences created on account of the differences in terms of physical makeup of the bodies. Individuals differ in height, weight, color of skin, color of eyes and hair, size of hands, arms, feet, mouth, nose, waistline, structure and functioning of internal organs, facial expression and mannerisms of speech, walk, hairstyle and other physical characteristics.
2.	Psychological differences	Psychological makeup generate differences among individuals in terms of varying intellectual potentialities, interests, attitudes, emotions, social and moral development, etc.
3.	Gender	Men and women are different in every organ of the body even their skin. They are different at the cellular level and these differences may influence the variations in disease, treatment like type and amount of medicine that is safe on the basis of gender.

Contd...

Contd...

Sl No	*Types*	*Description*
4.	Race	Racial differences can add up to significant group differences. Many factors are involved like socioeconomic factors, lifestyle behaviors, social environment and access to preventive health services as well as treatment among other environmental differences.
5.	Age	Age is an important factor, which decides the treatment and diagnosis of a disease in an individual. The mental, physical and intellectual abilities and the maturity level determine the individual variability according to the different age groups.
6.	Intelligence	Individuals have difference in their general intelligence. For example, it is not possible to send children with an intelligence quotient of below 50 to school.
7.	Nationality	Studies showed that the individuals of different nations differ in respect of nature, physical and mental differences, interest and personality.
8.	Personality	Personality is the total quality of an individual's behavior as is depicted in his habits of thinking, attitude, interest and his manner of acting and his personal philosophy of life. Personality is the sum total of an individual's traits and characteristics, which is expressed through his behavior.
9.	Abilities	Abilities will determine the individual for special professional and specialized fields of vocation.
10.	Psychomotor activity	The individual's movements of the hand and feet and other physical abilities are seen to be very different and do not resemble to one another to a great extent.
11.	Learning	Learning can be seen in children of different ages, but also among those in the same age group. It depends on their maturing and educational background.
12.	Social background	Individual difference occurs based on types of family, culture, neighborhood and class, which manifests individual variations.

Contd...

Contd...

Sl No	*Types*	*Description*
13.	Economical status	Economic background creates differences in interest, tendencies and character, etc.
14.	Development	It is evident not only among those of different ages but also in the individuals of same ages.
15.	Mental differences	People differ in intellectual abilities and capacities like reasoning and thinking, power of imagination, creative expression, concentration, etc.
16.	Differences in attitudes	Individuals are found to possess varying attitudes toward different people, groups, objects and ideas. Their attitudes may be positive, negative or somewhat indifferent in nature.
17.	Emotional differences	The individuals also differ in the manner they express their emotions. Some are emotionally stable and mature, while others are emotionally unstable and immature.

CAUSES OF INDIVIDUAL DIFFERENCES

There are many factors that make a person unique from others. These factors are related to family, trait, social life, situation, emotion, culture, etc. Person with different traits possess different personalities, this includes heredity, intelligence, physical traits. Individual differences are also caused by hereditary and environmental factors. A child comes to this world with certain traits, which determine his individual capabilities and thus he differs from others on account of hereditary.

Heredity

Heredity refers to the process of transmission of certain biological and psychological characteristics from parents to their children through genes. The hereditary decides the path of progress and development of an individual. Hereditary provides the limits of one's growth and development in various dimensions and aspects of one's personality and thus variations in hereditary characteristic causes differences between individuals.

Environment

Environment refers to such factors, in and around the individual and brings about changes in the individual physically and psychologically. The environment covers all the outside factors that act on the individual, since he begins the life. The first environment for a child is the mother's womb. The fetus gets its nourishment from the bloodstream of its mothers. After birth, the child is expected to numerous environment factors, such as food, water, climate, physical atmosphere at home, school, village, parents, members of the family, friends, neighbors, teachers, society, mass media, recreation, religious places, etc.

MEASUREMENT OF INDIVIDUAL DIFFERENCES

To measure individual differences, different tests are given in Table 7.2.

Table 7.2: Measurement of individual differences

Sl No	*Measurement*	*Description*
1.	Intelligence test	• Stanford-Binet test • Raven's progressive matrices • Bhatia's battery of performance test of intelligence
2.	Aptitude test	Differential aptitude test (DAT) • Achievement tests • Term-end examination
3.	Personality test	• Self-reported or open reports • Rating scales • Questionnaires (Minnesota multiphasic personality inventory, Cattell's 16 personality factors test, Eysenck's personality test) • Projective tests [Rorschach inkblot test, thematic apperception test (TAT)] • Performance test • Situational tests • Interviews

HEREDITY

Heredity is considered as 'the sum total of inborn individual traits'. Biologically, it has been defined as 'the sum total of traits potentially present in the fertilized ovum'. According to Douglas and Holland "one's heredity consists of all the structures, physical characteristics, functions or capacities derived from parents, other ancestry or species."

All organisms possess a life cycle, which includes growth, development, reproduction and decline. Though there is essential unity in life, the ways by which each organism exercises its capacities are different. These individual qualities of organisms and their basic properties are transmitted by means of heredity.

There is a popular notion that life begins at birth. But, biologically life begins at the moment of fertilization (conception), i.e. when matured sperm of a man fuses with matured ovum of women. It is most crucial events in the life of an individual, because the biological substances present in the sperm and ovum determine the sex, biological, physiological and psychological characteristics of the emerging individual. Thus, biological hereditary by interaction with the prenatal and postnatal environment, determine the potentialities of the individual. The knowledge of such hereditary factors and their functions help us to understand the growth, development, similarities and differences in physical, physiological and psychological makeup of an individual. Similarly the knowledge of the environment, which shapes the growth and development pattern of hereditary potentials, is necessary to understand the individual.

1. *Genetic diversity:* It is the amount of variation seen in a particular population. The differences occur in different communities, races or ethnic groups that lead to individual differences among population. The genes have an impact on the characteristics of human being. Like the Japanese and Chinese have significant appearance than Whites and Indians.
2. *Genetic variability:* It is a measure of the tendency of individual genotypes in a population to vary from one another. The genetic variability describes the susceptibility of organisms to disease and sensitivity to toxins or drugs.

Mechanism of Heredity

The life cycle of an individual begins with the fusion of a sperm and ovum. The origin of every human life can be traced to a single cell called zygote. When a sperm unites with an ovum, zygote is produced. The genes, which are the carriers of distinctive traits, are present both in the sperm and the ovum. In the fertilized ovum, there are 23 pairs of chromosomes, half of which are given by the father and the other half by the mother. While, females have 23 pairs of XX chromosomes, males have 22 pairs of XX chromosomes plus two single chromosomes represented by X and Y. X and Y are called sex chromosomes.

Occasionally, through some unfortunate bodily error, aberrations in chromosomes appear. If an extra chromosome appears making the total 47 rather than the normal 46, mongolism (Down syndrome or trisomy 21 anomaly) results. A child with mongolism suffers from deceleration of growth during the prenatal period, which results in a highly complex, multidimensional disorder in which every organ is involved.

When chromosomes are studied under a microscope, bands of markings appear, representing an entity called genes which appear to be the actual determiners of traits. Each chromosome is made up of many genes. Man has probably not less than 2,000 and not more than 50,000 genes in the chromosomes. Each gene is the determiner of a specific characteristic, such as straight nose or a deep lobed ear. At present, it appears that there is no simple one -to-one relationship, between genes and traits that are one gene may influence many characteristics or traits or conversely many genes may combine to determine one characteristic.

Action of the genes on the cytoplasm changes, the shape and other characteristics of the cells. The heredity basis of individual differences lies in the unlimited variety of possible gene combinations that can occur. No two siblings get an identical heredity, as they do not get the same genes from the parents. Fraternal or dizygotic twins born to the same parents are different from each other because of different pairs of germ cells. However, identical or monozygotic twins develop from the same sperm and ovum, hence have exactly the same set of genes and therefore, resemble each other completely.

Determination of traits is not only due to combination of genes but also due to their dominant or recessive nature. In the color of the eye, for example, brown is dominant over blue, if one parent carries only brown and the other only blue, their offspring will have brown eyes. Many people, however, carry both; and if two recessive blues happen to matchup in the assorting process of meiosis and fertilization, the child would have blue eyes even though parents and all the immediate relatives have brown eyes.

Some characteristics are sex linked, i.e. one sex shows the characteristics, while the other sex not apparently affected is the carrier. One such trait is color blindness. For example, the sons of a color blind man and normal woman do not inherit the defect, but the daughters may be carrier of the disorder to another generation of males, their sons. Another example is hemophilia; a bleeding disorder, which rarely occurs in women, but is transmitted by them to their sons (Stern, 1960).

Occasionally, in the reproductive cells of any living thing a change occurs, which causes the introduction of completely new traits in the next generation. Such changes are called mutations. Mutant plants and animals might have characteristics that breeders can use to improve existing varieties. In human beings, mutations are almost always undesirable. Their causes are not clear, but are known that they can be induced by atomic radiation.

Genetics and Behavior

Heredity is the basis for the development of human personality. It is like the raw material in the hands of the artist out of which the potter or tailor prepare the specific objects. Any amount of molding and treatment with special processes will still retain the basic properties of the raw material.

Many aspects of human behavior and development ranging from physical characteristics, such as height, weight, eye and skin color, the complex patterns of social and intellectual behavior are influenced by person's genetic endowment. They also include physical deficiencies and the nature of glandular functioning. Heredity is a source of both similarities and differences among individuals.

Identity

'Like begets like' the principle states that, children have a tendency to be like their parents; the children of bright parents tend to be bright and those of dull, tend to be dull. But this law is not universally true. It has exceptions. Sometimes we see white parents having black children. Such occurrences can be explained by the 'law of variation'.

Variation

The law of variation explains the causes of differences in the children of the same family. As the germ cells of the parents have genes, which unite in various ways, each combination produces a different quality of offspring, i.e. there will be as many variations as there are possible combinations of genes. We sometimes find the same parents having children who are very different from one another. It is because of the different combinations of genes, that different types of children are born, e.g. one combination would produce a white child, the other a dark one. We must remember that though the child of the same family is different in intellect, etc. yet they show a greater tendency to be like each other, than the children who are not related.

Regression

According to Sorenson, "the tendency for the children of very bright parents to be less bright than parents and a comparable tendency for the children of very inferior parents to be less inferior is called regression.

Sources of Variability in a Population

Sources of variability and its description are given in Table 7.3.

Table 7.3: Sources of variability in a population

Sl No	*Sources*	*Description*
1.	Genetic recombination	During meiosis, two homologous chromosomes from male and female crossover one another and exchange gene sequences. The chromosomes, than split apart and are ready to form an offspring. The crossover is random and is governed by its own set of genes that code from where crossovers can occur.
2.	Immigration, migration and translocation	Each of these is the movement of an individual into or out of a population. When an individual comes from a previous genetically isolated population into a new one, it will increase the genetic variability of the next generation, if it reproduces.
3.	Polyploidy	Having more than two homologous chromosomes allows for even more recombination during meiosis and allowing for even more genetic variability in one's offspring.
4.	Diffuse centromeres	Being diffuse causes the chromatids, to split apart in many different ways allowing for chromosome fragmentation and polyploidy, hence creating more variability.

Contd...

Contd...

Sl No	*Sources*	*Description*
5.	Genetic mutations	Contributed to the genetic variability within a population and can have positive, negative or neutral effects on the individual's fitness.
6.	Correlated traits	Although, some genes have only an effect on a single trait, many genes have an effect on various traits, so the change in a single gene will have an effect on all those traits.
7.	Resemblance between relatives	A child has a father and mother, the child and father share 50% of their alleles, as do the child and the mother. However the mother and father normally do not share genes as a result of shared ancestors. Similarly two full siblings share on average 50% of alleles with each other, while half siblings share only 25%.

Chromosomal Abnormalities

Anomalies and description for chromosomal abnormalities are given in Table 7.4.

Table 7.4: Chromosomal abnormalities

Sl No	*Anomalies*	*Description*
1.	Cleft palate	Cleft palate is an abnormal fissure in the palate of the mouth that is present at birth. It is caused by faulty development of the facial structure of the fetus. Very often, a cleft palate is accompanied by a similar division in the upper lip called harelip. In the normal development, separate tissues fuse together to form the palate, i.e. upper lip and upper jaw. Cleft palate occurs because the roof of the mouth does not develop completely and there will be a vertical gap (fissure) in the roof of the mouth.
2.	Lobster claw	Lobster hand is a rare congenital deformity of the hand. Here, the middle digit is missing. Lobster claw is an inherited condition. It often, occurs both in males and females equally. The chance is 1 in 90,000 babies. It can be treated surgically to improve function and appearance, genetic counseling is given to parents who have genetic load. It is called by different names: lobster claw hand, lobster hand, split hand deformity, cleft hand, etc.

Contd...

Contd...

Sl No	*Anomalies*	*Description*
3.	Polydac-tyly or syndactyly	It is webbing between the fingers and toes. In most cases the condition is inherited. It usually affects both hands and feet. Syndactyly of the toes does not require treatment, but fingers can be corrected by surgery. Polydactylism is nothing, but having one or more extra fingers and or toes. It is probably a most common abnormality of development found at birth. It occurs in about 2 per 1,000 children.
4.	Hemophilia	It is a congenital disorder, where the blood clotting is very slow. Due to this condition any wound or injury, even if it is a minor one, gives rise to prolonged bleeding. This individual will have a risk of anemia and dangerous loss in blood volume. Hemophilia is due to deficiency in one of the factors in blood plasma, which helps blood clotting normally. Hemophilia occurs almost exclusively in males (sex-linked trait); it is due to genetic defect, transmitted only by women.
5.	Down syndrome	Down syndrome is also known as mongolism, it is also known as trisomy 21. It is called Down syndrome because this kind of mental retardation was first traced and studied by Dr John Langdon Down and hence, it is named after him. It is called mongolism because, these mentally retarded individuals will have the features of Mongolian race, i.e. short, broad face, round head, small lowest ears, flat nose, large tongue that protrudes from small mouth, a fold of skin at the inner corners of the eyes, short fingers, weak muscles. The child exhibits a marked degree of mental retardation with an intelligence quotient of 50 or below.

ENVIRONMENT

Man cannot remain untouched by the environment in which he lives. If the environment is favorable, the impact is positive whereas in an unfavorable environment, man's development may be hindered or he may have to do more effort for adaptation. Environment is an extensive and broader concept, everything around us is environment. But for physical scientists, environment means only nature and physical conditions.

Any and every influence with which an individual comes into contact after the hereditary pattern has been received to the germ plasma. It includes the effects of training, trial and error learning influences of the home, school, neighborhood, hospital, church, playground, climate, geographical location and anything else that stimulates the senses in any way. Thus, the heredity plays its game only at the time of conception. What happens afterwards (i.e. after conception in the game of environment)? It affects the individual, his bodily structure and all of his personality makeup and behavior.

Definitions

1. Total environment includes physical and social aspects.
   —*McIver*
2. The environment can be explained as natural environment and sociocultural environment.

Types of Environment

According to Landis, environment can be divided into three parts: natural, social and cultural.

Natural environment: Physical environment, all natural life conditions, forces and objects, which influences life are included.

Social environment: It consists of social organization, institutions and social relationship.

Cultural environment: It includes customs, tradition, usages, pattern and values.

Environmental forces can be categorized into internal and external environments.

Internal Environment

Internal environment refers to the prenatal environment. The nucleus with its chromosomes and their genes is surrounded by a jelly like substance known as cytoplasm. Cytoplasm is considered as an intercellular environment. This environment influences the genes and thereby the triads they carry. In fact, what the organism becomes is determined by its cytoplasm and its heredity. Further the cells press upon one another and influence their neighboring cells chemically and electrically. This intracellular environment has an effect on the developing embryo. The cells in each area will develop into the respective organ.

1. The environment received by the individual from his conception till his birth in the womb of the mother, i.e. a period of about 9 months is called an internal environment.

2. In this environment, the embryo receives the nutrition through the bloodstream of the mother. The physical and mental health of the mother including her habits, attitudes and interests, etc. all constitutes the inner surrounding or internal environment that affects the growth and development of the fetus along with the emerging behavior in future.
3. External environment: After the birth, what the child gets in terms of environmental influences is purely external in nature. These can be physical and social or cultural influences.
4. The physical environment includes earth, river, mountains, weather and climatic conditions, food, water, etc.
5. The parents, family members, friends, classmates, teachers, members of community and society, the means of mass communication and recreation, religious places, etc. include with social and cultural environment helping to shape the personality and behavior.
6. The role of heredity and environment in the development of personality and behavior has been extensively searched, in the form of twins and family studies and on experimenting selective breeding. The results have failed to establish a clear cut role of either presence of particular behavior or trait in an individual.

   What behaviors are learned or what are inherited is a controversial question that can only be answered through a reasonable understanding that one's behavior or development of a specific personality trait is always a result of the interaction of the environmental process on the genetically inherited characteristics.

External Environment

The environment after birth is more complex and powerful. It involves immense variety of physical and social contacts. This is what we customarily call the environment. The social environment includes language, customs, tradition and many cultural aspects like values, moral, religion, etc. further schools, community, family, peer group, neighborhood also influence the individual. The physical environment involves stimuli like the food we eat, the drinks we take, the cloths we wear, the shelter we live in, light, sound, smell, taste, etc. will have their own impact on the individual.

RELATIVE IMPORTANCE OF HEREDITY AND ENVIRONMENT

The relative importance of hereditary and environment is rather disputable because both hereditary and environmental factors are equally important in the individual. They interact in such a way that influence of each factor is dependent on the contribution of the others. Any single hereditary factor operates differently under different environmental conditions. In the same way, the environmental conditions differ in their relative influences depending upon the hereditary factors involved. However, hybrids and certain abnormalities prove the importance of hereditary; monsters prove the importance of environment. Hybrid is a product of two different species, which are similar to each other.

INTERACTION BETWEEN HEREDITY AND ENVIRONMENT

Each individual enters the world with certain hereditary characteristics transmitted through the parents. He grows up in a certain environment with its human, social and material surroundings. Everything he does as a child or adult results from the complex interactions between heredity and environment.

1. The relative influence of heredity and environment differs from one individual to another and from one human trait or condition to another.
2. Heredity and environment are interdependent forces. Inheritance is an important factor in the development of the artistic abilities like music. Heredity supplies the potential talent, while favorable environment brings it out.
3. Heredity and environment are equally important in shaping the temperament of the child. Heredity lays down the essential foundations, while environment can change these foundations for better or worse.
4. Heredity provides the raw material from which a person is made. How the material is molded and what he becomes depend chiefly on the environment. Good materials placed in good hands result in a fine-finished product. Poor material, no matter how carefully fashioned can never become a first-rate product.

5. Our inheritance prescribes the limits beyond which it may not be possible for any individual to develop, however wholesome and stimulating the environment may be.

Today, no one believes that nature or nurture alone, completely determine the course of our development. Psychologists, agree that the development is shaped by the interaction of heredity and the environment. Within this interaction, our genetic endowment for many characteristics provides us with a reaction range of possible levels that we may ultimately reach depending on the quality of our experience in the environment. Heredity and environment are interdependent forces. The influence of heredity and environment are so inter-related that they are practically inseparable.

The knowledge of the mechanism of heredity and the influence of environment on the personality development is important for a nurse to understand the behavior of a patient.

INDIVIDUAL DIFFERENCES IN HEALTH AND ILLNESS

Understand Child's Abilities

Individual Differences in Intelligence

It is not possible to send children with an IQ of below 50 to schools. Children with a higher IQ can go to school. Children with IQ's between 50 and 70 can learn only the simplest tasks. Even the small schools trouble children whose IQ varies between 70 and 80. Children with IQ varying between 115 and 120 are considered brilliant or intelligent. Very low and high IQ's children have difficulty in learning with those having average IQ. Generally, 40% to 60% of the children in school have IQs varying between 95 and 105, being the children with average intelligence who form the basis for the formulation of the syllabus and curriculum, as well as the method of teaching.

1. Individuals with special abilities are helpful to judge special professions and specialized fields of vocation.
2. Mental ages and education are intimately related. The child's level of education is determined according to his mental age.
3. Children's interests, tendencies and character can also be seen influenced by economic situation, which would affect the learning and special abilities.

Understanding Patient's Health

1. Individual differences are useful for explaining and predicting behavior and performance.
2. People vary on a range of psychological attributes. Thus, it is possible to measure and study these individual differences.
3. It helps to understand the behavior, feeling, thinking and attitude of patients during sickness.
4. The gene-environment interaction means some people carry genetic factors that cause susceptibility or resistance to a certain disorder in a particular environment. It may be significant public health benefits in using genetic information, to decide environmental interventions that prevent disease.

Preventive and Treatment Measures

1. It can assess the health promoting or treatment behaviors, such as medication taking, proper diet and engaging in physical activity through patient perceptions of health and threat of disease, and barriers in a patient's social or cultural environment.
2. It helps in evaluating, the effectiveness of a new therapy on the group.
3. The treatment with drugs can be made safer and more effective when the patient's genotype is known. Pharmacokinetics, studies the genetic variation that causes people to respond differently to drugs.

CONCLUSION

Thus, the individual from the time of conception to death is subjected to environmental influences. So, we find that the continuous interplay of the heredity endowments and the environment factors are in determining the physical, physiological, social and psychological growth, and development of the individual. So, man is a product of the interplay of heredity and environment.

SUGGESTED READING

1. Brody Nathan, Ehrlichman Howard. Personality Psychology: Science of Individuality; A Thoughtful Introduction to the Broad Field of Personality. Prentice Hall Press; 1997.

2. Cooper C. Individual Differences: A broad Overview of the Field that Includes a Review of Measurement Methodologies. London: Arnold; 1997.
3. Eysenck HJ, Eysenck MW. Personality and Individual Differences: A Natural Science Approach. New York: Plenum; 1985.
4. Eysenck HJ. Personality: Biological foundations. In: Vernon PA (Ed). The Neuropsychology of Individual Differences. London: Academic Press; 1994.
5. Gale A, Eysenck MW. Handbook of Individual Differences: Biological Perspectives. Chichester: Wiley; 1991.
6. Galton F. Measurement of character. Fortnightly Review. 1884;36: 179-85.
7. Goldberg LR. The structure of phenotypic personality traits. Am Psychol. 1993;48(1):26-34.
8. Hogan R, Johnson J, Briggs S (Eds). Handbook of Personality Psychology. San Diego: Academic Press; 1997.
9. Jensen AR. The G Factor: The Science of Mental Ability. Westport: Conn. Praeger; 1998.
10. Loehlin JC. Genes and Environment in Personality Development. Newbury Park, Ca: Sage Publications; 1992.
11. Maltby J, Day L, Macaskill A. Personality, Individual Differences and Intelligence. London: Prentice Hall (Pearson Education); 2007.
12. Saklofske DH, Zeidner M. International Handbook of Personality and Intelligence. New York: Plenum; 1995.
13. Tyler LE. The Psychology of Human Differences. New York: Appleton-Century-Crofts; 1965.

REVIEW QUESTIONS

1. Define individual differences. Explain the types of individual differences.
2. Explain the causes of individual differences.
3. Define heredity. Discuss the mechanism of heredity.
4. Define chromosomal abnormalities; discuss in detail.
5. Define environment. Explain different types and importance of environment in individual difference.

CHAPTER 8 Intelligence and Abilities

LEARNING OBJECTIVES

1. Definitions.
2. Intelligence and abilities during sickness.
3. Measurements of intelligence and abilities.

INTRODUCTION

The term intelligence is derived from Latin word *intelligence* coined by Cicero, used to cover all mental process. The individuals differ from one another in their ability to understand complex ideas, to adapt effectively to the environment, to learn from experience, to engage in various forms of reasoning, to overcome obstacles by taking thought. Owning to his/her intelligence, man is considered to be better than other animals. Some people are very intelligent, while others do not have that ability. Intelligence is not a single trait or character; rather it is combination of many traits. It is a composition of capabilities that makes a person rational, able to think correctly, act purposefully, person can learn through signs and symbols and can adjust effectively with his/her environment. Most of the people have an intuitive notion of what intelligence is and many words in English language distinguish between different levels of intellectual skills—bright, dull, smart, stupid, clever, slow and so on. It is necessary for a nurse to learn about intelligence because difference in the amount and quality of intelligence make their ability to adjust the situations around them. Intelligent patients want more explanations for their treatment they are getting, whereas less intelligent patients will be satisfied with a little or no explanations.

MEANING OF INTELLIGENCE

Intelligence is one of the most studied and debated personal qualities of the human being. It is invisible, cannot be directly seen, yet it is studied at greater length and is considered to be one of the most important qualities. The study of intelligence has made psychology a more interesting subject, but still psychologists are not unanimous about the nature of intelligence. Many aspects of intelligence are included in intelligent behavior because intelligence is a conceptual structure with many characteristics. It is difficult to perceive intelligence in physical form, but intelligent behavior can be assessed by the practicality, success in examinations and objectives, mental maturity and ability to adjust, etc. Other than these, ability to express himself/herself, sharpness of memory, ability to perceive, foresight, ability to forecast results, etc. also help in determining the intelligent behavior of a person. Potential to accept challenges and passing the examinations with good division, behaving as per one's age, position, prestige and social status are also the indicators of intelligent behavior.

DEFINITIONS OF INTELLIGENCE

1. Intelligence is the potential or ability of a person to adjust to new conditions. —*William Stern*
2. Intelligence can be defined as the ability of a person to act purposefully, think rationally and deal effectively with his environment. —*DL Wechsler*
3. Intelligence is organized around an ideal portiere. One's intelligence is defined by the degree of resemblance to this prototype. Since, there exist multiple prototypes; there would be no validated concept of intelligence. —*Nesser*
4. One's adaptation to the environment is called intelligence. —*Piaget*
5. Intelligence is defined as a biological mechanism by which the effects of the complexity of stimuli are brought together and given a somewhat unified effect in behavior. —*Peterson*
6. Intelligence is the capacity to learn and adjust to relatively new and changing conditions. —*Wagnon*
7. An individual is intelligent in proportion as he is able to carry on abstract thinking. —*Terman*

8. Intelligence means intellect put to use. It is the use of intellectual abilities for handling a situation or accomplishing any task. —*Woodworth and Marquis*
9. Intelligence is defined as a mental activity consisting of grasping the essentials in a situation and responding appropriately to them. —*Heim*
10. Intelligence defined as the effective all-round cognitive abilities to comprehend, to grasp relations and reasons. —*Vernon*
11. Intelligence is the capacity to learn and adjust to relatively new and changing conditions. —*Wagnon*
12. Intelligence is the property of recombining the behavior patterns, so as to act better in a novel situation. —*Wells*
13. Intelligence is an ability to demand to solve the problems, which require the comprehension and use of symbols. –*Garret*
14. An intelligent person uses past experience effectively, is able to concentrate and keep his attention focused for longer periods of times, adjusts himself to a new and unaccustomed situation rapidly, with less confusion and with fewer false moves, variability of responses, is able to see distinct relationships, can carry on abstract thinking, has a great capacity of inhibition or delay and is capable of exercising self-criticism. —*Richard Wellington Husband*
15. Intelligence may be defined as the power of good responses from the point of view of truth or facts. —*Thorndike*

NATURE OF INTELLIGENCE

1. Nature of intelligence is an innate mental ability, which grows and is influenced by the environment.
2. It shows the capacity to adapt to new or changed situations quickly and correctly.
3. It consists of the ability to carry on the higher mental processes such as reasoning, criticism, application and judgment.
4. It implies the capacity to learn difficult tasks and the ability to solve increasing difficult problems.
5. It shows the capacity to observe the relationships and detect absurdities.
6. Intelligence may be regarded as a sort of mental energy (in the form of mental or cognitive abilities) available with an

individual to enable to handle his/her environment in terms of adaptation and facing novel situations as effectively as possible.

TYPES OF INTELLIGENCE

According to Sternberg's triarchic theory of human intelligence (1995), intelligence is of three types:

1. *Analytical intelligence:* It is academic problem-solving skills, based on combined operations of execution, performance and knowledge. These three operations will enable to encode stimuli, hold information in short-term memory, make calculations, perform mental calculations and mentally compare different stimuli, retrieve information from long-term memory.
2. *Creative intelligence:* It involves insights, synthesis and the ability to react to novel situations and stimuli. It consists of ability, which allows people to think creatively and adjust creatively and effectively to new situations. Novel task or situations are good measure of intellectual ability because they assess an individual's ability to apply existing knowledge to new problems.
3. *Practical intelligence:* It is the intelligence, which operates in the real world. People with this type of intelligence can adapt to or shape their environment. It is influenced not only by mental skills but also by attitudes and emotional factors.

Eight Types of Intelligence—Gardner (1999)

1. *Linguistic intelligence:* It is involved in reading, writing, listening and talking.
2. *Logical-mathematical intelligence:* It is involved in solving logical puzzles, deriving proofs and performing calculations.
3. *Musical intelligence:* It is involved in playing, composing, singing and conducting. Furthermore, Gardner believes that auto mechanic and cardiologists may have this kind of intelligence in abundance.
4. *Spatial intelligence:* It is involved in moving from one location to another or to determine one's orientation in space.
5. *Intrapersonal intelligence:* It is involved in understanding oneself and having insight into one's own thoughts, actions and emotions, e.g. self-understanding.

6. *Bodily-kinesthetic intelligence:* It is involved in using one's own body (or parts of it) to perform skillful and purposeful movements, e.g. dancer, athletes and surgeons.
7. *Naturalistic intelligence:* It involves the ability to understand and to work effectively in the natural world, e.g. biologists and zoologists.
8. *Interpersonal intelligence:* It is involved in understanding of others and one's reaction to others. Being high in social skills, psychologists, teacher and politicians are supposed to be high in this type of intelligence.

FACTORS INFLUENCING INTELLIGENCE

Biochemical Factors

From the recent studies it is found that the disturbances of biochemical balances of the body may underlie various disorders of learning and intelligence. For optimum functioning of the nervous system, sufficient supply of oxygen and various nutrients are necessary. Apart from these, body temperature, pH balance and hormones also influence neural activities and thereby affect intellectual performances.

1. It is found that the defective genes may lead to defective enzyme functioning and this in turn produces a rare condition known as phenylpyruvic oligophrenia, a type of feeble mindedness.
2. Cretinism is another type of mental deficiency caused by underactivity of the thyroid gland in childhood.
3. Mongolian idiocy is caused by defective cerebral metabolism. If the mother becomes pregnant nearing to menopause, the biochemical imbalances in her during pregnancy may cause Mongolian idiocy. Thus, various factors affect the growth of intelligence.

Sociocultural Factors

All the intelligence tests, to some extent or the other, are subjected to the influence of sociocultural factors because the test items are drawn from the culture from whom the test is developed. The tests reflect the cultural experiences and reveal how well an individual deals with cultural factors.

Parent's occupation: It is found from the studies that there are pronounced difference in the IQs of children, whose parents belong to different occupational groups. The children of professional parents have a mean IQ of about 115; children of day laborers have a mean IQ of 94 and of intermediate occupational groups range between these two extremes. The rationale behind this is that only higher intellectual ability can reach higher occupation.

Socioeconomic status: This is more comprehensive factor than occupation. It includes factors like education, source and level of income, ethnic and residential area, etc. The socioeconomic differences in IQ are attributed to the factors, which account for occupational differences. In any society, more intelligent man tend to rise up in the socioeconomic scale and remains there, while the less intelligent man comes down and remains in the lower strata.

Regional influences: Regional location is correlated with performance on intelligence tests. According to McNemar, the mean IQ of urban children was 108; of suburban children was 107 and of rural children was 96. City offers better schools, better educational facilities, and affords wide variety of extracurricular and recreational facilities. This provides a greater challenge to the growing child.

Environment: The environment wherein the educational facilities are poor and outside contacts are rare, will reduce the IQ as they grow older. In short, the poor environment will have progressively adverse effect as the age increases. On the other hand enriched environment is provided to the children. But it will have more beneficial effect if it is provided very early in life. If it is provided after 7 years of life, it will have no effect. Thus, various biochemical and environmental factors contribute their share to the intellectual growth of the individual.

INTELLIGENCE QUOTIENT

The intellectual capacity of the person can be assessed through IQ. This works as a guide in the future, but it is essential to know the stability and limits of IQ. IQ of 80 percent of people is either 100 or around 100. According to modern concept, IQ is a measurement of quality and assessment of intelligence. Stanford-Binet had invented the method of quantifying or measuring intelligence. IQ can be obtained by multiplying the ratio of mental age and chronological age by 100. This can be explained by the following formula:

IQ = Mental age/chronological age × 100.

Mental age: This represents the development of performance level of a child at certain age. In other words, if 5-year-old child is able to do the tests, which is meant for a 6-year-old child, mental age would be counted as 6 years. Failures in the tests meant for a particular age group reduces the mental age.

Chronological age: This is the physical age of the child that is based on his/her date of birth.

Distribution of IQ: Psychologists have described level of intelligence in many ways. The different levels of IQ have been explained in Table 8.1.

Table 8.1: Levels of intelligence

Sl No	*Intelligence quotient (IQ)*	*Description*
1.	140 and above	Genius
2.	120–139	Very superior
3.	110–119	Superior
4.	90–109	Normal
5.	80–89	Low normal
6.	70–79	Borderline
7.	50–69	Moron
8.	25–49	Imbecile
9.	0–24	Idiot

Intelligence quotient is determined by both hereditary and the environment. Hence, level of intelligence may change as result of environment. Similarly, repeated tests and using different types of tests may show a change in intelligence level.

INTELLIGENCE TESTS

History of Intelligence Tests

In the beginning, mental tests were devised to study individual differences among college students. These tests were used to measure the speed of reaction, sensory acuity and other simple psychological processes. The primary interest was to study the extent of individual differences and not to assess the level of intelligence of the individual.

In 1896, Binet, a French psychologist who was studying process of school suggested special classes for children showing poor progress in classwork. Eight years later the French Government requested Binet to discover children in public school who were not having sufficient intelligence to benefit themselves by usual instruction.

Measurement of Intelligence Tests

Measurement of intelligence tests can be categorized in the following categories.

Individual intelligence tests: These tests measure the intelligence of one person at a time. These are used to measure the intelligence of retarded children or to provide treatment and guidance. Major limitations of these tests include the skills of examiner and problems of qualification. Financially, these tests are more expensive. These tests can be administered not only individually but also a group at a time. For example, Alexander battery of performance test, Bhatia tests of intelligence, form board test, Stanford-Binet, Wechsler tests, etc.

Group intelligence tests: This method of measuring intelligence is used to measure the intelligence of more than one person. These tests are very popular. Group intelligence tests were also used in World War I, to measure the intelligence of the literate and illiterate soldiers. These tests can be administered to a large number of individuals at a time. For example, for army alpha, army beta and Raven's progressive matrices (RPM).

Verbal intelligence test: In this test, intelligence of a person is measured on the basis of his/her answer or reactions to the given questions. This is a reliable test and is useful for both the individuals and group, but the examiners should have the knowledge of language or words. Examiner should be highly skilled to get maximum results from these tests.

Non-verbal performance tests: These involve no language, but require duplication of block patterns, completion of jigsaw puzzle, arrangements of pictures, drawing, etc. Goddard form board, Link form board, Alexander battery of performance tests, RPM, etc.

Verbal, non-verbal combined tests: These include both verbal and non-verbal items. For example, Wechsler test for children and adults,

Bhatia tests of intelligence, army alpha and beta test of performance, army general classification test (AGCT), armed forces qualification test (AFQT), etc.

Power tests: These tests allow sufficient time to the subject to try most or all the items he/she can do. The score obtains as an indicator of his/her achievement, e.g. RPM.

Uses of Intelligence Tests

Intelligence tests are used in many ways of life to determine the levels of IQ of an individual, which is of utmost importance for success in any walk of life. Hence, innumerable tests have come into existence and these reveal its importance in life. Some of the areas in which intelligence tests are useful are mentioned as follows:

1. Intelligence tests have helped us to understand fully the nature of the intelligence.
2. As intelligence plays a very significant role in the determination of personality, intelligence tests are used as a part of personality assessment.
3. Intelligence tests are useful to dispel the wrong notions of racial differences, sex differences, caste differences, etc. These tests have ruled out the superiority of any race, sex or caste in intelligence over others.
4. Intelligence tests are useful in educational guidance of children. By determining the IQ of a child he/she may be guided to take up a particular course of study for which he/she is studied.
5. Intelligence tests are used in many educational institutions to select the students for admission. If the student is found below the required level of intelligence for the courses they offer, may be rejected.
6. Intelligence tests are also used as a part of vocational guidance. The success in any vocation partly depends upon intelligence in addition to aptitude and interest.

Other Uses

1. Studying the individual differences.
2. Identifying the retarded children and treating them.
3. Help in the field of education.
4. Finding the solution of disciplinary problems.
5. Use in business skills.
6. Use in armed forces.
7. Help in research work.

THEORIES OF INTELLIGENCE

The theories and description of intelligence are shown in Table 8.2.

Table 8.2: Description of the theories of intelligence

Sl No	*Theory*	*Description*
1.	Monarchic theory or unitary theory	The theory holds that intelligence is one power or energy, which affects all the activities of the individual. According to Victoria Hazlitt, intelligence is a general ability, which determines the various specific abilities. The theory has been proved to fallacious. Prominent people show a less than average ability in many activities. The theory has been proved to be fallacious. Prominent people show less than average ability in many activities. For example, Darwin had a very bad handwriting.
2.	Oligarchic theory	This theory postulates that intelligence is an aggregate of mutually independent powers. Binet believed this theory. Experiments disproved this theory by showing that the mental powers are interdependent.
3.	Multifactor or anarchic theory or group factor theory (Thurstone, 1933)	Thorndike is the most prominent among those who believed this theory. This theory holds that intelligence is the mean of undetermined independent rudimentary elements. But Spearman has criticized this theory.
4.	Two-factor theory (Spearman, 1927)	This theory was conceived by Spearman who holds that intelligence has two parts: a. General intelligence or G. b. Specific intelligence are confined to specific activities. General intelligence is found in lesser or greater degree in every one. Specific intelligence is of various types; the several types being independent of each other. They differ from individual to individual. This intelligence of a person depends on his/her general intelligence.
5.	Structure of intellect model (Guilford, 1959)	In structure of intellect model, Guilford postulated many factors of intelligence. He categorized these factors under three broad dimensions: a. The process or operation performed. b. The kind of product involved. c. The kind of material or content involved. He then subclassified under each of these dimensions five operations, six types of products and four types of contents.

Spearman's Two-factor Theory

Charles Spearman has proposed two-factor theory of intelligence. According to Spearman, intelligence constitutes two factors, these two factors are:

1. General intelligence factor called G factor.
2. Specific or special factor called S factor.

He further said the G factor varies from person-to-person. Depending upon the amount of G they possess, people are described as generally brought bright or generally dull. Intelligence tests measure the amount of G factor, which individual possesses. The amount of S factor varies within the same individual. For example, a student may be very good in mathematics, but poor in spatial relations.

Louis Thurston, another psychologist, objected to Spearman's two-factor theory. Thurston said that "human intelligence could broken down into a number of primary abilities." His statistical studies lead to the following primary abilities (Table 8.3).

Table 8.3: Types of primary abilities obtained from statistical studies by Louis Thurston

Sl No	*Primary abilities*	*Description*
1.	Verbal comprehension	The ability to understand the meaning of words; vocabulary test intelligence measures this factor
2.	Word fluency	The ability to think words quickly
3.	Number	The ability to work with numbers and perform computations
4.	Space	The ability to visualize space from relationships, e.g. recognizing the same figure presentation in different orientation
5.	Memory	The ability to recall verbal stimulus such as parts of words or sentences
6.	Perceptual speed	The ability to grasp visual details and to see similarities and differences between picture objects
7.	Reasoning	The ability to find a general rule on the basis of presented instances

Group Factor Theory

Thurstone LL, an American psychologist, while working on a trust of primary mental abilities, came to the conclusion that certain mental operations have a primary factor in common, which gives them psychological and functional unity and differentiates them from other mental operations. These mental operations constitute a group factor. So, there are a number of groups of mental abilities each of which has its own primary factor (Table 8.4). Thurstone and his associates have differentiated nine such factors.

Table 8.4: Primary factors of mental abilities

Sl No	*Factors*	*Description*
1.	Verbal factor (V)	Concerns comprehension of verbal relations, words and ideas
2.	Spatial factor (S)	Involved in any task in which the subject manipulates an object imaginatively in space
3.	Numerical factor (N)	Ability to do numerical calculations, rapidly and accurately
4.	Word fluency factor (W)	Involved whenever the subject is asked to think of the isolated words at rapid rate
5.	Inductive reasoning factor (RI)	Ability to draw inferences and conclusions on the basis of specific instances
6.	Memory factor (M)	Involving the ability to memorize quickly
7.	Deductive reasoning (DR)	Ability to make use of general results
8.	Perceptual factor (P)	Ability to perceive objects accurately
9.	Problem-solving ability factor (PS)	Ability to solve problems with independent efforts

The weakest link in the group factor theory was that it discarded the concept of common factor. It did not take Thurstone very long to realize his mistake and to reveal a general factor in addition to group factors.

MENTALLY HANDICAPPED PERSON

Mentally handicapped person is one whose mental ability develops at a very slower rate than normal children of his/her age. He/she does not achieve the full intellectual functions of normal adult. He/she finds difficulty in learning social adjustment and economic productivity. He/she will have physical and anatomical peculiarities and will be physically inferior.

General Characteristics

1. They have difficulty in learning useful information and skills. They are poor in adaptation to new problems and conditions of life and profitless from experience. Abstract and creative thinking is nil. Critical judgment is absolutely poor. Reading, writing and arithmetic are so poor that are excluded from normal school. They forget soon unless reinforced by reviewing.

2. They are incapable of self-care, self-support or self-management in society. Need a lot of assistance during childhood. They must be fed, dressed, taken care against accidents and need supervision, while playing. They are incapable of personal and social affairs even during adulthood. If not guided and controlled, they may engage in delinquent acts. In short they are incapable of adjusting to social environment by themselves.
3. It is difficult to draw and hold their attention, interests are few, memory span is limited and thinking is strenuous and hence avoids it.
4. The development of drives and emotions vary greatly with the degree of feeble-mindedness. Laughing and giggling for no reason is common.
5. No two feeble-minded are exactly alike in personality, but individual differences are less compared to normal. They are rarely dynamic, charming, forceful, etc. They are submissive and easily subjected to influence, usually stable and apathetic.
6. They are very poor in physical resistance to illness and hence mortality is more.
7. They learn to walk and talk very much later than normal children. Their speech is defective, i.e. speech is pedantic and they walk with shuffling gait. Their visual and auditory defects are common at all levels. They are seemingly deaf, poor eye contact, unusual body language. These are some of the characteristic features of mentally handicapped.

Causes of Mental Retardation

There are more than 200 known causes and many more unknown causes. Some of the causes operate before birth, some during birth and some other after birth.

Prenatal Risk Factors

1. If the mother's age is under 15 years or over 40 years at the time of pregnancy, there is an increased risk of chromosomal abnormalities or prematurity.
2. History of difficult previous pregnancy like miscarriage, still-birth, premature birth, etc.
3. Mother with chronic health diseases like diabetes mellitus, syphilis and hypertension.

4. Parents with family history of congenital abnormalities like phenylketonuria (PKU), muscular dystrophy, etc.
5. Parental risk of biological origin, i.e. infections contacted during first 3 months of pregnancy—rubella, toxoplasmosis, cytomegalovirus (CMV), etc.
6. Subjecting pregnant lady (within 3 months) to frequent X-ray treatment.
7. Excessive drugging.
8. Taking certain drugs like carbon monoxide, antitetanus serum, typhoid vaccine, etc. affect brain growth and development and cause mental deficiency.

Perinatal Hazards (During Birth)

1. Injury to head at the time of birth.
2. Anomies (no respiration immediately after birth).
3. Deficiency of thiamine and glutamic acid.
4. Ineffective fevers like encephalitis or meningitis and brain tumor.
5. Prematurity and low birth weight (intrauterine growth retardation) may cause congenital malformation and biological dysfunction.
6. Low blood pressure.
7. Premature separation of placenta.
8. Compression of cord.
9. Postmaturity glycemia and polycythemia.
10. Preeclampsia (toxemia of pregnancy).
11. Rhesus (Rh) incompatibility along with kernicterus.

Postnatal Conditions

1. Meningitis.
2. Chronic lung diseases.
3. Meconium aspiration.
4. Persistent pulmonary hypertension.
5. Drugs.
6. Poisoning.
7. Poor nutrition or malnutrition.
8. Trauma during first 2 years of life.
9. Parent child separation.
10. Very poor environment, which is not stimulating during babyhood and childhood.

11. Encephalitis, etc. affect the growth of intelligence and cause mental deficiency.

Classification of Mental Retardation

Borderline mental retardation: Their IQ is 68 to 83. These are slow learners and cannot understand complex ideas. Verbal training is slower than motor learning. They can make adequate adjustment to society and sometimes they require help of others.

Moderate mental retardation: Their IQ is between 36 and 51, which is equal to 4- to 7-year-old boys. They read and write a little, but very slow in learning. They look clumsy and suffer body deformities and motor coordination. With parental help and training, can take care of themselves and economically useful.

Severe mental retardation: These will have an IQ of 20 to 35, their motor and speech developments are severely retarded. Sensory defects and motor handicaps are common. They can develop limited personal hygiene and self-help skills. They can perform simple occupational tasks under supervision.

Profound mental retardation: These will have an IQ of a child of 2 years. They are absolutely deficient in adoptive behavior. Speech is very rudimentary. They will have severe physical deformities, retarded growth, convulsive seizures, mutism, deafness, etc. They largely depend on others. Resistances to disease are very low and are short lived.

Clinical Types of Mental Retardation

Cretinism is a condition of mental deficiency and lack of physical and mental development caused by thyroid deficiency during prenatal and postnatal growth period.

Down syndrome (mongolism): The term Down syndrome given to certain type of amentia who have Mongolian features like eyes are narrow, slant and upward, and poor muscular coordination. Mongoloids are particularly susceptible to circulatory, respiratory and gastrointestinal disorders.

Hydrocephalus: It is a rare condition in which the accumulation of an abnormal amount of cerebrospinal fluid within cranium causes damage to the brain tissues and enlargement of the cranium. So, the skull looks very large. The head is either already enlarged at birth or begins to enlarge soon afterwards. This may be due to prenatal disturbances in the formation, absorption or circulation of the cerebrospinal fluid. The clinical picture depends on the extent of neutral damage. This in turn, depends on the age at which the onset, and duration and severity of the disorder. The degree of intellectual development varies depending upon the amount of pressure exerted on the brain tissue and damage caused to it.

Macrocephalus (sclerotic amentia): It is a condition of enlarged head due to excessive development of glial cells or cells, which support the active nerve cells. Here both skull and the face are grossly enlarged. On the basis of the shape of the head and skull, this can be differentiated from hydrocephalus. The main symptoms are pronounced mental defect, convulsions and fatty tumors of the face. Intelligence is below the level of imbecile. The mental age ranges between 3 and 7 years.

Microcephalus: The term microcephaly means small headedness. The head is usually small and cone shaped and they are called pin-headed people. The circumference is usually less than 17 inches, as against normal 22 inches. The chin and forehead recede, hair is coarse, thick and wiry. The brain is small in size and less in weight. The convolutions are less and simpler than the normal. They are below average in stature and have a relatively short span of life. Microcephalics are uninhibited in their emotional expressions. They are restless and hence, quick in movement and repetition is much.

Phenylketonuria: This is a rare metabolic disorder. They constitute 1 percent of the mentally retarded population. The baby appears normal at birth, but lacks an enzyme needed to breakdown phenylalanine, which is an amino acid found in protein foods. If this condition is not detected, the phenylalanine accumulates in the blood and damages the brain. This appears between 6 and 12 months after birth with symptoms of vomiting, a peculiar odor, infantile eczema and seizures. The extent of retardation depends upon the degree of the disease progressed.

Congenital syphilis: Children born to syphilitic mothers are sometimes infected with disease through placental circulation, while still in uterus. Many of these are terminated in abortion or stillbirth.

Of those born alive many have normal mental development, but others are mentally retarded. These children will have generally physical handicaps, paralysis of the limbs, epilepsy, blindness and deaf-mutism. Some children, who are infected show normal mental growth until puberty and then deteriorate, are diagnosed to have juvenile paresis.

Amaurotic family idiocy: This is also known as Tay-Sachs disease, which is very rare. This essentially a neurological disorder characterized by diffused degeneration of brain cells leads to progressive blindness, wasting the limbs and mental enfeeblement. The mode of transmission is through mating of persons who are free of overt symptoms or carriers of the defective genes. This is more with the offspring of pedigrees of consanguineous mating.

Traumatic amentia: Brain injuries account for 5% to 10% of mental retardation. The cerebral damage may be inflicted before, during or after birth. Many cases are due to intracranial lesions and hemorrhages occurring during birth. In the later cases, there is always a history of difficult labor, with or without instrumental delivery. Severe head injuries occurring before or after birth sometimes result in mental deficiency. The degree of mental deficiency present in traumatic amentia ranges from idiocy to high-grade morality.

Pseudodementia: The ability is present, but not used. He/she is an extreme introvert. External response is inadequate because the patient is preoccupied with subjective problems. The mental ability is present, but is undeveloped because of inability to see or hear.

Treatment, Rehabilitation and Prevention

Mental retardation is not an illness and hence the question of treatment and cure does not arise when it sets in. It is a lifelong condition. No amount of training or medical care will transform a mentally retarded child into normal child. However, certain condition contributory to mental retardation can be improved or cured. For example, deafness, poor vision, emotional disturbances, poor living condition, deficiency of nutrition, glandular imbalance, etc. make child appears retarded. Early detection can help to lessen the degree of handicap. It is mainly a problem of education and rehabilitation. The treatment for mentally retarded individuals lies in the stimulation and education from the earliest possible moment to develop their limited potentialities to the maximum possible extent. Mental ability grows when nourished by love and care.

Parent education: The parents of the mentally retarded must be educated to accept the child's limitation and the permanency of mental retardation. Generally parents refuse to admit that something is wrong with their child. Even when they realize that the child is subnormal, they believe that special education and good medical attention can make them normal and hence spends a lot of money, but will be disappointed. So it is essential to provide intensive parental counseling to enable family to provide love and security to the retarded child.

Home training: Home is the natural place for the beginning of training. Almost all mentally retarded remain at home during infancy and even during adulthood. Here, mother's emotional attitude is of major importance. Some mothers reject and ignore their mentally retarded child and some are overprotective, even at the cost of normal children. In spite of the fact that a mentally retarded child is slow in learning and has poor memory, following things to be considered.

1. The mother should make every effort to teach the child to feed and dress himself/herself, talk, walk and acquire habits of personal cleanliness.
2. As he/she grows up, should be given responsibilities and duties to his/her mental abilities.
3. Special attention must be given for moral and personality training.
4. Misdeeds and temper outbursts should be checked and pleasant disposition must be encouraged.
5. The sibling and other children in the family should be encouraged to accept the sibling as less intelligent, but an equal member of the family.
6. Opportunity to play with other children in the neighborhood should be permitted, but care must be taken to see that other children do not ridicule or exploit the defective child.

School training: Idiots and imbeciles cannot be sent to school because they cannot be educated. Only morons can be sent to school at the age of eight and not earlier because of slow growth of mental ability. It is better to put them with other feeble-minded of the same age to special classes. This has many advantages as follows:

1. He/she need not have to compete with bright children and avoid ridicule and humiliation for failure.
2. In special classes, the competition will be with equals and hence can experience some measure of achievement and success.
3. The curriculum of the special classes can be fitted to the capacity of the defective children.
4. The class can go slow with more emphasis on developing motor coordination, speech and desirable social traits.
5. The teacher can devote more time and attention to each pupil, which is very essential.

Institutionalization: Generally these are overcrowded. Children sent to these schools are of two groups. One group is chiefly of idiots and imbeciles, who are generally handicapped. The parents are unwilling or unable to care for them at home. The second group consists of morons. These children (older), due to undesirable or delinquent behavior, necessitate segregation from society. A large number of these are discharged after a period of social and occupational training, but the former group remains in the institution till their death.

Vocational training and rehabilitation: Higher grade defectives can be taught a variety of occupations, which will make them work in sheltered workshops or in open employment and can become self-supporting. Imbeciles can be trained for simple farming, laundry, dairy and kitchen work. Morons can be trained to assist carpenters, bakers, tailors, shoe makers, electricians, etc. They can also be trained to do complex farm work, poultry and livestock, operate various kinds of machines, etc. Thus they can be made self-supporting.

Family care: This is more economical and desirable way of segregating the mentally retarded, by putting them under families in rural homes. This is better than keeping them in institution.

Legal facilities, insurance and trust schemes: These facilities for the retards must be provided to make them economically independent.

Child guidance clinics: Clinics to help diagnose the handicap and assess the children must be set up, so that necessary action can be taken to improve their lots.

Home nursing and parent counseling program: These must be established to help the parents care for their children and to manage day-to-day problems.

Trained personnel: Like teachers, psychologists, occupational therapists, specialists concerned in the medical fields and social worker must be provided to cater to their special needs.

Specialized diagnostic facilities and special wards: These must be provided for them in all major hospitals and specialty in children's hospitals.

Government: It should recognize their functional rights.

Prevention of Mental Retardation

Sterilization: All the imbeciles and morons on social ground is desirable and especially to girls. Defective boys rarely marry or produce children because they cannot compete with normal boys for female attraction.

Institutionalization: If not sterilized, promiscuous defective girls must be institutionalized for the entire period of reproductive years. However, sterilization as a social measure is found to be useful.

Routine health measures: For the pregnant mother, precautions against possibility of intrauterine or birth damages and use of various diagnostic measures to detect and correct abnormalities early, can help to prevent such births.

After detecting the defect early: If normal stimulating environment is provided, many kinds of mental retardation, which were once thought to be hereditary and inevitable, can be prevented to a great extent.

Genetic counseling: It is realized now that chromosomal anomalies lead to faculty development. Tests are developed to identify parents who have these anomalies and to provide them genetic counseling, which will help in prevention of such births.

Alleviation of social culture: Another way of prevention is alleviation of sociocultural conditions, which deprive children the necessary stimulation, motivation and opportunity for normal learning and mental development.

Applications of Intelligence in Nursing

1. Hospitalized children who are in the sensorimotor stage have not achieved object permanence and therefore, suffer from separation anxiety. They are best off, if their mothers are allowed to stay with them overnight.
2. Children at the preoperational stage, who are unable to deal with concepts and abstractions, benefit more from role playing for medical procedures and situations than by having them verbally described in detail, e.g. a child who has to receive intravenous (IV) therapy is helped by acting out the procedure with a toy IV set and dolls.
3. As the children could not understand the cause and effect, they may interpret physical illness as punishment for bad thoughts or deeds.
4. Adolescents thinking may appear abstract. Nurse can explain the procedure to an individual on the basis of his/her intellectual ability. She knows to what extent she can explain. Otherwise she educates the parents/relatives about necessary details of the patient. During any nursing procedure, the nurse must always understand the particular age and his/her cognitive ability.

Nurse's Role in Intelligence

1. Knowledge about the nature of intelligence and its measurement is useful to the nurse in understanding herself, her colleagues as well as her patients.
2. Nurse's explanations or guidance to the patient would be according to the patient's intellectual level.
3. As a student and later as a teacher, the knowledge of intellectual function is useful for a nurse. Teaching method, content of the subject matter and expectations from students should be based on student's intellectual functioning.
4. Knowledge regarding intelligence helps the nurse in diagnosing a patient with mental subnormality or with very superior intelligence.
5. In diseases related to neuropsychiatry disorders, epilepsy, psychiatric disorders and some of the endocrinal disorders, assessment of intelligence is of great assistance in their management.
6. Knowledge about abnormalities in newborns and development of their intelligence helps the nurse in providing suitable care.

7. Aging patients, though physically slow, retain their levels of intelligence. Respect and encouragement with the right mix of nursing care has to be ensured.

Every individual is unique, especially when intelligence is the judging factor. A nurse in the course of discharging her duties has to heavily rely on verbal and non-verbal communication patterns. He/she may have to interact with the patient, his/her family members, explain and clarify procedures and medications. The intelligence level of the patient and family members decides how effectively the nurse is able to communicate and discharge her duties. Lower the levels of intelligence, more the time and patience the nurse will have to invest in caring for the patient. The instructions may have to be simple and repeated more often. However, where the patient is more intelligent he/she can be expected to take an active part in his/her own health care in the future.

CONCLUSION

The term intelligence is a very popular term used widely to mean many things—quick understanding, fast learning, accuracy in learning, clever talking, quick doing, good memory, etc. Intelligence is generally mistaken for intellect. The concept of intelligence is defined by psychologists in different ways. There is little agreement regarding the suitability of the definition of intelligence. The most general definition stresses versatility or flexibility of adjustment. Alfred Binet, the pioneer in this field, defines intelligence as something, which sensory acuity tests or reaction time experiments measure. As child grows older, his/her intelligence also grows correspondingly. Under normal conditions, both chronological age and mental age increases proportionately up to 13th year. According to the studies, the growth of intelligence in the early childhood is rapid. It begins to slow down around the age of 12 or 13. The yearly increment becomes smaller and smaller until the growth ceases.

SUGGESTED READING

1. Sreevani R. Psychology for Nurses, 1st edition. New Delhi: Jaypee Brothers Medical Publishers (P) Ltd; 2009. pp. 88-100.
2. Jocob A. Psychology for Graduate Nurses, 4th edition. New Delhi: Jaypee Brothers Medical Publishers (P) Ltd; 2007. pp. 168-88.

3. Mangal SK. General Psychology. New Delhi: Sterling Publishers Pvt Ltd; 2006.
4. Thompson RF. Introduction to Psychology. New Delhi: Harper and Row; 1975.
5. Clifford T Morgan. An Introduction to Psychology. New Delhi: Tata McGraw-Hill Publishing Co Ltd; 1978.
6. Gross R. Psychology: The Science of Mind and Behavior, 4th edition. London: Hodder and Stoughton; 2001.
7. Clement I. Psychosocial Foundation of Nursing, 1st edition. New Delhi: Jaypee Brother Medical Publishers (P) Ltd; 2010.

REVIEW QUESTIONS

1. Define intelligence. Explain the nature and types of intelligence.
2. Enumerate the various factors influencing intelligence.
3. Discuss the various types of intelligence test.
4. Explain the various theories of intelligence.
5. Define mental retardation. Explain the causes and classifications of mental retardation.
6. Describe the various methods of treatment, rehabilitation and preventive measures of mental retardation.

CHAPTER 9

Learning

LEARNING OBJECTIVES

1. Definitions.
2. Conditions of learning.
3. Laws of learning.
4. Learning during health and sickness.

INTRODUCTION

An individual begins to learn soon after his/her birth and goes on learning throughout lifetime. An infant is quite helpless at birth, suit slowly to learn to adapt himself/herself to the environment around him. There are usually two factors involved in his/her learning this adjustment to the environment; they are maturation and the ability to profit by experience.

Learning occupies an important position in the life of an individual. Most of one's behavior shows evidence of some type of learning or the other. It is learning that makes an adequate adjustment of life situations possible. Learning implies cumulative improvement. The nature of improvement can be clearly gauged by the changes, which take place, while learning is progress.

MEANING OF LEARNING

1. Learning is a change in behavior; it is a change that takes place through practice or experience.
2. Learning is not a reflex action, it means that winking or withdrawal of leg when knee is struck is not learning.

3. Learning may be for conscious purpose or it may be for biological and social adjustments.
4. Through learning, in a person, permanent or temporary changes are produced.
5. It can be for adjustment or maladjustment. It can create a socially adjusted individual or it may give rise to antisocial behavior.
6. Learning is a self-active process, which takes place in a social setup or environment.
7. Learning is a process that is purposeful and goal-directed. It also consists in establishing the right stimulus-response connections.
8. Learning is universal and continuous; it is a continuous never-ending process that goes from womb to tomb.
9. Learning prepares an individual for the necessary adjustments and adaptation.

DEFINITIONS

1. The more or less permanent modification of an individual's activity in a given situation, due to the practice in attempts to achieve some goal or solve some problem. —*Bernhardt*
2. Learning is a change in the individual following upon changes in his environment. —*Peel*
3. Learning is the process by which behavior is originated or changes through practice or training. —*Kingsley and Garry*
4. The term learning covers every modification in behavior to meet environmental requirements. —*Gardner Murphy*
5. Learning is the process by which an activity originates or is changed through reacting to an encountered situation, provided that the characteristics of the changes in activity cannot be explained on the basis of native responses, tendencies, maturation or temporary states of organism. —*Hilgard*
6. Learning defined as an expected and permanent change in the behavior, brought about as a result of practice. —*Hilgard and Atkinson*
7. Learning is acquiring new activities or enhancing or improving the old activities. —*Underwood*
8. Comparatively, learning is the serial or gradual change of the behavior. This is a special process, which takes place as a result of observation or training. —*ML Mann*

DETERMINANTS OF LEARNING

1. *Kind of material:* It is observed that certain type of material is more easily mastered than some other type. The meaningful material is more easily learned than the matters that lacks meaning. Verbal learning takes place at an ideational level. When one tries to understand the concept of specific gravity, he/she learns with the help of ideas.
2. *Method of learning:* There are certain methods of learning, which are found to be effective than certain others. These methods are related to the way he/she breaks up the learning material and the time spent in learning.
3. *Practice:* Repetition in terms of trials is necessary for all learning activities. All learning is based upon some amount of practice.
4. *Motivation:* Effective learning is directly related to the strength of the motives. Educationists try to utilize different motives to make the pupils learn better. Out of all the external goals with which motives can be connected, the inner goals like interest and curiosity are bound to be strong motivating forces.
5. *Intelligence:* Learning cannot take place effectively without intelligence. Intelligence enables to understand things, to see relationship between things, to reason and judge correctly and critically.
6. *Maturation:* Learning and maturation contribute to the development of the person. Those two actually are so interlinked that any line of separation is hardly visible. Maturation is growth, which takes place regularly in an individual without special condition of stimulation, such as training and practice.
7. *The learner:* Besides these situational factors, the learner himself is the most vital factor in deciding the efficiency of learning. The learner's intelligence, age and experience make considerable difference in learning effectiveness.

STEPS IN LEARNING PROCESS

1. Motivation within the learner.
2. Goal or goals become related to the motivation.
3. Barriers or difficulties are perceived and experienced, which may lead to tension. Strong barriers may cause excessive

tension, which may altogether discourage and confuse the learner.

4. The search for an appropriate solution to the problem or an appropriate line of action to reach the goal.
5. The most appropriate line of action is selected and practiced and inappropriate behaviors dropped.

LAWS OF EFFECTIVE LEARNING (THORNDIKE)

The laws of effective learning were put forward by Edward L Thorndike.

Major Laws of Learning

Law of Readiness

1. Learning takes place best when a person is ready to learn. If a person is ready to act, acting gives him/her satisfaction.
2. Some sort of preparatory attitude or the mindset is necessary. The learned should be stimulated to learn new things in such a way that he/she obtains satisfaction out of learning.

Law of Exercise, Use and Disuse or Practice

1. Learning takes place through, exercise and repetition. We learn skills in games, music, craft, typing or in nursing by constant exercise and practice.
2. An activity, which is not used, practiced or exercised for sometime tends to be forgotten by disuse.
3. The learner should be provided with opportunities of practicing and repetition. But repetition should be continual rather than continuous.
4. Most of the nursing skills and procedures are learned through practice on the wards and in the public health field.

Law of Effect or Satisfaction and Dissatisfaction

1. We learn things and do things that give us satisfaction and we learn not to do things, which annoy us.
2. The connections between stimuli and response become strong when we derive satisfaction from those responses, but remain weak or unformed when we are annoyed.

3. Activities, which are accompanied by a feeling of pleasure or satisfaction, are more readily and effectively learnt than activities, which are unpleasant or annoying.

Minor Laws

1. The law of maturation.
2. The law of purpose.
3. The law of selection.
4. The law of association.
5. The law of recency.
6. The law of multiple learning.

TYPES OF LEARNING

Verbal Learning

1. Learning of this type helps in the acquisition of verbal behavior.
2. The language we speak, the communication devices we use, etc. are the result of such learning.
3. Rote learning and rote memorization, which is a type of school learning is also included in verbal learning.
4. Sign, pictures, symbols, words, figures, sounds and voices, etc. are employed by the individual as an essential instrument for engaging him/her in the process of verbal learning.

Motor Learning

1. The learning of all types of motor skills may be included in such type of learning.
2. Learning how to swim, riding a horse, driving a car, flying a plane, playing piano and handling various instruments are the examples of such learning.
3. The art of these skills can be acquired through a systematic and planned way of the acquisition and fixation of a series of organized actions or responses by making use of some appropriate learning methods and devices.

Concept Learning

1. A concept in the form of a mental image denotes a generalized idea about the things, persons or events.

2. The formation of such concepts on accounts of previous experiences, training or cognitive process is called concept learning.
3. Such type of concept learning proves very useful in recognizing, naming and identifying the things. All of our behaviors, verbal, symbolic, motor as well as cognitive is influenced by our concepts.

Problem-solving Learning

1. In the ladder of learning and acquisition of behavior, problem-solving denotes a higher type of learning.
2. Problem-solving learning requires the use of the cognitive abilities like reasoning, power of observation, discrimination, generalization, imagination, ability to infer and draw conclusions, trying out novel ways and experimenting, etc.
3. Problem-solving learning has essentially caused human being to contribute significantly to the process and improvement of society.

Serial Learning

1. Serial learning consists of such learning, in which the learner is presented with such type of learning material that exhibits some sequential or serial order.
2. Children often encounter such a learning situation in schools where they are expected to master lists of material such as the alphabet, multiplication tables, the names of all the states in their country, etc.

Paired-associate Learning

1. In this learning, learning tasks are presented in such a way that they may be learned on account of their associations.
2. The name of a village like Krishnapur is remembered on its association with the name of Lord Krishna or a girl's name Ganga by learning it in the form of making paired association with the river Ganga.
3. The practice with such procedure then helps in building what is known as associate learning.

GOALS OF LEARNING

1. The goals in learning can be classified into two broad categories: the acquisition of knowledge and the acquisition of skill.
2. The acquisition of knowledge means the bringing up of intellectual and emotional modification and control in the individual through learning.
3. The acquisition of skill refers to the sensory motor modification and control through learning.

Acquisition of Knowledge

Perception

1. Perception refers to the acquisition of specific knowledge about objects or events, directly stimulating the sense at any particular moment.
2. A young child sees a woman; in the past, the woman had fed him/her. On the basis of that experience, he/she comprehends that the woman is his/her nurse or mother. The type of learning at perceptual level is known as perceptual learning.

Conception

1. Conception means the acquisition of organized knowledge in the form of concepts or general ideas, which transcend any particular percept.
2. The child gets the perception of orange, apple, banana, etc. and is able to locate certain general qualities in them.

Associate Learning

1. Associate learning corresponds to memory both as the deliberate recall and recognition, past experience and a habit or automatic memory due to association.
2. Associate learning is fundamental to all other learning.

Appreciation

1. Appreciation is the acquisition of ideas, attitudes or dispositions characterized by an emotional tone.

2. In our knowledge this factor is present as the effective or feeling element. When we talk about an ideal, we are talking about a concept, which is colored by appreciation.

Acquisition of Skills

1. Under skill are included the sensory motor process: writing, reading, musical performance, language acquisition in its vocal aspect, drawing and the arts generally.
2. True learning is enrichment of experience; it is because of this view of learning process that today we find an emphasis on activity programs, learning by doing the project method, self-activity, etc. rather than on book learning.

THEORIES OF LEARNING

Classical Conditioning

Classical conditioning gets its name from the fact that it is the kind of learning situation that existed in the early 'classical' experiments of Ivan P Pavlov (1849–1936). In the late 1890s, this famous Russian physiologist began to establish many of the basic principles of this form of conditioning. Classical conditioning is also called respondent conditioning or Pavlovian conditioning.

Concept

1. The dog salivated not only upon actual eating but also they saw the food, noticed the man.
2. In every animal and person, there are a number of innate stimulus-response association-connections wired in at birth, before any learning occurs.
3. Classical conditioning is constructed upon these inborn neurological connections.
4. Through learning, a previously neutral stimulus can come to acquire some of the same properties as unconditional stimuli. In this case, the previously neutral stimulus is called conditioned stimuli (CS) and the response it produces is called a conditioned response (CR).
5. Pavlov described the process by which associations are acquired and become the source for more general behavior or

more complex ones, as well as the ways in which the learned responses could be unlearned or extinguished. These processes include acquisition, higher-order conditioning and extinction.

Principles

Acquisition: It is the process by which a stimulus comes to elicit a condition response. To see how this occurs, Pavlov performed an experiment to see whether he could produce salivation to previously neutral stimuli.

Extinction: This process related with the gradual disappearance of the CR on disconnecting the stimulus-response (SR) association is called extinction.

Stimulus generalization: It is referring to a particular state of learning behavior in which an individual, once condition to response to a specific stimulus, is made to respond in the same manner in response to other stimuli of similar nature.

Stimulus discrimination: It is the opposite of stimulus generation. Here in sharp contrast to response in a usual fashion, the subject learns to react differently in different situations.

Association: Repetition of the CS, followed by the unconditioned stimulus (UCS) and consequent response must occur without exception.

Reinforcement: It is not only the association of two stimuli and a response that is essential but also what works in conditioning is the effect of reinforcement. Food in this case, which has a reinforcing effect strengths and bond between the condition stimulus and the unconditioned response (UCR) changing it ultimately in the form of a CR.

Pavlov's Experimentation

1. Pavlov began to study this phenomenon, which he called 'conditioning'. Since the type of conditioning emphasizes was a classical one, quite different from the conditioning emphasized by other psychologist at the later stage. It has been renamed as classical conditioning.
2. Pavlov kept a dog hungry for a few days and then tied him on to the experimental table, which was made comfortable and distractions were excluded as far as it was possible to do.

3. The observer kept himself hidden from view of the dog, but was able to view the experiment by means of a set of mirrors. Arrangement was made to give food to the dog through automatic devices.
4. Every time the food was presented to the dog and the bell was rung, there was automatic secretion of saliva from the mouth of the dog. The activity of presenting the food accompanied with a ringing of the bell was repeated, several times and the amount of saliva secreted was measured.
5. After several trials, the dog was given no food, but the bell was rung. In this case also the amount of saliva secreted was recorded and measured. It was found that even in the absence of food (the natural stimulus) the ringing of the bell (an artificial stimulus), caused the dog to secrete saliva (natural response).
6. The above experiment thus, brings into the picture the four essential elements of conditioning process. They are natural stimulus or UCS, UCR, CS and CR.
7. The theory of conditioning as advocated by Pavlov, thus considered learning as a habit formation and is based on the principle of association and substitution.

John Watson Theory of Conditioning

1. Watson (1878–1958), the father of behaviorism, supported Pavlov's ideas on CR. Watson tried to demonstrate the role of conditioning in producing as well as eliminating the emotional response such as fear.
2. When a child receives his/her first injection at the doctor's dispensary, he/she cries when the needle is pricked. On receiving some more injections from the same doctor and at the same dispensary on following days, the child would start crying on seeing the doctor and later, even on passing by the dispensary along the road.
3. Most of our attitudes toward persons and situations, early language responses, numerous components of complex skills and a number of emotional responses can be common examples of CR.

Operant Conditioning

Definition

Operant conditioning refers to a kind of process whereby a response is made more probable or more frequent by reinforcement.

1. Operant conditioning also known as instrumental conditioning, an action of the learner's instrumental in bringing about a change in the environment that makes the action more or likely to occur again in the future.
2. An environmental event that is the consequence of an instrumental response and that makes the response more likely to occur again is known as reinforce.
3. A positive reinforce is a stimulus or event, which when it is contingent on a response, increases the likelihood that the response will be made again.
4. A negative reinforcement is a stimulus of event, which when its cessation or termination is contingent on a response, increases the likelihood that the response will occur again.
5. In instrumental or operant conditioning, the term shaping refers to the process of learning a complex response by first learning a number of simple responses leading up to the complex one.
6. Each step is learned by the application of contingent positive reinforcement and each step builds on the one before it until the complex response occurs and is reinforced.
7. In instrumental or operant conditioning the procedure of not reinforcing a response is called extinction. If after learning, reinforcement is no longer contingent on a response, the response will become less likely to occur.
8. In instrumental or operant conditioning, reinforcement following every occurrence of a particular response is called continuous reinforcement.
9. But reinforcement in operant conditioning is often given according to certain schedules, not every occurrence of the response is reinforced. Fixed-ratio (FR), fixed-intervals (FI), variable-ratio (VR) and variable-interval (VI) schedules are described to illustrate the concept of reinforcement schedules.

Skinner's Operant Experimentation

1. In operant conditioning experiments conducted by BF Skinner, a specially devised box called the Skinner box was used.
2. There was an iron bar inside the box. In order to get food, the rat had to press the iron bar. For every such pressing a food pills was dropped through a chute into the pallet.
3. Here, the rat after a few trials learns to press the bar and then run to the pallet to secure food.

4. Unless the animal presses the bar, it cannot get the reinforcement and habit cannot be learnt. But the basic factors involved in both these forms of learning are identical.

Differences between classical and operant conditioning are shown in Table 9.1.

Table 9.1: Differences between classical and operant conditioning

Sl No	*Classical conditioning*	*Operant conditioning*
1.	It helps in the learning of respondent behavior	It helps in the learning of operant behavior
2.	It is called type-S conditioning because of the emphasis on the stimulus	It is called type-R conditioning because of the emphasis on the response
3.	In this, beginning is being made with help of specific stimuli that bring certain response	Here, beginning is made with the responses as they occur naturally or unnaturally, shaping them into existence
4.	Strength of conditioning is usually determined by the magnitude of the condition response	Here, strength of conditioning is shown by the response rate

Schedules of Reinforcement

Continuous reinforcement schedule: It is 100 percent reinforcement schedule where provision is made to reinforcement or rewards every correct response of the organism during acquisition of learning.

Fixed interval schedule: In this schedule, the reinforcement is given after a fixed number of responses.

Variable reinforcement schedule: When reinforcement is given at varying intervals of time or after a varying number of responses, it is called a variable reinforcement schedule.

Implication of Operant Conditioning

1. The principle of operant conditioning may be successfully applied in the task of behavior modification.
2. The task of the development of human personality can be successfully manipulated through operant conditioning. According to Skinner, "we are what we have been rewarded for being."

3. The theory of operant conditioning does not attribute motivation to internal process within organism.
4. Operant conditioning lays stress on the importance of schedules in the process of reinforcement of the behavior.
5. The theory advocated the avoidance of punishment for unlearning the undesirable behavior and for shaping the desirable behavior.
6. In its most effective application, theory of operant conditioning has contributed a lot toward the development of teaching machines and programmed learning.

Laws of Learning by Thorndike

Law of frequency: When an activity is repeated a number of times; it requires a tendency to be permanently established. Any response that is repeated either some strength in its favor.

Law of recency: In a series of activities, those at the close of the series would be more freshly retained in the repertoire of the animal so that when put to a similar situation it shows a tendency to respect them.

Law of effect: This is perhaps the most important among all the laws. It says that the response that gives the organism the satisfaction of success is the one that is most likely to be fixed. On the other hand, when the response does not lead to such a satisfaction is tends to be discarded.

TRIAL AND ERROR LEARNING

The theory of trial and error learning propagated by Thorndike emphasizes that we learn through a trial and error mechanism. In trying for a correct behavior, one tries hard in so many ways and may commit so many errors before a chance success. On subsequent trials he/she may learn to avoid erroneous ways, repeat the correct ones and finally learn the proper way.

Concept of Trial and Error

1. When we are placed in a new situation or face a new problem we have to seek solution, which we are not able to perceive in the beginning.

2. This made of learning is slow, wasteful and unintelligent. It requires more time and greater energy than higher types of learning.
3. Learning implies establishment of new connections between the stimulus and response. These new connections are gradually established blind process of trial and error.
4. In this kind of learning, which is very common in animals, there is assumed to be at first nothing, but random, aimless reaction, but in which there emerges after a time a chance correct response that finally is stamped into the neuromuscular system of the animal.
5. There are random movements in the beginning, gradually the number of random movements is reduced along with error and finally the goal is reached. Thus, improvement takes place through repetition.
6. The principles involved in the process as to how the learner stabilizes the new response pattern, gives the clue to the understanding of learning by trial and error.

Thorndike's Trial and Error Experiment

1. In the typical experiments of Thorndike, he made use of a puzzle box that could be opened by some mechanical contrivance, e.g. pressing a button on its floor.
2. When a hungry cat was placed inside this puzzle box and food like fish was placed outside the box within the sight of the animal, the cat would struggle hard to come out of the box.
3. In this process, it went through a series as random activities that could not bring about the solution for the problem.
4. It may try to squeeze itself out of the bars, bite them, scratch the floor with the claws or run about. In the course of the new response pattern, cat's paw may accidentally fall on the button and the door is opened for it.
5. Out of all the series of responses given by the cat a single one proves to be the correct response, e.g. keeping the paw on the button and pressing it.
6. Immediately following this response the cat comes out and can take food that has a reinforcing effect. Its success during the first trial may be due to sheer chance.
7. But when the animal is put to the same situation next time there is a definite reduction of the random responses and the successful solution of the problem requires less time than before.

8. This way with practice the errors or wrongs responds are gradually eliminated and the correct response is strengthened.
9. When a person learns to swim or to ride on a bicycle, the initial pattern of behavior displays a large number of random responses. With practice, all the wrong movements are gradually eliminated.

Stages of Trial and Error Learning

Drive: In the present experiment it was hunger, which was intensified with the sight of the food.

Goal: To get the food by getting out of the box.

Block: The cat was confined in the box with a closed door.

Random movements: The cat, persistently, tried to get out of the box.

Chance success: As a result of this striving and random movement, the cat, by chance, succeeded in opening the door.

Selection: Gradually the cat recognized the correct manipulation of the latch. It selected the proper way of manipulating the latch out of its random movements.

Fixation: At least, the cat learned the proper way of opening the door by eliminating all the incorrect responses and fixing only the right responses. Now, it was able to open the door without any error or in other words, learned the way of opening the door.

Background of the Theorist

1. Edward L Thorndike, a famous psychologist (1874–1949), is known as the propagator of the theory of trial and error learning.
2. Thorndike has written; learning is connecting. The mind is man's connection system.
3. Thorndike named the learning of his experimental cat as trial and error learning. He maintained that the learning is nothing, but the stamping in of the correct responses and stamping out of the incorrect responses through trial and error.

Implication of Trial and Error Learning

1. Whatever we want to learn or teach, we must first try to identify the things that are to be remembered or forgotten.

2. What is being taught or learnt at one time should be linked with past experiences and learning on the one hand and with the future learning on the other for utilizing the benefits of the mechanism of association, connection or bonds in the process of learning.
3. The learner should try to see similarities and dissimilarities between the different kinds of responses to stimuli and with the help of comparison and contrast should try to apply the learning of something in one situation to other similar situations.
4. The learner should be encouraged to do his task independently. He must try various solutions of the problem before arriving at a correct one.

LEARNING BY INSIGHT

The gestalt psychologist has offered an altogether different explanation of the learning process. They do not believe that learning is a process of blind habit formation. The learning process studied by Thorndike or the behaviorists occurs, according to Kohler, in a very unnatural and restricted situation, where the animal is denied all possibility of a clear perception of the whole situation.

Definition

Insight may be defined as sudden awareness of the relationships among various elements that had previously appeared to be independent of one another.

Background of the Theorist

1. Insight learning introduced by a group of German psychologist called gestalts. Wolfgang Kohler, in particular, originated a learning theory known as insight learning.
2. The nearest English translation of gestalt is configuration or more simply an organized whole in contrast to a collection of parts. Gestalt psychologists consider the process of learning as a gestalt, an organized whole.
3. In practical sense, gestalt psychology is primarily concerned with the nature of perception.
4. Gestalt psychologists tried to interpret learning as a purposive, exploratory and creative enterprise instead of trial and error or simple stimulus-response mechanism.

Concept of Insight Learning

1. It involves mental exploration and understanding of what is being learned. It implies some insight, some awareness of the consequences of performing an act.
2. The learner perceives the reactions, which the problem involves or the significant characteristics of the situation and connects the right response with the solution by using intelligence.
3. The uses learner past learning and the ability to generalize from one situation to another.
4. The principles involved in any learning process depend upon the nature of the learning situation.
5. Kohler, in his experiments on learning, offered different types of situation and eventually arrived at totally different conclusions regarding the principles involved in the learning process.
6. Insight involves a perceptual reorganization of elements in the environment such that new relationships among objects and events are suddenly seen.
7. It is goal directed and oriented toward the solution of a problem. When the organism is put to a problematic situation, it starts to tackle it. Such tackling involves the perception of the problem.

Kohler's Insight Learning Experimentation

1. Some of the well-known experiments of Kohler performed on chimpanzees had the following plan. The hungry chimpanzee was kept in a cage and a bunch of bananas was hung from the ceiling.
2. A number of wooden boxes were lying about. The chimpanzee tries to jump high to reach the bananas. When it was impossible to reach the highest it tries to jump from a ceiling.
3. When this also was found to be failure, the chimpanzee gave up the efforts for some time. All of a sudden it got some new idea and started putting one box upon the other.
4. Finally by getting up on the topmost, it could successfully grab the bananas.
5. In the situation described above, there was no evidence of a blind trial and error procedure where the corrected responses occurred gradually.

TRANSFER OF LEARNING

Learning one skill sometimes influences the acquisition of other skills. This influence may be positive that can facilitate the new learning. It can also be negative when it interferes with the acquisition of new learning. In the first case we have positive transfer of training, often referred to as merely 'transfer of training' or transfer of learning. In the second case we have what is commonly called habit interference.

Definition

According to Sorenson, transfer refers to the transfer of knowledge, training and habits acquired in one situation to another situation.

Meaning of Transfer of Learning

1. Transfer of training or learning influences to carry over the learning from one task to another. The learning or skill acquired in one task is transferred or carried over to other tasks.
2. Transfer of training is the carry-over of habits of thinking, feeling or working of knowledge of skills from one learning area to another usually is referred to as the transfer of training.
3. One of the simplest examples of positive transfer is to be found in experiments showing improvement in performance with the left hand as a result of practice with the right hand. This is called bilateral transfer or cross education.

Characteristics of Transfer of Learning

1. *Transfer to a similar activity:* Learning one activity sometimes easier the learning of another activity.
2. *Transfer in verbal learning:* Transfer is also evident for several verbal skills. When comparable lists of nonsense syllabus are learned one after the other, there is a gradual reduction in the trials required to learn successive list.

Types of Transfer

Positive transfer: Transfer is said to be positive when something previously learned, benefits performance or learning in a new situation.

Negative transfer: When something previously learned hinders performance or learning in a new situation, we call negative transfer.

Zero transfer: In case the previous learning makes no difference at all to the performance or learning in a new situation, there is said to be zero transfer.

Principles of Transfer

Similarity of Contents

A person familiar with several card games will learn the rules of new card game readily. This is possible as the rules are like those he already knows. Learning to drive one model of car, a person soon master the control of another, since many of the activities involved in driving cars are identical.

Similarity of Techniques

When subjects were given practice to toss a ball in air and then catch it in a cup with their right hand, there was bilateral transfer when they performed the same task with their left hand.

Similarity of Principles

Transfer of principles is not always different from transfer of techniques because the use of techniques may involve the application of principles.

Formal Discipline

Transfer was once sought to be explained on the basis of the doctrine of formal discipline of mental faculties. The mind was supported to be a bundle of independent faculties of reasoning, memory imagination, etc. Transfer of training was thus supposed to be automatically achieved through the exercise of mental faculty.

Bagley's Transfer of Training

1. The transfer of training or learning can also be explained on the basis of the theory of ideals put forward by WC Bagley.
2. According to this theory, transfer of learning or training takes place in the form of ideals.

3. The experience we have, the generalization or conclusions we arrive at, all do transfer, if they are imbibed as ideals of some value or desirable by the individual.
4. Bagley (1922) developed the ideals of neatness on the basis of stress laid on doing things quite neatly in school, is likely to transfer in performing all other activities in a quite neat and clean way.
5. If we wish to seek positive transfer from one situation to another, we must strive for the formation of general attitude for an ideal.

NURSE'S ROLE IN LEARNING

1. Learning is fundamental to the development and modification of behavior, thus knowledge of the learning process may be usefully applied to many clinical situations and academic work.
2. Many of our subjective feelings, emotions and attitudes are probably conditioned responses. Through generalization it becomes difficult to identify the origin of our emotional responses. Both our adaptive emotional responses as well as unadaptive responses are learned and can be unlearned through principle of learning.
3. Learning methods have wide applications in educational setting. In programmed learning the material to be learned is broken up into small easy steps, so that the learner can accomplish without frustrations. Also with programmed learning, learner can master the task at his own pace; with versatile and flexible learning, the learner can improve learning style.
4. Applications of reinforcement principles can often increase productivity both in studies as well as in vocation.
5. A nurse should understand the nature of learning and the factors, which will affect learning. As learning modifies our behavior, it is necessary for a nurse to learn only the right things so that modification takes place in the right direction.
6. She must have a well-defined purpose and goal in all learning situations.

CONCLUSION

Learning is universal and continuous. Every creature that lives learns. In human being it is not limited to any age, sex, race or culture. It is a continuous never-ending process that goes from womb to tomb.

Learning process requires the learner to pay attention, observe, memorize, understand, set goals and assume responsibilities, which can be realized when they are build on their natural desire to explore. Motivated learners have a passion for achieve so that they take a great deal of efforts in their learning besides being determinant and persistent.

Extrinsic motivation viz. rewards increase the frequency of desired behavior among the learners, while intrinsic motivation promotes active participation without any expectation. Intrinsically motivated learners believe that efforts are importance for success.

SUGGESTED READING

1. Anthikad Jocob. Psychology for Graduates Nurses, 4th edition. New Delhi: Jaypee Brothers Medical Publishers (P) Ltd; 2007.
2. Bhatia BD, Craig Margaretta. Elements of Psychology and Mental Hygiene for Nurses in India. Chennai: Orient Longman; 2005.
3. Clement I. Psychosocial Foundation of Nursing, 1st edition. New Delhi: Jaypee Brothers Medical Publishers (P) Ltd; 2010.
4. Hilgard RE, Atkinson CR. Introduction to Psychology, 6th edition. New Delhi: Oxford and IBH Publishing Co Pvt Ltd; 1975.
5. Khan MA. Psychology for Nurses. New Delhi: Academia Publications; 2004.
6. Mangal SK. General Psychology. New Delhi: Sterling Publishers Pvt Ltd; 2006.
7. Morgan T Cifford, Kind A Richard. Introduction to Psychology, 7th edition. New Delhi: Tata Mc Graw-Hill Publishing Company Limited; 2004.
8. Thompson RF. Introduction to Psychology. New Delhi: Haper and Row; 1975.
9. Zwener J Ann. Basic Psychology for Nurses in India. Chennai: BI Publications Pvt Ltd; 2003.

REVIEW QUESTIONS

1. Define learning. Explain the meaning and determinants of learning.
2. Explain the laws of effective learning.
3. Discuss the types and goals of learning.
4. Describe the theories of learning in detail.
5. Define trial and error learning.
6. Discuss the learning by insight.
7. Enumerate transfer of learning. Explain the characteristics of transfer learning.
8. Explain the roles and responsibilities of a nurse in learning.

CHAPTER 10 Memory and Forgetting

LEARNING OBJECTIVES

1. Definitions.
2. Nature of memory.
3. Memory during health and sickness.
4. Forgetting during health and sickness.

INTRODUCTION

The problem of retention is an important problem for a student of learning. He/she is curious to know as to how much amount of learning is retained by him/her. He/she also wants to know why he/she forgets, at times, certain common things. Remembering and forgetting are the opposite sides of the same coin. What can be directly measured is only the amount that is retained. But this has a reference to the amount that is forgotten. Our concept of memory is somehow associated with verbal memory. No doubt, we have to memorize a majority of verbal facts; but in actual life situation, all forms of memory need not involve verbalization. Thus, we remember someone's looks, we remember places and we remember the taste of a particular food, which requires no verbalization, moreover, our concept of memory indicates that it is a single function. Memory denotes the ability or a power of mind to retain and reproduce learning. This ability helps in the process of memorizing. Memory consists of remembering what has previously been learned. Thus, the process begins with learning and ends with its retrieval and reproduction.

MEANING OF MEMORY

Memory is a general word, which includes several mental activities like recall, recognition. We see indications of memory all around us. A person or animal experiences ease in relearning any activity, which he/she had learnt previously, but had forgotten. This proves very obviously that the previous learning had not been wiped out completely, but had left an impression on the mind or a change in the nerves, which facilitated relearning. People do not completely forget the story of any motive they have seen, but recount it with ease when they are requested to do so by a friend.

Memory can be called structural mental process in which the person brings the learned material to the conscious mind and then tries to recall it. To remember or memorize, it is essential to first learn the subject and then retain it. The meaning of memory in Latin and Greek words is to be mindful or to remember. Effective memory is not a function of how much time is spend on the material to be remembered, but is directly influenced by the kind of strategy and method of organization imposed on the material to be remembered.

DEFINITIONS

1. Memory means showing the signs of earlier learned activities in present activities. —*Hilgard and Atkinson*
2. Memory is the capacity of a person to represent the information in response to the collection of previously learned activities and specific stimuli. —*HJ Eysenck*
3. Memory is defined as the power where we have to store our experiences and bring them into the field of unconscious sometimes after the experiences have occurred. —*Ryburn*
4. Memory is the ideal revival, so far as ideal revival is merely reproductive. This productive aspect of ideal revival requires the object of past experiences to be reinstated as far as possible in the order and manner of their original occurrence. —*Stout*
5. Memory consists of remembering what has previously been learned. —*Woodworth and Marquis*

QUALITIES OF GOOD MEMORY

1. Good retention power of the person.
2. Representing the facts quickly.

3. Quick and clear recognition.
4. Learning the subject matter quickly and immediately.
5. Using the facts and thoughts at suitable time.

COMPONENTS OF MEMORY

Memory operates through four important components, which are registration, retention, recall and recognition.

Registration

Registration is the short-term storage of the sensory input. Most of the information briefly held in the sensory register is lost. However, we pay special attention to some of the information in the sensory register. When we do this the attended information is passed on to the short-term storehouse. The sensory register holds information for such a brief time that some psychologist prefers, to discuss it as related to perception rather than memory.

Retention

Retention refers to a performance of what was learnt. When the active process of learning ceases, comparatively passive process of retaining takes place. The material is retained when we are not thinking about it. People differ in their retentive capacity, which is largely due to genetic constitution.

Recall

Recall is the third aspect of memory. Things are learned in order to recall them whenever need arises. Recall is affected by a number of conditions as interference, set, attitude, etc. Failure to recall does not necessarily indicate the absence of retention. Without retention there is no recall; but there can be retention without recall.

Recognition

Recognition is closely related to recall. It is the act of affirming that a particular object or situation has been seen or experienced before. During the process of recalling, our cognitive effort is more obvious and hence we may think that recall is an active process, whereas recognition is a passive state. But, in fact recognition is also an active phenomenon.

FACTORS OF MEMORY

We feel that a certain person has good memory, whereas some other person has a bad memory. Experiments in memory show that although there is a general factor of memory, the actual functioning of memorizing is seen through specific operation that differ from person to person. People may differ in their visual memory, auditory memory or olfactory memory. The following factors are influencing on memory.

Learning

Learning will be quite good in keeping with the context to give a brief description of each of these activities. As it has been mentioned above, the first step or activity is learning. If learning is good, memory will also be good. Thus the methods that assist learning do the same for memory. Learning creates memory traces on the mind on the basis of which recollection is affected.

Retention

Retention means making permanent the remains of experience. The remains of experiences are left on the mind in the form of memory traces, where they are safe though they are acted upon the interest and other mental states. The proofs of retention are recollection, recognition and relearning.

Observation

Correct observation gives us correct and accurate information. Observation keeps us alert and informed of latest events happening, which helps in remembering.

Attention

Attention here denotes concentrating our mind on the purpose, which helps in collecting information. Therefore, if we pay attention it will help in retaining.

Sense Perception

Sense perception is the process by means of which we become aware of our environment. Sense perception is necessary for accurate observation of object, event, thing, person, etc.

FAVORABLE CONDITIONS OF COMPONENTS

In Retention

Duration: A sensation, which continues for a longer time can be retained in mind for a longer period. A sensation of a shorter duration will be, respondingly, retained for a shorter duration.

Amount of material: If the subject being pursued is long it will be retained for a longer time, while a shorter subject will take less time before it is forgotten. The amount of material to be learnt has favorable effect on its retention.

Nature of material: Intensity, distinctness, meaning help in its retention to a large extent.

Amount of learning: The extent of retention is directly proportional to the amount of learning that is to say that retention will be more, if the amount of learning is large. A subject studied more stays longer in the mind, while studied less will remain in the mind for a shorter period. Over learning has a favorable effect on the retention.

Methods of learning: Learning by the whole method instead of the part method, the spaced method and the active method instead of the passive method result in better and longer retention.

Speed of learning: The faster the learning, the better the retention. This is the principle in accordance with which people learning faster seem to retain the subject learned for longer periods as compared to the slow learners.

Feeling: Freud and other psychologist assert that we retain pleasant experiences for a longer time, whereas we forget painful experiences quickly.

Attention: While studying a subject, if greater attention is paid to the subject the retention will be better. On the contrary, retention will be weakened by inattention.

Sleep: Sometimes elapses after study, before the subject is retained in the mind and if this time of strengthening and retention is used for sleep, the memory traces get a good opportunity to be attached upon the memory.

Mental review: If some experiences are incessantly contemplated upon its retention, then it is better than the one about which the mind does not trouble itself. Really speaking by mental review, a repetition of the subject is caused, which strengthen retention.

Mental set: A person retains those things for a longer period, which coincide with mental inclinations. A religious person remembers ideas relating to religion for longtime and a sensuous man remembers things of sexual interest.

Apperception: Apperception means the assimilating of learned subjects with the knowledge already present. The retention of a newly learned subject is greatly facilitated if it is assimilated with the present store of knowledge to start with. And on the other time is needed for retention if this assimilation is not affected.

Intention: If the subject is learned with the express intention of being retained, the aim will be fulfilled with extraordinary success. But, if there is not such retention, the subject removes itself from the memory of the person after sometimes. Learning gathered with a view to appearing in the examinations is remembered better and things picked up here and there, in the ordinary course, are easily forgotten unless the person has a special inclination toward them.

Massive experience: The retention will be more if the experience is massive. If a person has ever loved, he/she never forgets it, because it affects his/her whole personality and it is a fact that we remember that thing longer, which affects us more.

In Recall

Suitable mental and physical conditions: Recall is comparatively easy when both the mind and the body are healthy and fresh. And, adverse and indifferent physical and mental conditions hinder recollection.

Perfection of clues: Recall is done with the help of clues, which are stimulators of recall. For example, if we learn a poem, we cannot recall it without the help of the title, the first line or the clue to some part of it and clues are necessary for the recall of anything in mind.

Mental set: The mental set of the individual, too, affect recall. A religious-minded person remembers religious subjects easily, while sensuous person will find it easy to remember things associated with sex.

Motives: When a person is under the extreme influence of a motive, he/she has such clear recollection of related incidents that, sometimes had hallucinated.

Feelings: Recollection is not immune to feelings of pleasure and pain. These feelings and experiences of pain and pleasure are recollected easily than indifferent feelings, while pleasurable experiences are comparatively easily recollected.

Effort: This has a very significant effect on recollection. Unless the extreme limit of effect has been passed, recollection generally increases with the effort.

Absence of inhibition: Recollection is better in the absence of any inhibition, because inhibition obstructs recollection and it may be caused by the conflict of the simultaneous arising of two activities or by repression and again by fear or other emotions.

In Recognition

Mental set: Recognition is helped by the mental set, in the manner in which other factors assists memory. Recognition is correct when the mental set is favorable and it is incorrect when the mental set is unfavorable.

Confidence: This, too, is an indispensable element in recognition. In its absence, even correct recognition becomes infested with doubt and mistake is the outcome.

TYPES OF MEMORY

Short-term memory is the immediate memory, which refers to storage of learning for a few seconds. LTM differs from it in that the information is stored for a long duration. The limited storage capacity of STM is seen from the fact that our memory span for a single repetition is not more than seven items long. Whenever it appears that one has a longer span, it is, because of recording the material in convenient chunks. Most of us learn to break the material and organize it in groups. Thus, even though the material retained is longer, the units retained are fewer. The six or seven digit telephone numbers have a reference to span of immediate memory. The main differences between STM and LTM is given in Table 10.1.

Table 10.1: Differences between short- and long-term memories

Sl No	*Short-term memory*	*Long-term memory*
1.	Short-term memory is carried by active neural process	Long-term memory on the other hand is carried by permanent structural changes in nervous system
2.	Short-term memory traces decay spontaneously	Long-term memory traces show resistance to such spontaneous decay
3.	The short-term memory storage capacity is limited. It is easily subjected to interference	A single exposure to stimuli is not seen to produce long-term retention in human verbal learning. Many trials are usually for longer term retention

Immediate Memory

Immediate memory or sensory memory is that memory, which helps an individual to recall something a split second after having perceived it. Immediate memory is needed when we want to remember a thing for a shorter time and then forget it. We enter the cinema hall; see the seat number given on our ticket. After occupying the seat, we forget the seat number. We lookup a telephone number from the directory and remember it. But after making the call, we usually forget it. In such type of memory, retentive time is extremely brief, generally from a fraction of a second to several seconds.

Short-term Memory

Short-term memory can hold items fairly well for the first few seconds. After 12 seconds however, recall is poor and after 20 seconds, the information has disappeared entirely unless we have kept repeating the material to ourselves. A phone numbers that we lookup and dial is often forgotten by the time the call is answered. STM is also called working memory.

Long-term Memory

Long-term memory is relatively permanent in which information is stored for us at a longer time. Material enters a storehouse of almost unlimited capacity. LTM seems to be much more complex, for it stores many different aspects of one's experiences. Remembering our identification data like our name, father's name, date of birth, date of marriage, etc. is the simplest example of our LTM.

Permanent Memory

Under permanent memory, it is possible to remember a thing permanently. Remembering of our name is the simplest example of our permanent memory. It may or may not involve understanding and insight.

Rote Memory

Under rote memory, the things are learnt without understanding their meaning. Some students have a good rote memory. They can mug up material and reproduce it at the time of examination. Although rote memory can serve the purpose well when it is needed to remember a thing for the time being, for a specific purpose, yet is unreliable and fails to bring an enduring and lasting remembrance.

Logical Memory

Logical memory is based on logical thinking. It takes into consideration the purposeful and insightful learning. Here instead of mechanical memorization, the learner tries to understand what he/she learns and why he/she learns.

Associated Memory

The individual having this type of memory is able to associate the previously learned things with so many related things and then establish multiple connections. It demands that the learning or memorization of a particular thing should not be in isolation. We must try to connect or associate it with as many other things as we can. It will help our memory to maintain multiple relationships. We can be able to have a memory of so many things at a time by adopting the principle of association of ideas and images and make maximum use of our memory.

Active Memory

In active memory, one has to remain active or make deliberate attempts for recollecting past experiences. In answering the question in examination hall we are required to make use of this type of memory.

Passive Memory

In passive memory, the past experiences are recalled spontaneously without any serious attempt or will. For example, when somebody comes from our native village the mere sight of him/her is enough to remain us about our fields, neighbors and so many other things.

MEASUREMENTS OF SHORT- AND LONG-TERM RETENTION

Short-term Retention

The subject is presented a stimulus in the form of non-sense syllable by a three digit number. He is given some task like counting the number in reverse or something similar to prevent further rehearsal on his part. He is then asked to reproduce the stimulus when a signal is given. Thus, recall was elicited after every 3 seconds. The recall was seen to drop down considerably till it was almost non-existent after 18 seconds. This effect of reduction becomes more permanent after first few trials. This shows that previous activity interferes with retention. It is known as proactive interference.

Long-term Memory

There are several ways in which long-term retention is measured.

Recall

The method of recall is used in studying retention of verbal material, e.g. a poem or paragraph from a book. The subject then has to reproduce what he/she has learnt without any clues. It is either estimated in terms of the amount that was initially assimilated or in terms of saving of learning in a relearning situation. This former type of examinations with essay type questions utilizes recall method for measuring retention.

Recognition

Another method of measuring retention is recognition. Recall and recognition are measured as two independent entities. We may fail to recall the face of the person we met at a certain social function. But, if we happen to see him/her, we may easily recognize him/her.

Between recognition and recall, the former is considered to be a more reliable criterion of retention. In most of the memory experiments, retention is measured by recognition rather than recall. After presenting a list of non-sense syllables, they are intermingled with new and unfamiliar non-sense syllables. The subject has to recognize from among this bigger list, those that were presented to them. Similar experiments are conducted by using photographs of persons or sceneries instead of non-sense syllables. The modern trend of examination with objective questions in place of the essay type questions is mainly based upon the belief that recognition is a better indication of memory than recall. In the essay type questions, where the pupil has to be recalled, it may happen that one with adequate retention may fail to recall due to a number of emotional and situational factors. If he/she is asked to recognize, as is done by the objective questions, there are less chances of the above mentioned factors affecting the expression of the level of retention. Actually, so far as the experience in life is concerned, we are more often required to recognize than recall.

Saving

The saving method is frequently used in psychological experiments. The subject is made to learn a certain task. The trials required to master the task are noted. He/she is again made to relearn the task after a lapse of sometime interval. The measure of retention is the difference in number of trails required in the original learning and relearning situations. Such a method is sensitive and reliable. The saving method can show the retention long after other methods have caused to show any degree of it.

THEORIES OF MEMORY

The theories and its description of memory are given in Table 10.2.

Table 10.2: Theories of memory

Sl No	*Theory*	*Description*
1.	Fading of the memory	The theory regards the memory trace as resembling the marks of a pencil on a piece of paper or a path worn into a plot of grass. It can be kept functioning through use as a pencil mark can be emphasized by tracing and retracing and a pathway can be kept clear by continuing to walk over it. But without use, the memory trace may vanish, as a pencil mark fades with time and pathway becomes over grown when abandoned. Memory theorists continue to believe that memory trace has some physical quality that changes with passage of time, thus reducing, the likelihood that it can be retraced or reactivated.

Contd...

Contd...

Sl No	Theory	Description
		Indeed they think of it as having two qualities. The first is its strength—meaning how likely it is to pop into mind. In this quality, the strength of the memory trace is at its peak immediately after learning and declines with the passage of time. The second quality is resistance to extinction, meaning how well the trace can manage to survive and become immune to fade
2.	Failure in retrieval theory	This theory believes that memory trace, once it has been established as part of LTM, probably persists for as long as we live. But, information held in memory is of no use to us unless it remains not only stored, but available. To remember it, we must be able to find it and call upon it when needed, a process called retrieval. If we cannot call upon it, we say we have forgotten it. Thus, forgetting may not be a failure in memory, but rather a failure in retrieval. As one psychologist has put it: In this respect, memory is like a huge ware house in which all sorts of things are stored, but is less than perfectly organized. So, that it is not always easy to find a given item upon demand, there is evidence that forgetting may be a failure in retrieval
3.	Interference theory	This theory holds that our memory for what we learn today is often adversely affected by what we have learned in the past and also by what we will learn in the future. The various pieces of information complete for attention and survival and not all of them can prevail. When old information causes us to forget new information, this process is called proactive interference the phenomenon of proactive interference can be demonstrated very strikingly through simple laboratory procedures. Such as, asking subjects to try to learn and remember several lists of words. A steady decline in the ability to remember new material was caused by more and more proactive interference from prior learning. In proactive interference, old information gets in the way of remembering new information. The opposite situation—when new information causes us to forget old information is called retroactive interference
4.	Motivated forgetting	The fact that we seem to forget something deliberately has already been mentioned in connection with the processes that take place in STM. Motivated forgetting has been widely studied by psychoanalysis, who have found it often plays a part in certain forms of abnormal or neurotic behavior.

FORGETTING

The term forgetting seems to be a part of our day-to-day speech. Forgetting is a spontaneous or gradual process in which old memories are unable to recall from memory storage. In other words, it refers to inability to recall.

Definitions

1. Forgetting is the loss, permanent or temporary of the ability to recall or recognize learned earlier. —*Munn*
2. Forgetting means failure at any time to recall an experience, when attempting to do so or to perform an action previously learned. —*Drever*
3. Forgetting is the failure of the individual to revive in consciousness, an idea or group of ideas without the help of the original stimulus. —*Bhatia*

Curve of Forgetting

The studies made by the psychologist Ebbinghaus (1885) present the earliest systematic works in studying the phenomenon of forgetting. He/she memorized a list of non-sense syllables and then test himself/herself at intervals from 20 minutes to a month to see how much of the list he/she remembered. The results in terms of the percentage of material forgotten with the lapse of time found in the following order (Table 10.3).

He/she tried to plot the above data on a piece of graph paper. The curve obtained on the graph paper by plotting the amount forgotten as a function of time was named by him/her as curve of forgetting.

Ebbinghaus Conclusion

Ebbinghaus concluded the following:

1. Amount of learnt material forgotten depends upon the time lapsed after learning.
2. The rate of forgetting is very rapid at first and then gradually diminishes proportionately as the interval lengthens.

Table 10.3: Amount forgotten as time elapsed

Sl No	*Time elapsed*	*Amount forgotten*
1.	20 minute	47%
2.	1 day	66%
3.	2 day	72%
4.	6 day	75%
5.	31 day	79%

Causes of Forgetting

Interpolated Activity

As far as behaviorists are concerned, it is the interpolated activity after learning, which causes forgetting; the extent of forgetting depends upon the divergence of these activities from the material learnt.

Disuse

The theory of disuse postulate says that any learnt activity or accumulated knowledge will gradually be forgotten, if it is not regularly practiced.

Retroactive Inhibition

Some learning tends to contradict some previous learning, a tendency entitled retroactive inhibition, meaning the fatal effect of interpolated activity on learning.

Repression

The psychologists believe that the major cause of forgetting is repression, i.e. the pushing of the experience or thoughts into the unconsciousness.

Deficiency of Thinking and Repetition

Mental thinking and repetition assist retention and recollection and in the same manner, these factors affect forgetting, i.e. in absence of these factors forgetting increases.

Deficiency of the Mental Set

Mental set is a factor assistance in the retention and recollection of a subject, so that its greater concurrences will reduce forgetting.

Brain Injury

Often when a person suffers a brain injury, he/she forgets many incidents and experiences, and the extent of the forgetting depends upon the seriousness of the injury.

Uses of Stimulants

Wine and other stimulants have a detrimental effect on the brain, because they weaken the memory traces. Thus, forgetting will be increased, if such intoxicants are used.

Altered Stimulus Condition

If there is an association between the stimulus and the situation of the stimulus, then forgetting is facilitated by any change in the situation or condition of the stimulus. People, who stay abroad for long, forget their correct dialect.

Zeigarnik Effect

According to Zeigarnik, completed tasks are forgotten more than the uncompleted task. Her theory is based on Lewin's field theory. According to this theory, when the individual undertakes a task, tension develops within him/her and it persists until the task is completed that motivates the learner. This enables the learner to remember the task. In case of completed task, the tension disappears and forgetting will be more.

Lack of Rest and Sleep

Continuous learning without rest and sleep may lead to greater forgetting due to inefficient consolidation. Experimental studies have shown that sleep following learning favors retention; it has been found that saving (retention) is definitely greater after sleep especially with 8 hours interval. Forgetting may slow during sleep.

Raise in Emotion

Emotions play an important role in learning and forgetting. Sudden raise of emotions blocks the recall. During the high emotional state, blood sugar level is impaired; to maintain the balance, adrenal gland produces cortisol that disturbs memory cells.

Types of Forgetting

Passive or Natural Forgetting

The kind of forgetting in which there is no intention of forgetting on the part of individual is called passive or natural forgetting. In this kind of forgetting, one has no need to make any deliberate efforts. In a quite normal way, with the lapse of time, the person gradually forgets so many things experienced and learned earlier.

Active or Morbid Forgetting

Active forgetting is also known as abnormal forgetting. In this forgetting, type of one deliberately tries to forget something. This kind of forgetfulness, as Freud explains, originates from expression. Under this process, the painful experience and bitter memories are deliberately pushed into the unconscious layer of the mind and are left there for forgetting.

It is seen that forgetting is a function of time as shown in the curve of retention. The other explanation of forgetting is also discussed, but the cause of forgetting frequently has an emotional background. We have already referred to the affective nature of memory. Overexcitement or nervousness is often seen to prevent recall. One facing a big audience for the first time may be well prepared with his speech, but also may not be able to utter a word on the stage.

Emotional blocking also results from repression. The defense mechanism or repression has already been discussed by us. It shows how the experiences that bring disgrace or a feeling of guilt to us are pushed to the unconscious. Facts that are in keeping with our attitudes or those that support our view better remembered than those of a contrary nature. Similarly, memories of happy events are seen to be more lasting than those of unhappy events.

When experiences are forgetting as a result of repression, not only that the said experience is forgotten, but any associated idea likely to call back the repressed experience to consciousness will also be clamped down. Sigmund Freud in his book psychopathology of everyday life has discussed the events of such forgetting at length. He has analyzed a number of memory lapsed of this kind showing, how recent events too can be easily forgotten due to emotional blocking.

One interesting thing to know about the process of forgetting is that it is not simply a passive progress involving gradual elimination of the facts retained. It is partly active too. While, the originally retained facts are eliminated, the gaps are filled up by entirely new details. So, whatever portion that is remembered goes through constant distortion. Our needs, interests, attitudes and prejudices play an active role in filling up the gaps of memory. Frederic C Bartlett has shown an interesting experiment on how to reproduce memory, though an outline is maintained, the details go through a number of changes. In his experiments, on memory to form, the subjects were shown some drawings and asked to reproduce them out of memory. A number of details were either seen to be changed or omitted in the reproductions.

It is this quality of memory that really facilitates the spreading of rumors. Since, rumors are circulated from person to person at every juncture, some of the details are omitted and some new filled in that is why there is a world of difference between the actual event and the rumor concerning it. The distortion is not intentional. It is the outcome of the nature of the memory process.

Theories of Forgetting

Trace Decay Theory

According to many psychologists, time is the cause of much forgetting, what is learnt or experienced is forgotten with the lapse of time. The cause of such natural forgetting can be explained through a process known as decay of the memory trace. It says that learning results in neurological changes, leaving certain types of memory traces or engrams in the brain. With the passage of time through disuse, these memory traces of learning impressions get weaker and weaker and finally fade away. It leads us to conclude that the older an experience, the weaker its memory and as time passes, the amount of forgetting goes on increasing.

This theory has proved a failure in many instances of forgetting. In LTM, such as learning to ride a bicycle, forgetting does not occur even after years of neglect. However, this theory has provided good results in explaining forgetfulness in the case of STM drill practice, rehearsal or repetition of learning always results in preventing decay.

Interference Theory

Mechanism of interference is responsible for forgetting. Interference is caused on account of the negative inhibiting effects of one learning experience on another. We forget things because of such interference. The interfering effects of things previously learnt and retained in our memory with the things of our recent memory can work both ways, backward and forward. The psychological term used for these types of interference is retroactive inhibition and proactive inhibition.

In retroactive inhibition, the acquisition of new learning works backward to impair the retention of the previously learned material. For example, a second list of words, formulations or equations may impair the retention of a first list.

Proactive inhibition is just the reverse of retroactive inhibition. Here, the old learning or experiences retained in our memory works forward to disrupt the memory of what we acquire or learn afterwards. For example, learning a new formula may be hampered on account of the previously learned formula in one's memory.

In both types of the above inhibitions, it can be easily seen that similar experiences when follow each other, produce more interference than dissimilar experiences. Because, in this case, all experiences are so intermingled that a state of utter confusion prevails in the mind of an individual and consequently he faces a difficulty in retention and recall.

Interference theory as a whole has been proved quite successful in providing adequate explanation for natural and normal forgetting for both the STM and LTM.

Repression Theory

The 'repression theory' is put forward by Freud's psychoanalytic school of psychology. Repression, according to this school, is a mental function that safeguards the mind from the impact of painful experiences. As a result of this function we actually push the unpleasant and painful memories into the unconscious and thus try to avoid at least consciously the conflicts that bother us. As a result of the repression we forget the things, which we do not want to remember.

People under a heavy emotional shock are seen to forget even their name, home, wife and children. Apart from causing abnormal forgetting, an impaired emotional behavior of an individual does also play its part in disrupting his/her normal memory process. For example, a sudden raise of emotions in excess may completely block the process of recall. When one is taken over by emotions like fear, anger or love, one may forget all he/she has experienced, learned or thought beforehand. During these emotions, one becomes so self-conscious that his/her thinking is paralyzed. That is why a child fails to recall the answer to a question in the presence of a teacher whom he/she fears very much.

ECONOMICAL METHODS OF MEMORIZATION OR REMEMBERING

The problem of having economy in memorizing something has persuaded many psychologists to devise various methods of memorization.

Recitation Method

In recitation method, the learner first reads the matter once or twice and then tries to recite and recall without looking at that material. In this way, the recitation method provides continuous self-appraisal. Learner evaluates himself from time to time and notes the points, which he/she has been unable to recall. To these points, due attention can be paid and thus he/she is saved of unnecessarily repeating the already memorized material. Moreover, the recitation method is more stimulating than the continued and avoids them by close attention.

Whole and Part Method

There are two methods of memorizing a thing, e.g. poem. One is to read the poem again and again from the beginning till the end as a whole. This is called whole method of memorization. The other method is part method, the poem is divided into parts and each part is memorized separately.

Spaced or Unspaced Method

In the spaced or distributed practice method of memorization, the subject is not required to memorize the assigned material in one continuous sitting. After memorizing for some time, some rest is provided and in this way, the principle of work and rest is followed in this method. For example, if one has to memorize a piece of poetry by this method, then in beginning he/she will be advised to go on repeating it. After sometime he/she will be given some rest, again he/she will memorize it and take rest. In this way with repeated intervals of work and rest, he/she will be able to have mastery over the assigned piece.

Active and Passive Methods

Memorizing by utterance is the active method, while mental repetition is the passive method. Many experiments have been carried out to measure the economy, which this method may affect.

Rote and Intelligent Methods

If a person is learning or memorizing something without understanding it, he/she is said to be using the rote or unintelligent method. There is no apperception in this. On the other hand, by the use of the intelligent method it involves the understanding of the subject and apperception does come about.

Grouping and Rhythm

Memorization is considerably facilitated by rhythm and grouping. It is easier to memorize poetry than prose, but by the rhythm scheme. One couplet contains enough meaning to be spread over several pages, but the rhythm makes their memorization easier.

Association

Association is a factor, which keeps memorization in no less importance than the other, suppose if we have to remember that the first step in the solution of arithmetical problems is the bracket and successive steps are of division, multiplication, subtraction and addition and in order to facilitate it.

IMPROVEMENT OF MEMORY OR MEMORY TRAINING

A person may at time worry that his/her capacity for memory is being deteriorated. He/she may be considered with the consideration, whether his/her ability to memorize can be improved. The answer to such question is that memory is not single faculty and moreover, it does not improve nor does it deteriorate. Psychology deals with process of memorizing and not with a composite faculty of memory. Experiments on the process of memorizing show that whatever assimilation is superior, retention is more durable and eventually recall or recognition is prompt. Since, assimilation is more closely connected with the process of learning, a thing better learned has more chances of being better memorized. Hence, to facilitate memory that entire one can happen to be in the field of learning. All devices that promote learning are seen to help memory. Nothing can be independently done in the field of memory alone, since memory is a counterpart of learning.

Factors

The factors bringing about more permanent learning are obviously contributory for superior memory.

Will to learn: There must be firm determination or strong will to learn for achieving desired success in learning. Where there is a will there is a way. Materials read, heard or seen without intention or mood are difficult to be remembered later.

Interest and attention: Interest as well as close attention is essential for effective learning and memorization. One who has no interest in what one learns, cannot give due attention to it and consequently, will not be able to learn it. Therefore, every care should be taken to create the desired interest in the material by making its purpose clear and link it with one's natural instincts and urges.

Adopting proper methods of memorization: There are so many economical methods of memorization, but all are not suitable on all occasions for all individuals. Therefore, a judicious selection should be made in choosing a particular method in a given situation.

To follow principle of association: It is always good to follow the principle of association in learning. A thing should never be learnt in a complete watertight compartment. Attempts should be made to connect it with one's previous learning on one hand and with so many related things on the other. Sometimes for association of ideas special techniques and devices are used, that facilitate learning and recall.

Grouping and rhythm: Grouping and rhythm also facilitate learning and help in remembering. Rhythms also prove as an aid in learning and memorizing. Children learn effectively the multiplication tables in the sing song fashion.

Utilizing as many senses as possible: Senses are said to be the gateway of knowledge and it has also been found that the things are better learned and remembered when presented through more than one senses. Therefore, attempts should be made to take the help of audio-visual aid material and receive impressions through, as many senses as possible.

Arranging better learning situation: Environmental factors also affect the learning process. Therefore, due care should be taken to arrange better learning situation and environment. A calm and quite atmosphere and stimulating environment proves an effective aid in learning.

Internal factors within the learner: Besides the external factors there are things within the learner, which affect his/her learning and reproduction. The physical and mental health and state of the mind at the time of learning, as well as reproduction counts a lot for memory.

Provision for change and proper rest: Adequate provision for change of work, rest and sleep should be made as it helps in removing fatigue and monotony. A fresh mind is necessarily able to learn more and retain it for a long time than a tired and dull one.

Repetition and practice: An intelligent repetition with full understanding, always help in making the learning effective and enduring. The things repeated and practiced frequently learning are effective and enduring and remembered for a long time. Therefore, due care should be taken for drill work, practice and review, etc. in the process of memorization and learning.

Pulling it all together: Organizing and ordering information can significantly improve memory. As learning a large amount of unconnected and unorganized information from various classes can be very challenging. By organizing and adding meaning to the material prior to learning it, you can facilitate both storage and retrieval.

Funnel approach: This means learning general concepts before moving on to specific details. When you understand the general concepts first, the details make more sense.

Vivid associations: When you are learning something new and unfamiliar, try pairing it with something you know very well. Such as images, funs, music, etc.

Active learning: Active learning facilitates your memory by helping you attend to the process information. All of the memory techniques require active learning.

Talk it out: Repeat ideas verbatim, repeat the ideas in your own words, repeating information aloud can help you encode the information and identify how well you have learned it.

Mnemonic: It is a memory aid and mostly serves as a learning purpose. It is a powerful technique that helps in remembering some specific things. One common mnemonic for remembering lists consists of an easily remembered word, phrase or rhyme whose first letter are associated with the list items. Mnemonic rely not only on repetition to remember facts, but also an associations between easy to remember constructs and lists of data, based on principle that the human mind much more easily remember data attached to spatial, personal or otherwise meaningful information that are occurring in meaningless sequences. The sequences must make sense.

AMNESIA

Amnesia is a condition in which memory is disturbed. The cause of amnesia is organic or functional. Organic causes include damage to the brain, through trauma or disease or use of certain drugs. Functional causes are psychological factors, such as defense mechanisms. Hysterical post-traumatic amnesia is an example of functional amnesia. Amnesia may also be spontaneous, in the case of transient global amnesia.

Types

The types of amnesia and its description are given in Table 10.4.

Table 10.4: Types of amnesia

Sl No	*Types*	*Description*
1.	Anterograde amnesia	New events are not transferred to long-term memory, so the sufferer will not be able to remember anything that occurs after the onset of this type of amnesia for more than few moments. The complement of this is retrograde amnesia, where someone will be unable to recall events that occurred before the onset of amnesia
2.	Dissociative amnesia	It is used to refer the inability to recall information, usually about stressful or traumatic events in person's lives. A common form of dissociative amnesia involves amnesia for person identity, but intact memory of general information
3.	Long-term alcoholism	It can cause a type of memory loss known as Korsakoff syndrome. This is caused by brain damage due to a vitamin B1 deficiency and will be progressive, if alcohol intake and nutrition pattern are not modified
4.	Lacunar amnesia	It is the loss of memory about one specific event
5.	Childhood amnesia	It is also known as infantile amnesia. It is the common inability to remember events from one's own childhood

Contd...

Contd...

Sl No	*Types*	*Description*
6.	Global amnesia	It is total memory loss. This may be a defense mechanism, which occurs after a traumatic event. This global type of amnesia is more common in middle-aged to elderly people, particularly males and usually lasts less than 24 hour. Post-traumatic stress disorder can also involve the spontaneous, vivid retrieval of unwanted traumatic memories
7.	Posthypnotic amnesia	It is where events during hypnosis are forgotten or where past memories are unable to be recalled
8.	Psychogenetic amnesia	It results from a psychological cause as opposed to direct damage to the brain caused by head injury, physical trauma or disease, which is known as organic amnesia
9.	Source amnesia	It is a memory disorder in which someone can recall certain information, but they do not know where or how they obtained it

CONCLUSION

In psychology, an organism's ability to store, retain and subsequently retrieve information is known as memory. The process of memory begins with learning or experiencing something and ends with its retrieval and reproduction. Therefore memory is said to involve four stages: Learning or experiencing something, its retention and finally its recognition and recall. Learning occupies a significant place in one's life. Whatever is learned, need to be stored in the mind, so that it can be utilized whenever required in the future. Memory denotes the ability or a power of mind to retain and produce learning. Thus, this process begins with learning and ends with its retrieval and reproduction. Forgetting has positive and negative values on life. It is a great blessing to mankind. Forgetting is the temporary or long-term loss in our ability to reproduce the thing that has been previously learned.

SUGGESTED READING

1. Bartlett FC. Remembering: A study in experimental and social psychology. New York: Cambridge University Press; 1932.

2. Bhatia HR. Elements of Educational Psychology, 3rd edition. Calcutta: Orient Longman; 1968.
3. Ebbinghaus H. On Memory. New York: Dover; 1964.
4. Ferguson ED. Motivation: An experimental approach. New York: Holt, Rinehart and Winston; 1976.
5. Hunter, Ian MR. Memory. London: Penguin Books; 1964.
6. Klatzky RL. Human Memory. San Francisco: Freeman; 1976.
7. Lindsay PH, Norman DA. Human Information Processing, 2nd edition. New York: Academic Press; 1977.
8. Morgan CT. A Brief Introduction to Psychology. New Delhi: Tata McGraw-Hill; 1975.
9. Morgan CT, King RA. Introduction to Psychology, 6th edition. New Delhi: Tata McGraw-Hill; 1982.
10. Morgan JB, Gilliland AR. An Introduction to Psychology. New York: Macmillan; 1942.
11. Munn Norman L. Introduction to Psychology. New Delhi: Oxford and IBH; 1973.
12. Robinson DN. An Intellectual History of Psychology. New York: Macmillan; 1976.
13. Townsend Mary. Psychiatric Nursing. Philadelphia: WB Saunders Company; 2005.
14. Wertheimer M. A Brief History of Psychology. New York: Holt, Rinehart and Winston; 1970.
15. Wickelgren WA. Learning and Memory. Englewood Cliffs, New Jersey: Prentice Hall; 1977.
16. Woodworth RS. Experimental Psychology. New York: Holt, Rinehart and Winston; 1954.

REVIEW QUESTIONS

1. Define memory. Enlist the qualities of good memory.
2. Discuss the components and factors influencing memory.
3. Describe the types of memory and explain the measurements of short- and long-term memories.
4. Explain the various theories of memory.
5. Define forgetting. Explain the causes of forgetting and types of forgetting.
6. Describe the theories of forgetting.
7. Discuss the economical methods of memorization or remembering.
8. Explain in detail about improvement of memory or memory training.
9. Define amnesia. Explain the types of amnesia.

CHAPTER 11

Attitudes

LEARNING OBJECTIVES

1. Definitions.
2. Development and modifications.
3. Role of attitudes in health and sickness.

INTRODUCTION

Attitudes are not innate or unlearned like our physiological motives or some emotional reactions. They are acquired by us. Some of them are built by us and by our effort. Others are absorbed by us passively and spontaneously from the social environment into which we are born and in which we grow. Many of our attitudes are the result of reflection and purposeful thinking or the outcomes of training and suggestion from others, especially our parents and teachers. Attitude is the evaluation of an object, person, behavior or event based on beliefs guiding behavior of an individual. Psychologists have defined an attitude in many diverse ways. Kimball Young defines an attitude as, "a predisposition to respond, in a persistent and characteristic manner," in references to some situation, idea, value, material objects or class of objects or person or group of persons. This can be positive, negative or neutral views of an attitude object, e.g. person's behavior or an event.

DEFINITIONS

1. An attitude denotes an adjustment of the individual toward some selected person, group or organization.

—*Kuppuswamy*

2. An attitude is the entire package of particular beliefs, feelings and response tendencies of the individual toward the appropriate object. —*Kerch and others*
3. Attitude is a mental structure of framework that includes motivational, perceptual, emotional and cognitive reactions. The positive or negative reaction of a person to his/her environment, other persons and objects are based on his/her attitude.
4. Attitude is a permanent disposition of a person toward an object, subject or thought that tends to react in accordance with interests.
5. Attitudes are the manifestation of a person's concepts, thoughts or imaginations, which directs his/her behavior toward a specific direction.

COMPONENTS OF ATTITUDES

Cognitive Component

Cognitive component is the opinion or belief segment of an attitude. It is made up of thoughts and beliefs people hold about the object of the attitude. It is therefore, what we have learned about something. It is what we believe to be true about it. For example, vegetarian food is healthy.

Affective Component

Affective component is the emotion or feeling segment of an attitude. The affective component is the matter of liking or disliking something. This consists of the emotional feelings stimulated by the object of the attitude. For example, I like vegetarian food.

Behavioral Component

Behavioral component is an intention to behave in a certain way toward someone or something. The action component of attitudes refers to a readiness to respond. Thus expressed attitudes usually have a consistent relationship to behavior. For example, I always eat vegetarian food.

NATURE OF ATTITUDES

Attitudes are universal; they are either positive or negative and are found toward social as well as non-social aspects of the environment. These attitudes are not innate, they are acquired. It implies subject-object relationship. Attitude of respect toward our elders is a positive attitude, whereas, an attitude of hatred toward a certain community is a negative attitude. It is a way we perceive, think and feel more or less permanently in relation to something. It is a sort of mental readiness or a tendency to react to certain situations in a more or less consistent manner. We have acquired certain set ways of reacting to religious rituals to political democracy, to social equality, to our parents and teachers, to various racial, communal and religious groups, to people exercising authority over us, to our colleagues who work with us, to our own profession and its prestige and to other professions.

1. Attitude is the evaluation expressed in terms such as liking or disliking, pro or anti, favoring or not favoring and positive negative. They are the feeling tone aroused by any attitude object.
2. Attitudes are thought to guide behavior, e.g. if a person shows unfavorable attitude toward smoking, he/she shows negative attitude toward smokers.
3. The expressions that one makes publicly to others are not always the same as the expressions one makes privately to one's self.
4. They are feeling tones aroused by any attitude object. Attitudes can be formed about many things. The object of attitudes can be entities (a lecture, a restaurant), people (parents, siblings, Prime Minister, myself) or abstract concepts (abortion, civil rights, foreign aid).
5. The attitude varies. The attitude may be similar toward some of the objects and different toward others.
6. Individuals are not fully aware of their attitudes; this accounts in part for possible inconsistency of attitudes with one another.
7. The attitude attempts to understand the motives they serve for the individual.
8. It provides a ready basis for interpreting the world and processing new information.
9. It is a way of gaining and maintaining social interaction.
10. Attitude is a hypothetical construct that represents an individual's likes or dislikes for an item.

11. Attitudes that are accompanied by strong feeling tones are called sentiments. These can be positive or negative. We may have sentiments of love for our country, a sentiment of respect for our elders or a sentiment of hatred for dishonesty and lying.

MOTIVATIONAL FUNCTIONS OF ATTITUDE

Katz (1960) has suggested four motivational functions of attitude; they are knowledge, social adjustment, value expression and ego defensive.

Knowledge function: People seek a degree of practicability, consistency and stability in their perception of the world.

Social adjustment function: It refers to the favorable responses the individual achieves from others by displaying socially acceptable attitudes.

Value expression function: The individual achieves self-expression with regard of cherished values in the value expressive function of attitudes.

Ego defensive function: The ego defensive function allows the individual to be protected from acknowledging personal deficiencies.

DEVELOPMENT OF ATTITUDES

Attitudes of a person are the permanent ways of one's behaving. These are the acquired characteristics of a person, which are reflected in his/her work and behavior. Many of our attitudes are the result of reflection and purposeful thinking or the outcome of training and suggestion from others, especially our parents and teachers. Children, whose parents show respect and courtesy to others, acquire attitudes of respect and courtesy to most human being without being specially told about it. They simply take suggestions from their parents unconsciously. Our motives, our emotional conditions, our schooling, our cultural norms, the type of parent-child relationships that obtains in childhood, the way we have been taught to perceive thing, propaganda—all these factors affect the growth of our attitudes.

Our attitudes are also influenced by the type and quantity of the factual knowledge that we acquire about situation, things and person. Many a time we may develop hostile attitudes toward a person because what we have been told about him/her does evoke hostility or aggression. Many of our attitudes are the result of wrong or false knowledge that is available to us. The best example is our prejudices and biases. We may have acquired this knowledge from newspaper, journals, books, the movie, or the political speeches. The cognitive components of attitude are assumed to be learned in the same ways as any facts, knowledge or beliefs. The basic processes of association, reinforcement and imitation determine this acquisition.

Association and Reinforcement

A child is exposed to certain things about the world. He/she is reinforced for expressing some cognitions or attitudes or for actual acting on the basis of them, thus he/she learns them.

Imitation/Identification

Imitation/identification is important in the learning process. A child spends a great deal of time with parents and after a while begins to believe as they do simply by copying them, even when they do not deliberately try to influence him/her.

Classical Conditioning

Classical conditioning involves involuntary response and is acquired through the pairing of two stimuli. When two events repeatedly occur close together in time, they will become fused in a person's mind; before long the person responds in the same way to both events. For example, pleasant and unpleasant experiences with members of a particular group could lead to positive or negative attitudes toward the group.

Social (Observational)

Learning is based on modeling. As we observe others; if they are getting reinforced for certain behaviors or expression of certain attitudes, we make it more likely that we too behave in the same manner or express the attitude.

Cognitive Dissonance

When two contradictory feelings, beliefs or behaviors exist, it creates a state of tension and the person tries to reduce tension by changing the feelings, beliefs or behaviors.

Unconscious Motivation

Some attitudes are held because they serve some unconscious function for an individual. For example, a person who is threatened by his/her homosexual feelings may employ the defense mechanism of reaction formation and become a crusader against homosexuals.

Rational Analysis

Rational analysis involves the careful weighing of evidence for and against a particular attitude. The nurse giving health education to slum people will influence their attitude for personal hygiene when informing about rationale of unhygienic conditions.

Other Factors

Even after a child develops attitude, he/she continues to be exposed primarily to information that supports it. At this stage, various socioeconomic factors determine what hears. His/her neighborhood, newspaper, school, church, friend's, etc. tend to be more homogeneous than the rest of the world.

CHANGE IN ATTITUDES

An individual's attitudes are formed during the childhood stages as a result of socialization and later on when he/she meets and interacts with the peer group in later childhood, adolescence and early childhood. For example, when an individual says a smoker is confronted with communication from the communicator that cigarette smoking causes lung cancer. Now, the stress is produced by the discrepancy between the individual's attitude and the attitude expressed in the communication. This stress has been called conflict, incongruity, imbalance or just inconsistency. Therefore, there is pressure on the individual to resolve the discrepancy. If the individual changes attitude in the direction advocated by the communication, the discrepancy is reduced. Hence the stress is resolved.

Types

The attitude change can be either congruent or incongruent.

Congruent Change

For example, already negative attitude will increase negativity or positive attitude will increase positivity, i.e. change in the same direction.

Incongruent Change

For example, the change in attitude from positive to negative or from negative to positive. In other words, the change will be in the same direction.

Factors

Once the attitudes and beliefs have been formed they have a tendency to persist or continue. It is therefore, difficult to change the attitudes that have been established. There are many reasons for our inability to change them easily. One of the reasons is that we do not want to change on account of the social support we have acquired for them.

In order to change attitudes and beliefs we should:

1. Change perceptions by new experiences and factual knowledge.
2. Control emotions and motivational factors in early childhood when most of our daily attitudes are formed.
3. Tab the various formative agencies.

CHARACTERISTICS OF ATTITUDES

1. Attitudes are related to the needs and problems of the person.
2. Unconscious mind plays an important role in the formation of attitudes.
3. A series of emotional experiences is attached to attitudes.
4. Attitudes direct the activities or actions of person.
5. The reaction of a person toward an object, issue or environment can be predicted by knowing his/her attitudes.
6. Attitudes are related to some thoughts, images and external objects.

EFFECTS OF ATTITUDE ON BEHAVIOR

Attitudes manifest the nature of person and they direct the behavior of person. Hence, favorable or positive attitudes (kindness, service and assistance) are the indicators of good behavior, while unfavorable or negative attitudes (hate, non-cooperation, selfishness, etc.) express the bad behavior of person. It is easy to provide nursing to the patients having favorable attitude toward hospital, while the behavior of patients with negative attitudes toward hospital and may create obstacles in their nursing treatment. Similarly, nurses and doctors should adapt a professional attitude toward the patients.

THEORIES OF ATTITUDE CHANGE

Balance Theory

1. Balance theory given by Heider (1946, 1958), emphasized the positive and negative valences of attitudes toward persons, which might not agree with one another.
2. There is always movement toward a balance state, a situation in which the relations fit together harmoniously and then there is no stress.
3. The basic concept of the balance is that, a tendency exists for individuals to restore balance to attitude, which are not of the same sign.
4. Heider's P-O-X model explains situations in which there are two persons, a perceiver P and another O, each of whom might have an attitude toward a given object X.
5. If P likes O, the assumption is that O's attitude toward X should be the same as P's. For example, two staff nurses might share a common positive attitude toward ward sister. If they differed on that issue, than an imbalance state would exist. In that case, they might try to persuade each other or also avoid the topic until their duties are over in order to retain least apparent balance.
6. These theory statements are shown by plus or minus signs. It predicts that when all signs are positive, a state of balance exists. If there is one negative sign or three negative signs, the outcome is negative leading to an imbalance state (just like multiplication of two minuses yields a plus). Therefore, balance occurs when there are either no negative sign or two negative signs.

Congruity Theory

1. Osgood and Tannenbaum (1955) postulates that imbalance between attitudes is resolved by summing the amount of their

positive or negative quality. There is a pair of attitudes on which one has a positive sign and one has a negative sign.

2. The greater the amount of the positive or negative quality of an attitude, the less likely it is to change when paired with something of an opposite sign. The valence goes from +3 to –3 on the usual attitude scale.
3. Suppose you dislike a public figure at the highest scale value of +3 and then learn that he/she favors a policy, which you dislike at the relatively moderate level of –1.
4. The prediction is that you are more likely to alter the attitude toward policy, in a more favorable, a positive direction rather than the attitude toward the political figure in an unfavorable direction.
5. However, the actual results may be a less negative or neutral attitude, rather than a positive one. Abelson and Rosenberg (1958) gave three rules of cognitive interaction; they are:
   a. A likes B and B likes C implies that A likes C also.
   b. A likes B and B dislikes C implies that A dislikes C.
   c. A dislikes B and B dislikes C implies that A likes C.

Cognitive Dissonance Theory (Festinger, 1957)

1. When related cognitions, feelings or behaviors are inconsistent or contradictory, it creates an unpleasant state of tension that motivates people to reduce their dissonance by changing their cognitions, feeling or behavior.
2. For instance a person who starts out with a negative attitude toward marijuana and finds themselves enjoys the experience.
3. The dissonance they experience is thus likely to motivate to change their attitude toward marijuana or to stop using marijuana.

MEASUREMENT OF ATTITUDES

Self-report Methods

1. Self-report methods include attitude scales, questionnaires, interviews and projective tests. When a person is asked to express the preferences, likes and dislikes to an interviewer or to write the evolution of something on a questionnaire.
2. Attitudes are measured by attitude scales, which deal with an issue or set of related issues. These depict the direction of an attitude, the degree or extent in that direction and the intensity of feeling that goes with the attitude.

3. Sometimes these components may be a part of questionnaire studies and interviews in which people are asked, first, how they feel about something (pro or con) and then how strongly they feel. Finally these rates are highly related.
4. Attitudes scales typically consist of a number of statements with which a person may agree or disagree with several scale points, usually ranging from highly agree or highly disagree. In this way, both the direction and the degree are indicated by the response to each statement or item.
5. Typically, these items relate to some common social thing, person, issue, person's overall attitude, etc.
6. Attitude scales commonly used are Thurstone scale, Likert scale and Bogardus social distance scale.

Thurstone Scale (Methods of Equal-appearing Intervals)

1. Louis L, Thurstone and Chave EJ (1929) in their classic study of attitudes toward the church, developed an interval scale by using the method of equal-appearing intervals.
2. Since the scale represents an evenly graduated series of attitudes as in the foot rule, the method is named so.
3. Every statement in Thurstone scale has a numerical value already determined.
4. The subject has to place a tick mark against each item with which he/she agrees. The attitude score is the mean of the scale value.

Likert Scale (Summated Rating)

1. For the Likert scale, various opinion statements are collected, edited and then given to a group of subjects to rate the statements on a five-point scale: strongly agree, agree undecided, disagree and strongly disagree.
2. The subject expresses the degree (1–5) of their personal agreement or disagreement with each of the statements.
3. The respondent's attitude score in the sum of his/her rating of all the statements. For this reason, the Likert scale is also known as the scale of summated ratings.

Bogardus Social Distance Scale

1. Bogardus ES developed an attitude scale in 1933, called the social distance scale, which become a classic instrument to measure attitudes toward ethnic group.

2. He was the first one to design a technique for the specific purpose of measuring and comparing attitudes toward different nationalities, particularly measuring tolerance of out-group.
3. The subject is asked to indicate the extent of his/her willingness to accept members of different social groups into various social institutions.

Observations of Behavior

1. Observation is a method of studying the behavior, consists of the perception of an individual's attitude under conditions by the other individuals and analysis of perceived attitude by them.
2. By this method, we can interfere with the mental processes of other persons by observing them.
3. For example, observing the actual overt behavior of students in natural situation.

Involuntary Behavioral Measures

Involuntary behavioral measures study body's physiological responses to attitude objectives involving.

1. Galvanic skin response (GSR), measures the electrical resistance of the skin.
2. Electromyography (EMG), measures major facial muscles movements.

ATTITUDE AND NURSE

While giving nursing services in the hospital, the nurse has to deal with patients having all kinds of attitudes; simultaneously nurse also has to adjust with personal and professional attitudes. A nurse should try to understand the patient's attitudes; some of them enter hospital with ready and willing to cooperate; others enter hospital with afraid or resentful or event definitely antagonistic to the ideas of receiving treatment and to the rigidity of ward routine.

Kempf and Averill list the following attitudes for a successful and efficient nurse:

1. Ambition to do task.
2. Conformity with the rules and regulations of the profession for which he/she is preparing.

3. Willingness to work and to work with effectiveness.
4. Cheerfulness and optimism.
5. Interest in the problems and difficulties of other people.
6. Cooperativeness, industriousness, respect for the opinion and judgment of others.
7. Interest in increasing the fund of knowledge underlying effective nursing care.
8. Determination to grow professionally.
9. Maintenance of poise and self-control in all professional situations.
10. Maintaining a consistent pride in their profession.
11. Arising to the unexpected, without undue panic.
12. Determination to make the patient comfortable by giving attention to small details that mean so much to the patient's well-being.

CONCLUSION

Attitudes are not inborn, but acquired. A person develops his/her behavior pattern in accordance with knowledge, experiences and emotions. Such behavior becomes a relatively permanent basis of his/her actions. Parents, teachers, religious leaders, literature and media, etc. have an extensive impact on the development of attitudes. Healthy attitudes like kindness, generosity, self-less service, etc. must be encouraged. The nurse needs to develop and cultivate professional attitude, which will contribute to nurse being successful in work. The nurse should try to find out the cause of the unfavorable attitudes and should change them to favorable ones because favorable attitudes help in treatment and recovery.

SUGGESTED READING

1. Banerjee JC. Fundamentals of Modern Psychology. Calcutta: Asia Publishing House; 1965.
2. Charles G Morris, Albert A Maisto. Understanding Psychology. New Jersey: Prentice Hall Inc; 2001.
3. Cifford MT, Richard KA. Introduction to Psychology, 7th edition. New Delhi: Tata McGraw-Hill Publishing Company Limited; 2004.
4. Clement I. Psychosocial Foundation of Nursing, 1st edition. New Delhi: Jaypee Brothers Medical Publishers (P) Ltd; 2010.

5. Jocob A. Psychology for Graduate Nurses, 4th edition. New Delhi: Jaypee Brothers Medical Publishers (P) Ltd; 2007. pp. 134-41.
6. Mangal SK. General Psychology. New Delhi: Sterling Publishers Pvt Ltd; 2006.
7. Sreevani R. Psychology for Nurses, 1st edition. New Delhi: Jaypee Brothers Medical Publishers (P) Ltd; 2009. pp. 140-5.

REVIEW QUESTIONS

1. Define attitude. Explain the components and nature of attitude.
2. Discuss the development of attitude. Explain in detail about change in attitude.
3. Explain various theories of attitude; discuss in detail.
4. Enumerate various measurements of attitude.
5. Discuss and describe the various roles and responsibilities of nurse in attitude.

CHAPTER 12 Concept of Mental Hygiene and Mental Health

LEARNING OBJECTIVES

1. Definitions.
2. Characteristics of a mentally healthy person.
3. Defense mechanisms.

INTRODUCTION

Mentally healthy person is the one who is able to make adjustments, fully mature, able to evaluate, leading a regular life, having balanced behavior, satisfied with job, etc. Mental health is the ability of a person to make personal and social adjustments. Actually, it is essential to be mentally healthy for optimum health and well-being. It is an important constituent of optimum health. Mental health is essential for a healthy and successful life. Mental health and physical health are inter-related and that is the reason behind the popularity of saying healthy mind lives in healthy body. Ancient saints of India have stressed the importance of emotional balance. It means, mental health is the balanced department of a person's personality and emotional attitudes because of which he/she becomes capable of living happily with his/her friends, relatives and environment.

MENTAL HEALTH

Nature and Meaning

1. Mental health is influenced by both biological and social factor.
2. Major importance of mental health is related to the ability of a person to develop pleasant relations with other. Also, it stresses

the constructive and positive contribution or participation in the changes of physical and social environment.

3. Mental health is the ability of a person to establish personal and social balance.
4. Mental health is the balanced development of a person's personality and attitudes, which makes him/her capable of living in harmony with himself/herself and relatives.
5. Mental health is that ability of a person through which he/she builds harmonious relations with others and participates or creatively contributes in the changes of the social, physical or spiritual environment.
6. Mental health is a state of the individual's mind, where he/she can adjust and adapt to the situations in a harmonious manner; body and mind work together in same direction in order to lead a happy and protective life.
7. A good mental health is the ability to respond to many varied experiences of life with flexibility and a sense of purposes.

Definitions

1. A mentally healthy person is the one who is comfortable with himself, lives peacefully with his neighbors, brings up his children to be healthy civilians and after completing his basic duties he has the energy and strength to do something for the welfare of society. —*PV Luken*
2. Mental health is a process of adjustment, which involves compromise, adaptation, growth and continuity. —*Bhatia and Craig*
3. Mental health is defined as the capacity in an individual to form harmonious relations with others and to participate in or contribute constructively to the changes in his/her social and physical environment. —*WHO*
4. Mental health concerns with the development of wholesome balanced personality, one who does not comfort himself like a series of compartmentalized selves—honest on Sunday, dishonest on Monday, generous today, crabbed tomorrow, reasonable and logical at times, at other times confused and inconsistent. —*Walton, JEW*
5. Mental health is the full and harmonious functioning of the whole personality. —*JA Hadfield*

6. Mentally healthy person is one who is happy, lives peacefully with his neighbors, makes his children healthy citizens and after fulfilling such basic responsibilities is still empowered with sufficient strength to serve the cause of the society in any way. —*PB Lewin*
7. Mental health is defined as the adjustment of human being to the world and to each other with a maximum of effectiveness and happiness. It is the ability to maintain even temper, an alert intelligence, socially considerate behavior and a happy disposition. —*KA Menninger*
8. Mental health is the ability, which helps us to seek adjustment in the different situations of our life. —*Cutts and Mosley*
9. Mental health is defined as simultaneous success at working, living and creating the capacity for mature and flexible resolution of conflicts between instincts, conscience. — *American Psychiatric Association*
10. Mental health is defined as a positive, but relative quality of life. It is a condition, which is characteristic of the average person who meets the demands of life on the basis of his/her own capacities and limitations. —*John Sutton and Webster*

Characteristics of Mentally Healthy Person

Mental health is also a state like physical health; this condition can be recognized by its characteristics.

Self-evaluation: A mentally healthy person is aware of his/her limits, accepts his/her shortcoming and tries to overcome these. He/she also introspects to reduce his/her problem and is able to estimate his/her potential accurately.

Adjusting capacity: A mentally healthy person lives in present not in the past dreams of future. He/she adjusts with the new condition with minimum pain and sorrow. He/she is well acquainted with the facts and change in the rules of life. Therefore, he/she is ready for every change.

Maturity: A mentally healthy person exhibits emotional maturity. He/she behaves in a responsible manner and expresses feelings and thoughts clearly. His/her sexual behavior is also mature.

Non-extremist: Excess of everything is bad, is the right principle for mental health. Excess of any behavior or desire has an adverse effect on health. Being excessively courageous, excessive speaking, lewd or ambitious does not let the person relax, which has an ill effect on health. Therefore, excessive (extremism) should be avoided for the development of mental health.

Regular life: Healthy habits are the basis of mental health. Regularity of habits, as those of living, eating, sleeping, walking, etc. are essential. Regular habits save time and energy. Mentally healthy people are able to accomplish all works of life in a natural and mature manner, without any problem.

Good social relationship: A mentally healthy person maintains good social relations with the people of society, colleagues and family members. Mutual cooperation helps in the building and development of personality. Goodwill and good behavior is more important for such people. Balanced relations in the society helps in the development of mental health.

Job satisfaction: Being satisfied with one's job or occupation is essential for mental health. Dissatisfaction with work gives birth to frustrations. Hence, one should increase interest in his/her job by making adjustments to achieve satisfaction and thus, the standard of mental health is increased.

Other characteristics: Mentally healthy person do not daydream, they expert in social etiquettes. They exhibit the capacity to tolerate stress and exhibit the ability to take decisions as per the situation. Mentally healthy person pay attention to make balance in every aspect of life, work and behavior. They take responsibility of their actions.

Personal worth/sense of personal security: Mentally healthy person has a sense of personal worth, feels worthwhile and important. He/she has self-respect and feels secure in a group.

Well-balanced life: He/she has a variety of interests and generally lives a well-balanced life of work, rest and recreation. He/she has the ability to get enjoyment and satisfaction of his/her daily routine job. According to Fromm, a mentally healthy person has developed a zest of living that includes a desire for activity, which reflects in an attitude of utilizing wherever possibilities he possesses in productive forms of behavior.

Rational attitude: He/she has a rational attitude toward problems of physical health. He/she maintains a daily routine of health practices, which promote healthful living. He/she practices good health habits with regard to nutrition, sleep, rest, relaxation, physical activity, personal cleanliness and protection from disease.

Philosophical life: He/she has developed a philosophical of life that gives meaning and purpose to his/her daily activities. This philosophy belongs to this world and discourages the tendency to withdraw or escape from the world. It makes him/her to something concrete about his/her problems as they rise. He/she does not evade responsibility or duty.

Faith in the ability: He/she has faith in his/her ability to succeed; he/she believes that, he/she will do reasonably well for whatever he/she undertakes. He/she solves problem largely by own initiative and effort. He/she feels confident of everyday life, more or less effectively.

Mental health is a dynamic concept: Mental health denotes a state of balance or equilibrium of our mind. This balance is not static, but is quite dynamic. The circumstances in our life are never static, they are changeable and so is our adjustment.

Factors Influencing Mental Health

Heredity: It provides raw material or the potentialities of the individual. It sets the limits for his/her mental health. What individual inherits are the potentialities in relation to growth, appearance, intelligence and the life. The development and utilization of these potentialities is determined largely by environmental opportunities. Investigations show that hereditary may predispose a person to the development of a particular type of mental illness, when placed under extensive stress. In the words of Wallin, defective heredity may furnish a fertile soil for the development of mental and nervous diseases, but as far as minor personality maladjustments are concerned, heredity supplies only a predisposing condition.

Physical factor: Physical health factors make a significant contribution to mental health. You will agree that an erect posture, a winning smile, color in the cheeks, a feeling of exhilaration, etc. promote a sense of personal security and have a marked influence on other people. People with greater strengths, better looks and robust health enjoy a social advantage in the development of personality characteristics. An individual with a feeling of physical well-being ordinarily enjoys a good disposition and is enthusiastic and intellectually alert. Sick people find it more difficult to adjust to new situations than healthy people. Vitamin deficiencies are found to be the causative factors in many personality difficulties.

Social factor: This pertains to the individual's society in which he/she lives, the interactional process and his/her social functioning with other persons. It is the social environment, which shapes the knowledge, skills, interests, attitudes, habits, values and goals that he/she acquires. Every individual is born into a society, which influences the content of his/her behavior. Of our social factors, the most important are home, school and community.

Satisfaction of fundamental or basic needs: From the discussion of the physical and social factor, it will be clear that mental health in childhood and later depends very much on the adequate satisfaction of our fundamental or basic needs. Our basic needs are physical, organic as well as emotional or psychological. The organic needs are to be satisfied for marinating physical well-being. Hunger, thirst, fatigue, lack of sleep, physical pain, exercise, heat or cold and the like set up certain tension in the individuals, which must be relived.

Environmental factor: It has now been the established account of various researches in the field of mental hygiene that environmental forces, family, school and society are more responsible for bringing mental illness than the hereditary or constitutional forces.

Principles Contributing to Mental Health

1. One should respect his/her own and other's personality.
2. One should be aware of the limitations of the self and others and should also have the knowledge of others' abilities.
3. This fact should be understood that every behavior has some reason.
4. Person should be evaluated according to his/her total behavior.
5. Important needs or drives should be recognized and efforts should be made to fulfill these.

Needs of Mental Health

To develop ideal mental health, one should pay attention to the important needs, which are given below:

1. Need for love and attachment.
2. Desire for being independent and self-sufficient.
3. Desire for achievements.
4. Need for recognition and respect.
5. Need for self-actualization.
6. Need for the identification of personality.

Major Foundations of Mental Health

1. Sound physical health.
2. Fulfillment of the basic needs of person like physical, psychological and social.
3. Development of healthy habits, education, philosophy of life, etc.
4. Various components related to hereditary and environment.

Skills Needed for Positive Mental Health

World health organization (WHO) has recommended some life skills, which may be used for promotion of mental health. These skills should teach every person to maintain the positive mental health.

Problem solving: Learning steps of problem solving and generating solutions to difficult problems.

Decision making: Learning basic steps for decision making.

Creative thinking: Developing creativity in thinking and developing adaptation behavior.

Critical thinking: Through making objective judgment about risks and choices.

Effective communication: Developing positive communication skills during the stress period.

Interpersonal relationship: Learning importance of interpersonal relations, making support groups for the need of time.

Self-awareness: Identifying one's own qualities, strengths and weaknesses.

Coping mechanisms: Understanding the emotions, their effects and coping with emotional distress and stressful situations.

Empathy: Through caring of people and avoiding prejudices and discriminations.

Nurses' Responsibilities in Promotion of Positive Mental Health

Nurses are responsible to provide mental health care to all sections of the people, community and hospitals. In this regard, some important activities of community health nurse are given below:

1. Educating the community about mental health, its importance and needs.
2. Educating the parents and other specific sections of society, this may be responsible for psychological development of children. It is necessary to caution against overprotection.
3. Preventing infection, trauma and poisoning before, during and after birth, which may lead to various mental health problems in the life span of a person.
4. Providing anticipatory guidance and counseling to prevent psychological problems.
5. Providing school-based mental healthcare services.
6. Avoiding misconceptions, superstitions about mental illness.
7. Educating the individuals about coping mechanisms.
8. Providing counseling services to parents of mentally and physically handicapped children.
9. Identifying the high-risk groups in the community and preventing them from forthcoming mental problems.
10. Providing mental healthcare services to sufferer of mental diseases.
11. Implementing the national mental health program.

Importance of Mental Health

Health is, rightly said, wealth. It involves one's physical as well as mental health. As said earlier, mental health has much wider scope than physical health, as it aims for the development of wholesome balanced and integrated personality.

Mental health helps in the development of desirable personality: Mental health helps in the development of a wholesome, well-balanced and integrated personality.

Mental health helps in proper emotional development: There is a close relationship between one's mental health and emotional behavior. Individuals who enjoy good mental health are supposed to demonstrate proper emotional maturity in their behavior.

Mental health helps in proper social development: One's mental health helps one in becoming quite sociable and establishing proper social relationships in the society.

Mental health help in proper moral development: The individuals who enjoy sound health are usually found to behave as a man of integrity and character by following the ethical standards of the society.

Mental health helps in proper esthetic development: Proper mental health helps the individual in the development of appropriate esthetic sense, artistic tastes and refined temperament.

Mental health helps in actualizing one's potentialities: Everyone of us has a fund of natural abilities and potentialities that can be actualizing through proper efforts. Exercising such effort and striving toward the actualization of one's mental health.

Mental health helps in seeking proper adjustment: A mentally healthy individual is an adjusted person. He/she is able to seek adequate adjustment with self and environment. He/she is able to adjust the needs to the demands of the situations and well-being of the society.

Mental health helps in seeking goals of life: Mental health helps the individual to strive properly for the realization of the goals of life. These goals may differ from person to person depending upon their lifestyles and philosophy of life.

Mental health helps in the progress of the society: Mental health helps the individual to develop as well-balanced useful citizens who are conscious not only for their rights but also for their responsibilities. They not only take essential from the society for their proper development and living but also ready to give something to the society for its progress and development.

Mental health helps in the prevention of mental illness: Mental health helps the individual in protecting self against abnormalities of behavior, maladjustment, illness and mental diseases. In the same way as physical health is helpful in saving the individual from physical illness, ailments and diseases. A sound mind and balanced personality has enough resistance for fighting with the odds of life and bearing the accidental stresses and strains of life in comparison to the people having impaired mental health.

Symptoms of Poor Mental Health

1. Emotionally unstable and easily upset.
2. Apprehensive, suspicious and insecure.
3. Lack of self-confidence and willpower.
4. No adequate adjustment with the self and environment—physical, social and professional.
5. Failure in setting a proper level of aspiration.
6. Suffering from frustrations, unresolved conflicts, strains and stresses.
7. Always remains in the state of over anxiousness and tension.
8. Lack of enduring power and tolerance.
9. Lack of decision-making ability.
10. Poor self-concept and achievement motivation.
11. Unrealistic attitude toward life and people.
12. Suffering from mental disturbances, disorder, ailments and diseases.
13. Always dissatisfied with achievements and tries to seek over-perfection in own or other's work.
14. Lives in the world of their own imagination and fantasy.

Mental Health in Different Age Groups

Mental health in different age groups is described in Table 12.1.

Table 12.1: Mental health in different age groups

Sl No	*Age group*	*Description*
1.	Prenatal and postnatal period	Emotional level of pregnant mother affects the mental behavior of the child. Some women are much tensed during pregnancy or pregnancy can be an existing and frightening experience for them. Therefore, along with the physical care of mother, she should also be given due emotional support. Maintaining a healthy and creative mental level by mother during pregnancy is very important for the mental hygiene of child. The psychiatric nurse should give health education to mother during antenatal and postnatal period about the importance of healthy living for healthy baby. After birth, the baby needs mother's protection, food, love, etc. for normal growth.

Contd...

Contd...

Sl No	*Age group*	*Description*
2.	Infancy (1 month to 1 year) and childhood (toddler to 12 year)	In the womb, the fetus feels more comfortable and enjoys warmth. But the newborn is full of fear when comes to this open world. Primary childhood is the foundation of mental health. It is essential that during this period, parents should have loving and close relations with children. Any incident that occurs in the school is imprinted in child's mind. Therefore, behavior of other children in the school, student-teacher relations and environment of school should be friendly and assisting in providing the emotional satisfaction to the child. Parents' responsibility is to provide happy and conductive environment for the child to grow. Understanding and sympathetic approach in meeting child's need is essential as adequate satisfaction of physical needs, which forms a basis for adequate mental health.
3.	Adolescence (13–18 year)	Adolescence is the most sensitive period from the point of normal health. Mental illnesses arising in adolescences, can be prevented by recognizing the needs of adolescence, proper adjustment with opposite sex, giving due importance to the freedom of teenagers and the balanced and understanding behavior of parents.
4.	Adulthood (20–40 year)	Adulthood is a period in which person should have complete mental health. But the tension of the responsibilities of family, social beliefs, financial limitations and other environment-generated stresses affect the mental health of the person.
5.	Old age (60 and above)	Mental problems of elderly have increased significantly owing to various factors. These include reduction in the importance of joint family system, changing moral and life values, industrialization and urbanization, financial dependence, physical disabilities, diseases, etc.

MENTAL HYGIENE

Mental hygiene is concerned with realization and maintenance of mind's health and efficiency or in other words, it deals with healthfulness of mind. Mental hygiene is concerned with the study of factors, which go against mental health and efficiency. Mental hygiene means the balanced and integrated development of personality. It is a science that deals with human welfare and pervades all fields of human relationships. The aim of mental hygiene is to aid people to achieve more satisfying and more productive lives, through the prevention of anxieties and maladjustments. According to dictionary, mental hygiene is the science or arts of maintaining mental health and preventing the development of maladjustment and neurosis.

Professor W Beers is called the Father of mental hygiene. Once, when he was suffering from some ailments, he realized that various ailments are caused due to failure of the individual to adjust him with situation and requirement of environment. This maladjustment also leads to the development of various mental ailments. It is necessary to do away with them. With this aim in view an international mental health society was established in 1908. The society believed in the slogan sound mind resides in sound body.

Definitions

1. Mental hygiene is concerned with the principle and practice in promotion, maintenance of the mental health and prevention of mental disorders. —*JA Hadfield*
2. The means by which the process of mental health is related; it is a way of life and involves that influences what one feels, says and does. —*HW Bernard*
3. Mental health defined as the realization and maintenance of the mind's health and efficiency. —*DB Klein*
4. It is an organized attempt to effort human adjustment through the application of principles and practices of living. —*Bhatia BD and M Craig*
5. Mental hygiene means establishment of environmental conditions, emotional attitudes and habits of thinking that will resist an onset of personality maladjustments. It is the study of principles and practices in the promotion of mental health and prevention of mental disorder. —*Dictionary of education*
6. Mental hygiene is defined as the application of a body of hygienic information and technique called from sciences of psychology, child study, education, sociology, psychiatric, medicine and biology for the purpose of observation and improvement of mental health of the individuals and the community; for the prevention and care of minor and major mental diseases and defects mental educational and social maladjustments. —*Wallace Wallin*

Spheres of Mental Hygiene

There are two spheres of mental hygiene, prophylactic hygiene and meliorative hygiene.

Prophylactic mental hygiene: It is oriented toward the prevention of diseases, breakdown, weakness, disaster and death.

Meliorative mental hygiene: It is oriented toward the acquisition of better health, more energy and abundant life. It stresses the normal and the ideal as opposed to the abnormal and pathological.

DEFENSE MECHANISMS

An individual is, as much, equipped with mental capacities to protect himself/herself against conflicts and frustrations as with physical energy and powers to safeguard against physical dangers or distress. These mental capacities give rise to protective devices known as mental mechanisms or adjustment mechanisms or defense mechanisms. This adjustment mechanism helps the individual in overcoming threats to own ego and thus, in maintaining inner balance or harmony. Mental mechanisms interact and overlap in our behavior. They are neither mutually exclusive nor generally operate as separate entities. Both well-adjusted and maladjusted individuals make use of these mechanisms in their daily behavior.

Definitions

1. Defense mechanism is a pattern of adjustment through which an individual relieves or decrease anxieties caused by an uncomfortable situation that threatens self-esteems.
2. Ego defense mechanism is consciously or unconsciously operating device to keep confliction issues out of consciousness of the individual to bring some protective measures.
3. Ego defense mechanisms are learned, usually during early childhood and are considered to be maladaptive when they become the predominant means of coping with stressors.
4. When psychological equilibrium is threatened by severe emotional trauma, frustrations or conflicts, the mind resorts to a variety of protective subterfuges and detours called mental mechanisms or dynamisms. —*Page*

5. An adjustment mechanism is a device resorted in order to achieve an indirect satisfaction of a need so that tension will be reduced and self-respect maintained. —*Carroll*
6. Certain patterns of behavior that are employed for protection against threat or anxiety are called defense mechanisms or adjustment mechanisms. Sometimes they are referred to as ego defense mechanisms, since they serve to defend the ego or the self from threat. —*Arkoff*
7. A defense mechanism is a strategy, unconsciously utilized, that serves to protect the ego from anxiety. —*Davison and Neale*

Functions of Defense Mechanism

1. Protecting individuals from dangerous situations.
2. To deal with minor hurt, pain, anger, anxiety, sadness and self-devaluation.
3. Removing anxiety and hurt.
4. Plays an important role in normal adjustment mechanism.

Characteristics

1. The purpose of defense mechanism is to reduce anxiety.
2. Defense mechanism is compromise solutions.
3. The pattern of defense mechanism depends on one's stability.
4. The same individual may use varied mechanisms he/she need.
5. Defense mechanisms may be used consciously, but usually act at unconscious or subconscious level.
6. Defense mechanisms are devised in the forms of certain pattern of behavior.
7. These mechanisms provide protection against whatever threatens our ego or self-esteem.
8. There are many situations in our environment and also within us, which threaten our psychological equilibrium.
9. Defense mechanism may be evolved by anything in conflict with minimum ideal of what the self must be.
10. Defense mechanisms are quite temporary defense against anxiety and inadequacies. By resorting to them one tries to deceive self more than somebody else.
11. Defense mechanisms are largely unconscious. They do tend to operate in a machine-like or automatic way. In fact, they are always, in corresponding degree, self-deceptive and thus aim

at softening or disguising what is unaccepted to us in terms of our failure or inadequacies.

12. Defense mechanisms should not be confused with symptoms of neuroses or other abnormal conditions. These mechanisms are purely psychic or mental devices or ways of perceiving and desiring.

Types

Defense mechanism is divided into four levels. Each level with its classification and description is given in Table 12.2.

Table 12.2: Types of defense mechanism

Sl No	*Classification*	*Description*
Level I Psychotic		
1.	Denial	It is protecting self from unpleasant reality by refusal to perceive it or face it. It is a defense mechanism in which a person is faced with a fact that is too painful to accept and reject it. The individual may deny the reality of the unpleasant fact altogether, admit the fact, but deny its seriousness or admit both the fact and seriousness, but denies responsibility.
2.	Distortion	A gross reshaping of external reality to meet internal needs. For example, mentally ill patients have no intact contact with reality. These patients may be suffering with psychosis.
3.	Delusional projections	Gross frank delusions about external reality, usually of persecutory nature. The delusions are the false beliefs of the person, which are not shared by race, age, educational background, etc.
Level II Immature		
1.	Fantasy	It is gratifying frustrated desires by imaginary achievements. It is the defense mechanism involving tendency to retreat into fantasy in order to resolve inner and outer conflicts.
2.	Projection	It is unconscious denial of unacceptable feelings and emotions in one, while attributing to others. It is primitive form of paranoia.
3.	Hypochondrias	The transformation of negative feeling toward others into negative feelings toward self, pain, illness and anxiety. Hypochondrias sometimes referred to as health phobia, refers to an excessive preoccupation or worry about having a serious illness.

Contd...

Contd...

Sl No	*Classification*	*Description*
4.	Passive aggression	Aggression toward others expressed indirectly or passively. Passive aggressive defense create or disorder known as passive aggressive personality disorder, is said to be marked by a pervasive pattern of negative attitudes and passive, usually resistance in interpersonal or occupational areas.
5.	Acting out	Direct expression of unconscious wish or impulse without conscious awareness of the emotion that derives that expressive behavior. This behavior is very common in children with temper tantrum, oppositional defiant disorder, truancy, etc.
6.	Regression	It is returning to an earlier stage of behavior when stress creates, problem at the present stage, involving less mature responds and usually lower level of aspiration. Regression is a mechanism of going from the present pattern to the past level of behavior. The individual returns to patterns of behavior that were successful in earlier stages of development.
7.	Idealization	Subconsciously choosing to perceive another individual as having positive qualities he/she may actually have.
Level III Neurotic		
1.	Displacement	Defense mechanism shifts sexual or aggressive impulses to a more acceptable or less threatening target; redirecting emotion to a safer outlet; separation of emotion from its real object.
2.	Dissociation	It is temporary drastic modification of one's personal identity or character to avoid emotional distress; separation or postponement of a feeling that normally would accompany a situation or thought.
3.	Isolation	It is separation of feelings from ideas and events. For example, describing a murder with graphic details with no emotional response.
4.	Intellectualization	It is avoiding unavoidable emotions by focusing on the intellectual aspects. It is separating from emotional contents of an event, focusing instead on the facts.
5.	Reaction formation	Converting unconscious wishes or impulses that are perceived to be dangerous into their opposites; behavior that is completely the opposite of what one really wants or feels; taking the opposite beliefs because of true, causes anxiety.

Contd...

Contd...

Sl No	*Classification*	*Description*
6.	Repression	Repression acts to keep information out of conscious awareness. Repression is more complicated mechanism in which unpleasant or unacceptable experiences, emotions or motivations are actively forced into the unconscious and kept there. Repression operates wholly on an unconscious level. Unacceptable feeling are unconsciously kept out of awareness. A man is jealous of his good friend's success, but is unaware of his feelings of jealous.
Level IV Mature		
1.	Altruism	This is constructive service to others that brings pleasure and personal satisfaction. Altruism loves others as oneself, behavior that promotes the survival chances of others at a cost to one's own. In other words, it self-sacrifices for the benefit of others.
2.	Sublimation	The transformation of negative emotions or instincts into positive actions, behavior or emotion is sublimation.
		Sublimation is a defense mechanism that allows us to act out unacceptable impulses by converting these behaviors into a more acceptable form.
3.	Suppression	Suppression is a device where a conscious effort is made by the individual to dismiss the impulses, feelings and thoughts that are unpleasant to the preconscious mind. So unacceptable feelings and thoughts are consciously kept out of awareness.
4.	Humor	Overt expression of ideas and feelings (especially those that are unpleasant to focus or too terrible to talk about) that gives pleasure to others.
5.	Identification	The unconscious modeling of one's self upon another person's character and behavior. Some individuals try to resemble with another person's character. A lonely teenager being copying the clothes and action of a popular peer.
6.	Introjections	It is identifying with some ideas or objects so deeply that it becomes a part of that person. It is complete acceptance of another's opinion and values as one's own.

ADJUSTMENT

The word adjustment means to fit, make suitable, adapt, arrange, harmonize, correspondence with. Adjustment is defined as the series of techniques, methods or processes by which an individual tries to meet the environmental, spatial or psychological changes and maintains a satisfactory equilibrium (balance) with the world. This is also called adaptation. There are different types of changes to which a person has to adjust himself. These changes can be environmental (e.g. change in temperature, humidity, oxygen level), spatial change (e.g. change of place) and psychological change (e.g. the husband leaves the job; family members face the problem of change of job of the head of the family).

Definitions

1. Adjustment can be defined in that form of social process in which two or more people or groups interact to end or reduce conflict. —*Fitcher*
2. Adjustment is that special process through which a person is able to develop the tendency of cooperation in his environment. —*MacIver and Page*
3. Any operation whereby an organism becomes more favorably related to the environment or to the entire situation, environmental and internal. —*Warren*
4. It is the establishment of satisfactory relationship, as representing, harmony, conformance, adoption, etc. —*Webster*
5. A continual process in which a person vary his behavior to produce a more harmonious relationship between himself and his environment. —*Gates and Jersild*
6. The process of finding and adopting modes of behavior suitable to the environment or the change in the environment. —*Carter V Good*
7. An individual's adjustment is said to be adequate, wholesome or healthful to the extent that he has established harmonious relationship between himself and the conditions, situations and persons who compromise his physical or social environment. —*Crow and Crow*
8. Adjustment is psychological survival. —*Von Haller*

Nature of Adjustment

1. *Continuity:* The process of adjustment is continued throughout life. Individual from birth to death has to adjust one way or the other. The individuals who are able to adjust themselves to

changing situations in their environment can live a harmonious, happy and continued life.

2. *Mental peace:* Conflict upsets a person, whereas adjustment provides peaceful.
3. *Universality:* Adjustment is prevalent in all the aspects of life, e.g. social, economic, political, religious, etc.
4. *Social necessity:* Adjustment is necessary to prevent society.
5. *Harmonious relationship:* A harmonious relationship between individual, their needs and environment is essential. The individual meets demand either by adopting, modifying previous ways of doing or facing the challenges.
6. *Day-to-day demand:* Adjustment will help the individual to change his/her way of life according to the demand of the situation and gives strength and ability to bring about necessary changes in the environmental conditions.
7. *Two-way process:* Adjustment is a process of not only fitting oneself into available circumstances but also changing the circumstances to fit one's own needs. In majority of cases, adjustment is compromise between two extremes.
8. *Conscious/unconscious activity:* To adjust in a society, the individual learns morals, traditions, etc. from birth to death in conscious and unconscious manner to adjust and accommodate the needs and demands of self and society.

Aims of Adjustment

1. To maintain harmonious and active relationship between structural components of society.
2. For social reform and social construction.
3. To lead a harmonious social life.
4. To perform functions effectively in relation to their culture, customs, values and beliefs.
5. To provide good interpersonal relationship.
6. To promote character building.
7. To develop orderly social unity.
8. To manifest collective behavior in terms of state, religion, economic agencies, organization and social group.

Measurement of Adjustment

Testing techniques: To assess the individual's characteristics at the unconscious level.

Projective techniques: To assess the individual's characteristics at the unconscious level.

Sociometric techniques: To measure social relationships and provide clues to the level of social adjustment.

Scaling techniques: Opinions, views are collected from other person about the adjustment pattern of a particular interval known to the respondents.

Inventory techniques: They may have many advantages to the techniques.

Methods of Adjustment

Direct Method

Improving efforts: To improve the behavioral process and to solve difficult situations in the environment; he/she will increase efforts to improve efficiency.

Compromising methods: Individual changes his/her efforts in a different direction to fulfill the aspiration.

Withdrawal and submissiveness: Accepts his/her own defeat and surrounding himself/herself to the powerful environmental forces.

Making proper choices and decisions: A person adapts himself/herself and serves harmony with his/her environment by making use of his/her intelligence for the proper choices and wise decision particularly when faced with conflicting situations and stressful moments/situations.

Indirect Method

By using defense mechanism/coping strategies, the individual will try to adopt himself/herself to the changing situation and accommodating new lifestyles.

Improving adjustments: It is very important to establish positive adjustment by finding out reasons of stress, hopelessness, frustration and maladjustments.

1. Find patterns of behavior that satisfy basic needs and solve problems effectively.
2. Assume conscious control on your behavior.

3. Use problem solving to find the best possible solution for a problem situation instead of acting impulsively.
4. Use emotion constructively when appropriate; express feelings at the time they are experienced.
5. Self-evaluation in a constructive sense. Look for ways to improve, but avoid feelings of guilt or inadequacy.
6. Avoid burnout: Perform effective stress management techniques such as yoga, meditation, exercises, etc.
7. Adapting to new situation when a change occurs in your life. Situation of your patterns of behavior in order to achieve a state of good adjustment in new situations.

CONCLUSION

Mental health is an important aspect of one's total health status. It is another word for adjustment or properly integrated living. A mentally healthy person feels, thinks and acts harmoniously. He/she is self-confident, adequate and free from continuous internal conflicts, he/she is able to make adaptations to a social setup. Waltin and Hadfield consider mental health as a means and measures for the development as well as functioning of a wholesome well-balanced and integrated personality. Considering this way, mental health has wider scope than physical health. It concerns with an all-round development of the personality of the child and not merely with the development of one's physical or bodily aspects. Moreover, it aims at the balanced personality, a personality like the balanced physical system who is able to stand firmly in the mildest of stress and strain and who can exhibit adequate emotional maturity and balance between his needs and circumstances.

SUGGESTED READING

1. Crow LD, Crow A. Educational Psychology. (3rd Indian reprint). New Delhi: Eurasia Publishing House; 1973.
2. Eysenck HJ. The Structure of Human Personality, 3rd edition. New York: Methuen and Co; 1971.
3. Garrett HE. General Psychology. Indian edition. New Delhi: Eurasia Publishing House; 1968.
4. Griffiths JH. The Psychology of Human Behavior. London: George Allen and Unwin Ltd; 1933.

5. Morgan, King. Introduction to Psychology. New Delhi: Tata McGraw-Hill Publishing Company Ltd; 1993.
6. Robert A Baron. Psychology. New Delhi: Prentice Hall of India Pvt Ltd; 2001.
7. Scheinfeld A. The New You and Hereditary. Philadelphia: JB Lippincott Co.
8. Sherman, Mandel. Psychology for Nurses. New York: Longmans, Green and Co.
9. Thurstone LL. Primary Mental Abilities. Chicago: University press; 1938.
10. Vernon PE. The Structure of Human Ability. London: Methuen; 1950.

REVIEW QUESTIONS

1. Define mental health. Explain the meaning and nature of mental health.
2. Enumerate the characteristics of mentally healthy persons.
3. Explain the factors influencing mental health.
4. Discuss the role and responsibilities of nurse in promotion of positive mental health.

CHAPTER 13 *Body-mind Relationship*

LEARNING OBJECTIVES

1. Definition.
2. Effects of body upon mind.
3. Theories of body-mind relationship.
4. Mind-body modalities.
5. Levels of consciousness.
6. Altered level of consciousness.
7. Nurses role and responsibilities.

INTRODUCTION

Psychology studies human behavior, which involves both the body and the mind. They are interrelated and interact upon each other. Mental function and physical status affect each other. Body and mind are two aspects of the living, dynamic and adjusting personality. Mind is regarded as a function of the body; it does not exist apart from the body. It is the sum total of various mental processes such as observing, knowing, thinking, reasoning, feeling, imaging, remembering, judging and others. Mind also grows just as the body grows.

BODY—THE INSTRUMENT OF THE MIND

The body is the most visible part; the physical presentation, the material medium; it is merely the instrument of the mind. The thought or idea that is consciously or unconsciously chosen and impressed upon the subconscious mind must move the body into action (Fig. 13.1). The action determines the results. Within the conscious mind, one have the ability to choose the thoughts and can choose any thoughts you want. The conscious mind has the power to either accept or reject any thought or idea that presents itself. So if has one that choice, why not choose to build those big, beautiful, wonderful pictures of everything you want in life instead of choosing to build a picture of all things, which is not required and all the reasons why something just is not going to work out. Consider the very worst of situations and choose to think something positive about it.

If the ability to replace the thoughts of an empty bank account with one full of what you need or the surrounded loving and caring friends or healthy and active life, then this is what gets pass to the subconscious (remember it does not have a choice) and that leads to the good results in life.

Either way, the thoughts you choose to accept, whether they may be positive or negative, are then impressed upon the subconscious mind and they dictate the way you feel. So if you think positive thoughts like 'everything always works out for me, life is great, I am grateful', than you are going to feel good and will actually attract more of those thoughts and feelings into life.

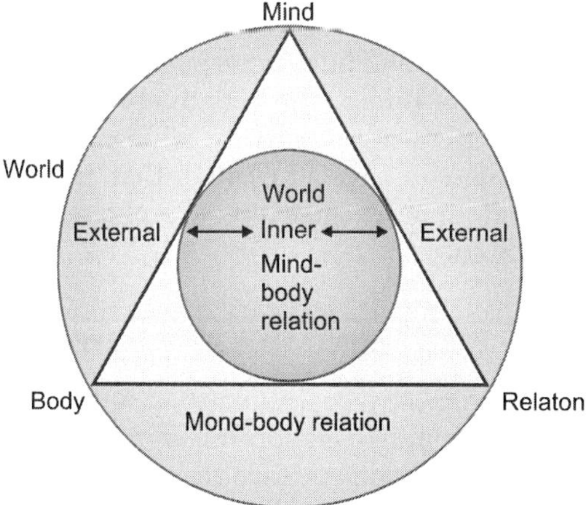

Fig. 13.1: The uniterity of living being

EFFECTS OF MIND UPON BODY

Every action of the mind produces a certain effect in the body. When the mental action is weak or superficial, the physical effect may be too slight to be noticed, but when this action is both deep and strong, the results will be so clearly in evidence that any one can detect them. These effects, however, are not simply functional, nor are the nervous system alone that is acted upon. The power of the mind can and does affect everything in the body, frequently producing chemical changes that we have believed were possible only through the use of most powerful drugs. But the action of mind on the body always follows exact law; therefore when one knows the exact physical effect produced by each mental state, physical conditions can be largely determined by the intelligent use of the mind.

Every thought you entertain, affects the body and emotions. For example, thinking about the favorite food, especially if you feel hungry, will cause the mouth to water. Every physical action affects the mood and the thinking. Walk around, very slowly so that you are almost dragging the feet, with the spine slumped forward and with head hanging down and notice how this affects the mood. It is pretty likely that it will drag you down emotionally.

You have no doubt recognized that when you feel physically tired or less-than-well, this affects the mood. It is very difficult, for example, to be cheerful and humorous when you have exhausted. Similarly this type of thinking affects the physical state. If you spend a while going around, silently telling yourself that you cannot cope or that you have a failure or that 'it is all too much' then this will undoubtedly cause you to feel tense, demoralized and physically tired.

THEORIES OF BODY-MIND RELATIONSHIP

This is the relationship between a human body and its unique mind. Theories of the body-mind relationship can be divided into two broad categories called monistic theories and dualistic theories.

Monistic Theories

These suggest that mind and body are not separate substances. Thinkers like Aristotle, Hobbes, Hegel and the behaviorists, collectively thought of as the materialists, postulated that the mind was nothing more than a body function. A mind is generally thought to be of a substance other than a physical substance. Berkeley, Leibniz and Schopenhauer, collectively known as the idealists, were monists of a different sort; they theorized that the body was simply a mental representation. Spinoza proposed that mind and body were the manifestations of some third property—what he considered God. This is the theory of double-aspectism, another monist view.

Dualistic Theories

According to the Dualist view, mind is thought to be a substance other than a physical substance. Popular dualists were Descartes, Locke and James, who collectively belong to the school of thought known as interactionism (Table 13.1). Other dualistic theories are as follows.

Table 13.1: Varied positions on the mind-body relation in psychology

Position	*Causal relation*	*Proponents*
Interactive-dualism	Both mind (soul) and body exist and causally interact. We are machines that think.	Descartes, La Mettrie
Epipheno-menalism	Mind real, but unimportant and not causal. Study bodily mechanisms or behavioral operants.	Hobbes, Skinner
Reductive materialism	Mind does not exist. Study bodily mechanisms, the nervous system, actions or behavior.	Hobbes, French materialists (e.g. Cabrini), mid-19th century physiology, Watson
Phenomenalism	Matter does not exist (theistic or logical immaterialism). Study sensations and habits.	Berkeley, Hume, Condillac
Vitalism	No 'soul', but mind, body, plus a 'life principle'. Mind/consciousness relies on, but not reducible to a material nervous system.	J Müller, early 19th century physiology
Double-aspect theory	Unity of body and mind, but not reducible. Did not have or use evolutionary theory. Study and measure the interaction of these aspects.	Spinoza, Fechner, CL Morgan, psychophysics

Contd...

Contd...

Position	*Causal relation*	*Proponents*
Parallelism	Mind (consciousness) and body separate—who cares why? Describe or measure each in own way.	British associationism, Wundt, structuralism, Gestalt and humanistic psychology
Pre-established harmony	Both run in parallel according to God's (or nature's) initial winding of two clocks. Study unconscious influences and character types.	Leibniz, phrenology, faculty psychology
Occasionalism	Active God	Malebranche
Emergentism	Non-reductive functional relation between substantive body and mind as a transformative process. Study the evolutionary development of the process.	James, Dewey, later CL Morgan, functional psychology; dialectical materialism; activity theory

1. *Double-aspectism:* Mind and body are distinguishable, but inseparable. Cognitive and experiential aspects can be distinguished from physical aspects, so there is a separate mind and body. The separate mind and body are two aspects of the state of being human. Spinoza explained it this way, "thinking substance (the mind) and extended substance (the body) are one and the same thing." For Spinoza, the single substance was God. This explanation of the mind-body connection may be the most difficult to understand, because it is perhaps the least clear.
2. *Epiphenomenalism:* The mind is really just a byproduct of the physical brain. Only physical events in the brain, (e.g. neurons firing) have causal power. Let us get clear about definitions before we go into this one. When we talk about the brain, we are speaking of a physical thing, so the brain is part of the body. This is very important to epiphenomenalism. If a human body were a television (TV) set, the mind would simply be the picture you see when it is switched on. In this view, the physical body affects (and even causes) the mind. However, because the mind is merely a byproduct, the mind does not affect the body. Huxley (1874) said that mental events are "like a steam whistle that contributes nothing to the work of a locomotive." According to James (1879), mental events do not affect the brain activity that produces them "any more than a shadow reacts upon the steps of the traveler whom it accompanies."

3. *Idealism:* According to idealism, what one knows to be real is in some way confined to the contents of one's own mind. Anything we experience through our senses is colored by how our mind perceives it. We therefore cannot have access to external reality. Only thoughts and ideas that originate in the mind can be immediately experienced. Idealism stands in stark contrast to the theory of materialism, which endorses the physical, spatial, factual domain as the ultimate reality. Plato's theory of forms/ideas has been compared to idealism, although the forms were not confined to the mind, but existed independently of it. It has also been argued that Descartes contribution in which access to the mind is prioritized influenced idealism. Idealism has been pervasive since the 18th century, but has been less popular in recent times.
4. *Interactionism:* Sometimes the mind affects the body and sometimes the body affects the mind. The body and the mind are separate and they affect one another. Descartes laid the groundwork here. We are physical beings because we are extended in space. We are mental beings because we think. In Descartes words, "I think, therefore I am" (Cogito Ergo Sum). Here is the problem we run into: The mind is not physical in any way and it exists separately from the body. So, how does the non-physical mind affect the physical body and vice versa? Descartes assumed that this interaction occurred in the pineal gland.
5. *Materialism:* This is the view that only physical matter is real. The body is governed by strictly material and non-mental causes. In as much as mental properties exist, they have no causal effect on the physical body. Strict materialists may hard-headedly deny that anything mental exists at all. Others may concede that the mind exists, but characterize it as being identical to the brain. The earliest exponents of something resembling materialism were the Greeks—Democritus and Aristotle. A specific type of materialism is epiphenomenalism, the view that the mind is a byproduct of physical processes. Another type of materialism is naturalism, the notion that nothing supernatural exists.
6. *Occasionalism:* It seems that God is following around us all day and when the mind gives the body, some instruction or vice versa, God makes it happen. Remember the problem we had with interactionalism? We could not explain how the mind and body affected one another. Well, we have that all solved here. When your mind decides that it would like your body

to be on the other side of the room, it gets some almighty intervention. Occasionalism was popularized in 17th century by French philosopher, Nicolas Malebranche. The problem with occasionalism is that it not only supposes that there is a God but he/she also has time to follow each and every one of us around.

7. *Parallelism:* Mind and body are separate, but they are perfectly synchronized. How do they affect one another? They do not affect, but they only appear. When your mind decides that it would like your body to be on the other side of the room it is just a coincidence that your body walks over there. Although the origin of this view can be traced back to GW Leibniz, he is also implicated in pre-established harmony, a view that implicates God in the correlation between mind and body.
8. *Pre-established harmony:* Mind and body, at the time of their creation, were perfectly synchronized by God, like two clocks set for exactly the same time. Although they appear to correspond and interact, there is no causal relationship between mind and body. Pre-established harmony was a theory expounded by GW Leibniz, to oppose the theories of parallelism, occasionalism and interactionalism. The problem with pre-established harmony is it presupposes that there is a God.

Relationship Between Consciousness and Mind/Body

The subconscious is that part of the body/mind that consciousness cannot access. As a person matures into adulthood, there is an intuitive sense that the subconscious grows. To state this differently, consciousness is gradually pushed out of more and more of the body/mind and into the head during maturation to adulthood. As this happens, it can be said that the subconscious mind grows as a person matures. It is not maturation itself that bring these changes about; rather it is the slow accumulation of difficult—and unresolved experiences. It is the core shifting, changing relationship between consciousness and the body/mind that this work is about.

MIND-BODY MODALITIES

Most people acknowledge that there is a mind and body connection knowing how this communication occurs, assists in the understanding of the mind and body modalities of relaxation, meditation and imagery.

Neuropeptides

Neuropeptides, the neurochemicals, are behaved to be the messenger molecules that connect body and mind. Neuropeptides have properties that allow them to affect neurological and physiologic tissue receptors as given below.

Relaxation

Relaxation is the state of generalized, decreased cognitive, physiological and/or behavioral arousal. The relaxation response is characterized by decreased heart and respiratory rates, blood pressure (BP), oxygen (O_2) consumption and increased alpha brain wave activity and peripheral skin comparatives. The long-term goal of relaxation therapy is for the person to continually monitor himself or herself for indicatives of tension and to consciously let go and release the tension contained in various body parts.

Imagery

Visualization technique is the conscious mind to create mental images to evoke physical changes in the body, improve perceived well-being and or enhance self-awareness. For example, the client may be directed to begin slow, abdominal breathing, while focusing to the rhythm of breathing and the client is then instructed to visualize waves coming to shoes with each inspiration, then seeding with each expiration. Next the client is instructed to take notice of the smells and sounds that he/she is experiencing. As the imagery session progresses, the client may be instructed to visualize warmth entering the body during inspiration and tension is leaving during expiration.

Meditation

Meditation seeks to change one's physiology to a more relaxed state and alter one's prescription to an increased acceptance of reality.

Nursing Considerations

Patients seeking inpatient case might have a meditation practice they want to continue. Nurses can provide the time necessary for this. Nursing is both an art and science that cares for the body, mind and spiritual unity of persons in relation to their environment. Nursing's caring perspective views human beings as persons in relation at every level of human existence and connection like individuals, families, groups and communities. The concept of human beings as persons in relation provides the framework from which nursing addresses the potential for promotion, maintenance and restoration of health. This framework underscores the importance of examining the political, economic and social forces that impact a person's agency and right to health. The infinite complexity of these forces creates a diversity of environments within which nursing seeks to maximize health at every level of human existence.

LEVELS OF CONSCIOUSNESS

The normal state of consciousness comprises either the state of wakefulness, awareness or alertness in which most human beings function, while not asleep or one of the recognized stages of normal sleep from which, the person can be readily awakened. The abnormal state of consciousness is more difficult to define and characterize, as evidenced by many terms applied to altered states of consciousness by various observers. Among such terms are clouding of consciousness, confusional state, delirium, lethargy, obtundation, stupor, dementia, hypersomnia, vegetative state, akinetic mutism, locked-in syndrome, coma and brain death. Many of these terms mean different things to different people and may prove inaccurate when transmitting and recording information regarding the state of consciousness of a patient. Nevertheless, it is appropriate to define several of the terms as closely as possible.

Three Levels of Consciousness

The totality of consciousness is comprised of three levels:

1. The subconscious.
2. The conscious.
3. The superconscious.

These levels of consciousness represent differing degrees of intensity of awareness.

Subconscious

The first level, the subconscious, is relatively dim in awareness; it is the stuff of which dreams are made. We may think of it as the repository of all remembered experiences, impressions left on the mind by those experiences and tendencies awakened or reinforced by those impressions. Every experience we have ever had, every thought, every impression of loss or gain, resides in the subconscious mind and determines our patterns of thought and behavior far more than we realize.

The subconscious, being unrestricted by the rigid demands of logic, permits a certain flow of ideas. This flow may border on intuition, but if the ideas are too circumscribed by subjectivity, they will not correspond with the external world around us. When we dream at night, we are mainly operating on the subconscious level.

The subconscious mind can all too easily intrude itself on our conscious awareness, tricking us into thinking we are getting intuitive guidance, when actually we are merely being influenced by past impressions and unfulfilled desires. The subconscious mind is in some ways close to the superconscious, where real intuition resides. Both represent a flow of awareness without logical obstructions. The subconscious is therefore more open to the intuitions of the superconscious and sometimes receives them, though usually mixed with confusing imagery. To be really clear in the guidance we receive is difficult, but very important. Calamitous decisions have been made in the belief that one was drawing on higher guidance, when in fact one was responding only to subconscious preconditioning.

Conscious

The next level of consciousness from which we receive guidance is the conscious state, the rational awareness that usually guides our daily decisions. When we receive input from the senses, analyze the facts and make decisions based on this information, we are using this conscious level of guidance. This process is also strongly affected by the opinions of others, which can cloud our ability to draw true guidance.

Dividing and separating the world into either category, the conscious level of awareness is problem-oriented. It is difficult to be completely certain of decisions drawn from this level, because the analytical mind can see all the possible solutions. But ultimately it does not have the ability to distinguish, which one is best. If we rely exclusively on the conscious mind, we may find ourselves lacking in certainty and slipping into a state of perpetual indecision.

Superconscious

Intuition and heightened mental clarity flow from superconscious awareness. The conscious mind is limited by its analytical nature and therefore sees all things as separate and distinct. We may be puzzled by a certain situation, but because it seems unrelated to other events, it is difficult to draw a clear course of action. By contrast, because the superconscious mind is unitive and sees all things as part of a whole, it can readily draw solutions. In superconsciousness the problem and the solution are seen as one, as though the solution was a natural outgrowth from the problem.

Altered Level of Consciousness

There is one more level of consciousness, altered levels of consciousness. In this level, the person needs a stimulus to respond. Without any stimulus, the person is unable to respond. It can be further classified into state of confusion, stupor, delirium, coma and obtundation. This level can be a result of some brain injury or brain disorders like inadequate supply of oxygen in the brain or extreme pressure from the skull, etc.

We all are at different levels of consciousness at different time so we possess different expressions and have a particular personality type. These levels sometimes become our identity. So we should always try to possess positive qualities. Negative qualities not only impact us, but also harm the sentiments of others. This is possible only when we always try to be in the state of consciousness.

Mnemonic for Causes of Altered Level of Consciousness

A – Alcohol, acidosis, anoxia
E – Epilepsy, environment
I – Insulin (diabetes)
O – Overdose
U – Uremia (metabolic), underdose
T – Trauma, toxins, tumors
I – Infection (sepsis)
P – Psychiatric disorders
S – Stroke cerebrovascular accident (CVA).

Altered Levels of Consciousness Include the Following Conditions

Confusion: A confused person cannot properly process all the information from their surroundings. Apathy and drowsiness are the most noticeable symptoms. The person may be disoriented, especially to time. A severely confused person is usually unable to carry out more than a few simple commands.

Delirium: This is a common and complicated problem, especially in the elderly. The signs of delirium include disorientation, which may be total. People with delirium may not remember who they are or may have delusions and hallucinations. People with delirium may also become drowsy or less alert at times.

Obtundation: A lower level of alertness typically characterizes this state. A person in this state often sleeps much more than usual and when awakened, remains drowsy and confused. Wakefulness can only be maintained by continuously talking to the person or through constant painful stimulation.

Stupor: Stupor is characterized by unresponsiveness from which a person can be aroused only by vigorous and repeated painful stimulation.

Coma: A person in a coma appears to be asleep, but cannot be awakened. Oftentimes reflexes are absent and the legs and arms may be rigid. The respiration rate is usually slowed for some persons in coma.

Causes

Trauma to the brain can cause impaired consciousness. Traumatic brain injury (TBI) is the leading cause of death and disability in young adults in the United State (US). Several types of head trauma may cause TBI. For example, a closed head injury—the most common TBI—can result, if the head rapidly accelerates or decelerates, causing the brain to move through the fluid in the skull and strike inside of the skull. Other causes include direct impact on the head or penetration by a foreign object such as a bullet.

Infections are common cause of impaired consciousness. The inflammation that accompanies infection is responsible for altered levels of consciousness (ALC). Encephalitis and meningitis are two nervous system specific infections that can cause ALC.

Defects in the metabolic system can lead to waste build-up that can cause ALC. As the body goes about, the normal processes needed to keep us alive, chemicals and other byproducts are produced. In most cases, byproducts get into the bloodstream and are filtered by the liver, kidneys and other organs. If one of these systems fails, waste products can build-up and act as a poison that interferes with the brain's ability to function. For example, the insulin/sugar imbalance of diabetes is a major metabolic problem that can cause impaired consciousness. Diabetes with low-blood insulin levels produce ketones, a toxic byproduct of fat metabolism. Conversely, when there is too much insulin, cells begin to starve to death. Either case can result in ALC.

Drug exposure is a common cause for ALC. Drug-induced ALC can result from an overdose of either over-the-counter or illegal drugs. Alcohol intoxication is probably the most common cause of drug-induced ALC. Similarly, exposure to certain readily available home or industrial chemicals can lead to changes in consciousness or even to death.

Structural abnormalities of the brain can lead to ALC. Tumors (benign or cancerous) can form and crowd out the normal structures of the brain. As a result, weakness in the walls of the blood vessels in the brain (aneurysms) may begin to swell or may even break, causing blood to pool inside the head and push the brain against the bony wall of the skull. The resulting damage can then cause ALC.

Pathophysiology

Although the neural science behind alertness, wakefulness and arousal are not fully known, the reticular formation is known to play a role in these. The ascending reticular activating system is a postulated group of neural connections that receives sensory input and projects to the cerebral cortex through the midbrain and thalamus from the reticular formation. Since this system is thought to modulate wakefulness and sleep, interference with it such as injury, illness or metabolic disturbances, could alter the level of consciousness.

NURSES ROLE AND RESPONSIBILITIES

Glasgow Coma Scale Measurement

Over the years, many assessment tools have been developed to improve neurological assessment. The most popular and universally used tool is the Glasgow coma scale (GCS), developed in 1974 by Teasdale and Jennett.

The GCS is divided into three sections: Eye opening, verbal responses and motor responses. The patient is assessed and scored in each area and the scores are added together to give the patient's GCS score—the highest possible score is 15 and the lowest possible score is 3. A patient who is fully aware and orientated score will be 15; a lower score will reflect the patient's level of consciousness (refer Table 13.2).

Pupil reaction is not included in the GCS, though it is often incorporated into locally adapted neurological observation charts.

Eye Opening

This should be spontaneous when the patient is approached. If the patient's eyes do not open spontaneously, determine whether they open to speech or painful stimuli. If the eyes are open, do not assume that the patient is fully aware and orientated to their surroundings. Some patients with head injuries may have spontaneous blinking and eye movement; this does not indicate full consciousness (Muxlow, 2000).

Table 13.2: Glasgow coma scale

Section	*Score*
Eye opening	
Spontaneous	4
To sound	3
To pain	2
None	1
Verbal response	
Oriented	5
Confused	4
Inappropriate words	3
Incomprehensible sounds	2
None	1
Motor response	
Obeys commands	6
Localizes stimulus	5
Withdrawal from stimulus	4
Abnormal flexion	3
(decorticate)	2
Abnormal extension	1
(decerebrate)	
Flaccid	
Total score possible	*3–15*

Verbal Response

This determines state of consciousness. Patients who are fully orientated will know their name, where they are, the date and year. A confused patient may be able to hold a conversation, but when asked questions may give replies, which are incorrect or inappropriate. They may use inappropriate words, which do not make sense to the assessor or they may make incomprehensible sounds such as moans or groans. Some stimuli may be required to obtain a response from the patient—this type of patient is not aware of their surroundings.

Motor Response

This is assessed by giving the patient some simple commands, for example, 'squeeze my hand (both sides)', 'lift your legs up off the bed' and 'show your tongue'. The strength of the patient's limbs should be noted—it is essential to observe for weaknesses. When a patient does not respond to simple commands, then response to painful stimuli is assessed.

The advantage of the GCS is that it is widely known and used and provides a standardized assessment of neurological observations. It is simple to use and requires only a pen torch with a bright beam and a copy of the assessment tool. However, Ellis and Cavanagh (cited in Woodrow, 2000) have noted that there may be variations in the recording of pupil size and motor weakness.

Inaccurate and inconsistent recordings could have a detrimental effect on the patient's well-being and may affect their care plan. Nurses therefore need to be educated in the correct use of the tool, in order to address potential irregularities.

CONCLUSION

The behavior is closely related to both physical and mental activity. Behavior means all the covert and overt activities of human being that cannot be observed. Both neural and chemical processes are important to understand the relationship between the brain and behavior. The state of mind can influence physical functioning and behavior, such as pain and stress. Therefore body and mind are interdependent on each other.

SUGGESTED READING

1. Adles C, Adles S. Biofeedback and Psychosomatic Disorders, 2nd edition. Baltimore: Lippincott Williams and Wilkins; 1989. pp. 10-89.
2. Carol Taylor, Carol Lillis, LeMone, et al. Fundamentals of Nursing, 5th edition. Philadelphia: Lippincott Williams and Wilkins; 2004. pp. 685-705.

3. Descartes René. Passions of the Soul (original French version published in 1649). Trans: Stephen Voss. Indianapolis: Hackett; 1989.
4. Dossey Montgomery B, Keegem L, Gazette Cathic. Holistic Nursing: A Handbook for Practice, 4th edition. Massachusetts: Janes and Basllett Publishers; 2004. pp. 5-898.
5. Edelman Gerald M. Wider than the Sky: The Phenomenal Gift of Consciousness. New Haven: Yale University Press; 2004.
6. Kim J, Honderich Ted. Problems in the Philosophy of Mind. Oxford Companion to Philosophy. Oxford University Press; 1995.
7. Kim J. Physicalism, or Something Near Enough. Princeton, NJ: Princeton University Press; 2005.
8. Lewith G, Kenyon J, Lewis P. Complementary Medicine: An Integrated Approach. Oxford University Press; 1998. pp. 36-8.
9. Lois White (Ed). Basic Nursing. Albany: Delmar; 2002. pp. 345-69.
10. Velmans Max, Susan Schneider (Eds). The Blackwell Companion to Consciousness. Malden, MASS: Blackwell; 2007.
11. Watson J. Applying the art and science of human caring. National League for Nursing Publ; 1994;42-2647:1-10.
12. William S. Theories of Consciousness: An Introduction and Assessment. London: Routledge; 1999.
13. Zelazo Philip David, Morris Moscovitch, Evan Thompson (Eds). Cambridge Handbook of Consciousness. Cambridge: Cambridge University Press; 2007.

REVIEW QUESTIONS

1. Explain 'body—the instrument of the mind'.
2. Discuss the effects of mind upon body.
3. Explain the theories of body-mind relationships.
4. Enumerate various levels of consciousness.
5. Define altered level of consciousness and explain the cause and pathology.
6. Describe the role and responsibilities of a nurse in care of altered level of consciousness.

CHAPTER

14 Biology and Behavior

LEARNING OBJECTIVES

1. To understand body and mind relationship.
2. To learn about behavior and neurosciences.

BEHAVIOR AND NEUROSCIENCE

Neuroscience is the field of study that examines the biological roots of behavior. This interdisciplinary includes the study of genetic factors, hormonal factors, neuroanatomy, drugs, developmental factors and environmental factors to team about brain-behaviors relations.

The human brain is the most complex of complicated structure in known universe. Scientists have estimated that the human brain is composed of about 180 million nerve cells, 50 million of which are devoted to processing information.

Major Activities of Brain

1. The brain monitors and controls our basic life-support system, such as breathing and digesting.
2. It directs our movements and maintains our balance and posture.
3. It receives and interprets information from the world around us.
4. It records significant and sometimes insignificant event into our memory.
5. It allows us to solve problems, use language and think of new ideas.

6. It enables us to feel materials such as soft cotton and to experience emotions such as happiness and snows.
7. Working together with the glands of the endocrine system and the rest of the nervous system.

Historical Review of Biology and Behavior

1. Early Greek and Roman physicians believed that behavioral problems were caused by imbalance of vital fluids that move through the body and brain. Only after the renaissance did, people accept the view that behaviors and thought were reduced by specific structures in the brain.
2. During the 19th century, neurologists performed autopsies on former patients and discovered the brain areas responsible for producing and comprehending speech. This work led to other discoveries that should the specific psychological functions were associated with specific brain areas.
3. Early in the 20th century, research on the physiological basic of behavior showed that when an area of the brain is destroyed, sometimes, remaining portions can take over its function. This view that different areas of the brain can be equivalent to one another is called equipotentiality theory.
4. According to integrationist theory, complex psychotic functions are based on number of basic abilities. These basic abilities may be involved in the same psychological function. Our thoughts and actions are a product of the functions of inter-related neural structures.
5. Today, neuropsychologists use a variety of procedures to learn about brain-behavior relation. Much of this work is based on studies of laboratory animals. They perform brain operations to see, how the removal or destruction of brain tissue in a particular area affects. Now, the medical imaging technique makes it possible to examine the living brain.

Relationship Between Mind and Body

The nervous system is the primary seat of the vibrating mind in the human body. The nervous system is pervasive throughout the body. There are even nerves in the walls of arteries; thus, there are few parts of the body that escape domination or at least contact by the mind. This means that the mind and body genuinely cannot be separated.

Thus, the relationship between them is that there is no relationship. They are the same thing—at least for as long as the body is alive. Once a body dies, then the nervous system is left to physically decay with mind long gone or dissipated depending on beliefs.

NEURON

The nerve cells called 'neurons' are the basic units of operation in nervous system. By themselves, though they cannot explain the complexities of thought and emotion. It is only when the nerves are arranged into complicated patterns by become of producing action and thought.

Basic Neural Processes

1. The nervous system is basically constellated from only two different types of cells, nerve cells; the neurons receive and transmit neural signals to other parts of the body.
2. Glial cells: the more numerous of the two, support and protect the neurons. Glial cells take their name from the French word for glue. They form a connective network that holds together the brain's billions of neurons.
3. The glial cells insulate non neuron from another throughout the nervous system and clear away cellular debris when neurons degenerate and die.
4. A continuous layer of glia surround the blood vessels in the brain to establish a blood-brain barrier, a protective shield that prevents many harmful chemical substances from passing the blood to brain.

Structure of Neuron

1. Neurons are of many different shapes and sizes, but they share certain anatomical features. Neurons have a cell body, dendrites and an axon.
2. The cell body consists of a membrane boundary that surrounds the nucleus and internal contents of the cell. The nucleus in the portion of cell that contains deoxyribonucleic acid (DNA) strands of protein that holds the genetic blueprint for the cells makeup and function. Neuropsychological—field of psychology that represents the convergence of this scientific discipline is called neuropsychology.

3. The cell also contains protoplasmic material that manufactures chemical substances used to communicate with other neurons.
4. Reaching out from the cell body like the branches of the tree, dendrites receive information from other neurons. The longer and more complex a neuron's dendrites, the greater number of connections it can make with other cells.
5. Neural signals are transmitted to other cells by the axon, a single fiber that emerges from the cell body. Axons in the brain are usually less than 1 mm long. But axons from the spinal cord to the brain can reach lengths of 3 feet or more.
6. The chemical substances can travel in both directions along on axon and more than one type of chemical messages can be passed to the receptors of an adjacent cell.
7. Myelin sheath—axons are usually coated with an insulating material called a myelin sheath that is produced by the glial cells. Myelin also helps to prevent the scrabbling of neural messages.
8. Nodes of Ranvier, periodic breaks in the myelin sheath, which cause the axon to resemble a beaded necklace, are called nodes of Ranvier. These nodes allow axons with myelin insulation to transmit neural signals faster than uninsulated axon can, because the signals can be transmitted along the axon by jumping from one node to the next.

Neural Impulses and their Transmission

1. When a neuron is sufficiently stimulated by another neuron, there is an electrical reaction in the walls of the axon that travels over the entire length of the walls of the axon terminals.
2. The electrical reaction is called the neural impulse, depending upon the diameter of the axon and the thickness of the myelin sheath, a neural impulse travels at a rate of approximately 2 to 2,000 miles per hour.

Neural Firing

1. Neural impulses are generated by electrochemical processes involving the cell membrane.
2. When a nerve cell is strongly stimulated by another cell, there is a chemical change in the cell membrane; the membrane becomes permeable causing positively charged ions from outside to enter and negatively charged ions from inside to exit.

3. This change quickly reverses the cell membrane electrical charge at the point of stimulation and causes the adjacent portion of the cell membrane to reverse its charge as well.
4. For a neuron to generate an impulse, it must receive a certain level of stimulation. This is called the threshold level, the neuron fires in a uniform and unchanging way.
5. Neuron can fire even without outside stimulation. There is a baseline level of spontaneous activity in each neuron as it lays waiting for new stimulation. That stimulation can come either in the form of excitatory influences that increases.
6. Drugs that have psychological effects often have an excitatory or inhibitory influence on neural firing. For example, the local anesthetic such as Novocain inhibits neural firing. Novocain blocks the conduction of the action potential along the axon.
7. Epilepsy itself provides a vivid example of the powerful influences that basic neural processes have on behavior. Dilantin is effective in berating firing of neurons.

Synoptic Transmission

1. Neurons not only fire but also they communicate with other cells to generate and to create an informational network that links the various parts of the body.
2. The billions of neurons in the brain produce at least 10 billion synoptic connections. A typical neuron may have several thousands of these synapses, small gaps separating the nerve cells.
3. The electrical impulse that has traveled down the axon of the transmitting cell must be converted into a chemical messenger that stimulates another neuron across the synaptic junction.
4. In neurological terms, the transmitting cell is called the presynaptic neuron, the receiving cell is called the postsynaptic neuron and the chemical messenger is known as the neurotransmitter. Since, neurotransmitter affects other cells chemically; this means the most drugs messengers that are transmitted from one cell to another.

NEUROTRANSMITTERS AND BEHAVIOR

Neurotransmitters are manufactured in the pragmatic neuron and stored in tiny sacs called vesicles, located in the axon terminals of the pragmatic neuron, it forces the vesicles to break, like cannon firing a burst of shells and the vesicles shoot their chemical contents, the molecules of the neurotransmitter, into the synaptic junction.

A receptor site is simply a portion of an adjacent neuron that receives the molecules of a neurotransmitter. Since, there are specific receptor sites, different types of neurotransmitters will key into a given receptor site.

Types of Neurotransmitters

Acetylcholine

1. Location: brain, neuromuscular junction and in the peripheral nervous system. It may be critical for normal thinking.
2. Effects: deficiency of acetylcholine (ACh) causes paralysis, Alzheimer's disease. Excess may cause violent muscle contraction. Drugs that increase ACh in cerebral cortex appear to help teaming and retention.

Amino Acids

1. Location: Brain, used by neurons for fast excitation and inhibition. Glutamic acid and aspartic acid for excitation. Gamma-aminobutyric acid and glycine for inhibition.
2. The effects of amino acids are linked to the control of anxiety. The deficiency causes mental deterioration (Huntington's chorea).

Catecholamine

1. Location: Brain and peripheral nervous system; it includes both dopamine and norepinephrine (NE).
2. Dopamine plays major role in the regulation of movement deficiencies causes Parkinson's disease; excess may cause major disturbances of thought, perception and emotion behavior.
3. NE affects arousal and mood; deficiency causes depression, excess causes agitation and manic condition.

Neuropeptides

1. Location: Brain—released during painful or stressful situation, end options.
2. Neuropetides causes pain reduction and may be involved in eating, memory, sexual behavior and mood.

Serotonin

1. Location: central nervous system (CNS), influences sleep and body temperature.
2. Deficiency of serotonin causes depression.

Action of Neurotransmitters

1. The excitatory or inhibitory influence can change a neuron's threshold for firing. These excitatory or inhibitory influences are determined by the synaptic cells.
2. Synaptic sites at dendrites tend to be excitatory, while synaptic sites at the cell body tend to be inhibitory.
3. Consequently, a neurotransmitter at an inhibitory synapse will make it less likely to fire. At any given time, a cell receives neurotransmitters from various receptor sites.
4. The postsynaptic neuron, analyzes the incoming excitatory and inhibitory signals and fires only if the net level of stimulation passes its firing threshold.
5. When this threshold is reached, the electrical to chemical, chemical to electrical transmission process is almost complete.
6. All that remains are for the neurotransmitter to be deactivated, to that the postsynaptic neuron can be stimulated again.

Deactivation or Reuptake

1. Deactivation can occur in one of two ways, first an enzyme at the synapse can breakdown the neurotransmitters.
2. Second, the neurotransmitter can return to the presynaptic neuron. This process is called reuptake and it is the most common form of deactivation.
3. Deactivation is crucial. Without it the nervous system would become overstimulated, this would lead to tremors and eventually death.
4. Some insecticides and nerve gases produce their deadly effects by blocking the deactivation of neurotransmitters at the neuromuscular junctions; thus, victims die due to uncontrolled muscle spasms.

Neurotransmitters and Diseases

Depression

A group of drugs called tricycles, among the most successful in relieving depression, are believed to increase the availability of both neurotransmitters in certain areas of the brain. The recent research that the antidepressant effects of these drugs may be related to increased sensitivity of the receptors for those two neurotransmitters (NE and serotonin) rather than a mere change in the actual levels of these brain chemicals.

Drug-related Behaviors

A wide variety of commonly used drugs have the effect of exchanging thought processes, emotional states or behaviors.

Extensive research has linked the brain opiates to an array of behavioral and mental processes, including a sense of well-being and euphoria, counteracting the influence of stress, modulating food and liquid intake, facilitating learning and memory and reducing anxiety.

ENDOCRINE SYSTEM AND BEHAVIOR

The endocrine system is a chemical communication network that sends messages throughout the nervous system and accretes hormone that affect body growth and functioning. Although the endocrine system is thought of a distinct form of the brain, nervous system and sense organs, it has important functional relationships with these statures.

Concepts on Behavior

1. About 300 years ago, the French philosopher René Descartes proposed that the pineal gland is the point of interaction between the soul and the body.
2. The endocrine glands are distinguished from duct glands. Also, they are said to be ductless because they secrete their products, chemical messengers called hormones, which directly enter into the bloodstream.
3. The duct glands secrete their substances into body cavities or the surface of the body. Examples of duct glands are the salivary, digestive and tear glands.

Pituitary Gland

1. The pituitary gland is located at the base of the skull, near the hypothalamus, as is about the size of a pea. It is sometimes,

called the master gland in view of the fact its hormones often play the role of triggering the activity of other endocrine glands.

2. One of the key hormones released by the pituitary is the growth hormone, which controls a number of metabolic functions, including the rate of growth of the bones and soft tissues.
3. The pituitary also produces a number of huge protein molecules called neuropeptides, the substances that control acts such as eating and drinking, sexual behaviors, sleep, temperature refutation, pain reduction, etc.

Thyroid Gland

The thyroid gland, located within the neck, responds to pituitary stimulation by releasing the hormone thyroxin.

The principle function associated with the thyroidal gland is the control of body metabolism, the rate at which a person burns glucose, circulating in the bloodstream.

The metabolism is in turn closely linked to motivational and mood states. The thyroid has important impact on behavior.

Parathyroid Glands

The four parathyroid glands are found behind the thyroid gland itself. They are small glands and they secrete a hormone that regulates the metabolism of calcium and phosphorus.

Disorders of the parathyroid glands could bring about defective above development during a child's early years of development.

Adrenal Gland

The adrenals are pair of glands; located just above each kidney that influences our emotional state, level of energy and ability to cope with stress.

They consist of two parts, an inner core called the adrenal medulla and outer layer called the adrenal cortex. The medulla produces epinephrine and NE; making the heart beat faster, diverting blood from the stomach and intestine to the voluntary muscles.

At times of stress, the hypothalamus causes the pituitary to release adrenocorticotropic hormone (ACTH), which in turn stimulates the adrenal cortex to increase its secretion of a number of hormones to influence metabolism.

Thymus Gland

1. The thymus gland is located below the thyroid gland and under the breastbone.
2. The thymus gland appears to play its major role in infancy and childhood.

Secreting a hormone associated with the body's capacity to resist infection. When a child has an infection, the thymus sends a message to the spleen and the lymph node. The message tells these structures that they should produce lymphocytes, cleaning cells that attack foreign organisms in the bloodstream. Once the body's immune system is developed, the thymus loses some of its functional role.

Pancreas Gland

The pancreas gland secretes two important hormones, insulin and glucagon.

Insulin is the hormone that induces the oxidation or burning of blood sugar. If a person's pancreas is defective and it is unable to secrete adequate amount of insulin, the person will suffer from diabetes or chronic high blood sugar.

Gonads

There are two types of gonads. These are the ovaries in female and testes in the male.

The ovaries are located in the vicinity of the uterus, one ovary on either side. In addition to producing egg cells, they also produce hormone. Estrogen is identified as playing a principle role in determining secondary female characteristics, such as breast development and lack of facial hair.

Progesterone cooperates with estrogen in the regulation of ovulation and in the preparation of the uterus for pregnancy.

Testosterone plays an important role in determining secondary male characteristics such as facial hair, voice depth and muscular development.

GENETICS AND BEHAVIOR

Genetics is the study of how traits are inherited or passed on from parent to child. The cells from which we started, contain genes that are the basic units of heredity. They determine our sequence of growth into a human baby. Genes determine our blood group, coloration and many other traits. In general, genes determine the resemblance between the newborn and the parents.

General Concepts of Genetics

1. Genes are located in the nucleus of every cell in the body. They are composed of DNA, which contains blueprints for life. Living organisms are made of protein and DNA controls the way in which protein chains are built.
2. Material for constructing protein surrounds cells and DNA sends out messenger molecules ribonucleic acid (RNA), to control how the material is fashioned into specific kinds of protein chains.
3. Every living cell contains 20,000 to 125,000 genes grouped together in cluster of a thousand or more. They are arranged in thread-like chains called chromosomes.
4. The cells in human body have 46 chromosomes, arranged in 23 pairs. We inherit one member of each pair from father and the other from mother.
5. Genes are transmitted from generation to generation by means of sex cells. A female gamete is called ovum and a male gamete is called sperm.
6. Ovum and sperm combine their chromosomes, when they unite to form one cell called a zygote. Thus, zygotes have 46 chromosomes, half from the father, which determine genotype or genetic inheritance for the rest of lives.

Genetic Errors

1. Errors are made occasionally in transmitting genes from one generation to the next. As a result, children are sometimes born with abnormal chromosome structures, which are called mutations.
2. Two Xs and a Y: People with an XXY mutation, often have characteristics of both sexes. They might have developed breasts and small testicles.
3. Two Ys and an X: Males with an extra Y chromosome (XYY) are often taller than other males. On the other hand, XYY males in the general population are no more aggressive than normal males.

4. Another kind of genetic mutation is one in which a person has 47 chromosomes, because of an extra one added to pair 21.
5. Children with chromosomal abnormalities suffer from Down syndrome, a disorder characterized by mental retardation and unique physical appearances, including folds on the eyelid corners, round face, head with a flattened back, short neck and small nose.

Causes of Mutation

1. Some people carry mutator genes that increase the rate of mutations in other genes.
2. High temperatures can increase mutation rate. Males generate sperm in their scrotum, a sac that is usually cooler than the rest of the body in mammals.
3. Radiation has been linked to mutation rate, X-rays are one source of radiation and pregnant women are advised to avoid them.
4. Radiation before pregnancy may also increase mutation rate. Recent evidence suggests, the exposure to radiation may explain the increased risk of having Down syndrome babies for older mothers.

Genetic and Behavioral Problems

Genetic Influences and Schizophrenia

While research and debate continue over the role of biological factors and life experience in schizophrenia, a consensus in forming on one major point. Genetic factors play a role. One of the studies that have convinced many people involves identical and fraternal twins. Identical twin pairs have identical heredity, fraternal twin pairs do not so, if schizophrenia is strongly influenced by genes.

Genetic Factors and Depression

The cognitive learning or life experience factors may be involved in depression; many investigations believe that biological factors also play a role. Some physiological deficit, either inherited or acquired in other ways, is thought to make some people, especially vulnerable, to depressive episodes. We have known for some time that hereditary factors play a role in some depression.

CONCLUSION

The term behavior is used extensively in psychology. Its scope is not limited to physical activities but includes all sense organs (eyes, ears, tongue, skin and nose), all activities of brain (concentration, imagination, thought, effort, memory, intellect, etc.). Thus, human behavior includes all activities and this indicates the concept of Woodworth that psychology is the science of activities. It is very important to study the health, behavior of man from the point of community health because human behavior is a result of complex interaction between body and mind. The inter-relation between physical and mental processes affects the total health of individual.

SUGGESTED READING

1. Arnold MB (Ed). The Nature of Emotion. Baltimore: Penguin; 1968.
2. Bandura A. Principles of Behaviour Modification. New York: Holt, Rinehart and Winston; 1969.
3. Carlson NR. Psychology of Behaviour. Boston: Allyn and Bacon; 1977.
4. Ferguson ED. Motivation: An Experimental Approach. New York: Holt, Rinehart and Winston; 1976.
5. Goddard FA. The Human Senses, 2nd edition. New York: Wily; 1972.
6. Hochberg JE. Perception, 2nd edition. Englewood Cliffs, NJ: Prentice Hall; 1978.
7. Korman AK. The Psychology of Motivation. Englewood Cliffs, NJ: Prentice Hall; 1974.
8. Lindsay PH, Norman DA. Human Information Processing, 2nd edition. New York: Academic Press; 1977.
9. Morgan CT. A Brief Introduction to Psychology. New Delhi: Tata McGraw-Hill; 1975.
10. Morgan CT, King RA. Introduction to Psychology, 6th edition. New Delhi: Tata McGraw-Hill; 1982.
11. Mueller CG. Sensory Psychology. Englewood Cliffs, NJ: Prentice-Hall; 1965.
12. Munn Norman L. Introduction to Psychology, New Delhi: Oxford and IBH; 1973.
13. Robinson DN. An Intellectual History of Psychology, New York: Macmillan; 1976.

14. Strongman KT. The Psychology of Emotion New York: Wiley; 1973.
15. Thompson RF. Introduction to Physiological Psychology. New York: Harper and Row; 1975.

REVIEW QUESTIONS

1. Define neuron. Explain the structure of neuron.
2. Define neurotransmitters. Explain the types of neuro-transmitters.
3. Explain endocrine system and behavior.
4. Discuss genetics and behavior.

CHAPTER

15

Educational Psychology

LEARNING OBJECTIVES

1. Educational psychology—meaning and definition.
2. Nature of educational psychology.
3. Importance of educational psychology.
4. Aims and objectives of educational psychology.
5. General categories of educational psychology.
6. Concept of education.
7. Values of educational psychology.
8. Elements of educational psychology.

INTRODUCTION

Educational psychology provides a base to education. It studies the problem, which crop up in the education of the children. Educational psychology has its primary concern with a viewpoint, with the organization of information and with group of techniques and activities for a sound education. It is an area of experiment, not a collection of specific subject matter.

Through this subject the contents, techniques and ways of functioning of psychology are applied in the solution of the problems of the classroom. It may be remembered that educational psychology is not merely general psychology applied to educational problems. The number of researches in various areas connected with educational psychology is increasing at a phenomenal rate.

NATURE

1. Psychology is a science, which studies all the aspects of human behavior. It concerned with the reasons of human behavior and with those principles, which may predict a behavior and bring modifications in it.
2. Education is mainly a social process. The chief aim of it is to modify behavior. In this sense, both education and psychology are similar. From the fusion of psychology and education, we get that branch of psychology, which we call educational psychology.
3. Educational psychology is the study of human behavior as it is influenced by the social process. It also studies those processes, which provide an understanding of the way in which the modifications are brought in the behavior.
4. Educational psychology has its own applied theory. This theory is as basic as the theory underlying the discipline of psychology.

DEFINITIONS

1. Educational psychology is that special branch of psychology concerned with the nature, conditions, outcome and evaluation of school learning, and retention. —*Ausubel*
2. Educational psychology is that branch of psychology, which deals with teaching and learning. —*Skinner*
3. Educational psychology describes and explains the learning experiences of an individual from birth through old age. —*Crow and Crow*

SCOPE

Scope of the subject implies its field of study. Speaking in specific terms, it means the areas of study that are included in a particular subject.

The scope of educational psychology is securing greater and greater importance in the field of education. Educational psychology is the combination of two, i.e. educational and psychology. So, educational psychology is the study of behavior of the teacher, taught and persons connected to educational environment.

Educational psychology is, therefore, that branch of educational content, which deals with human behavior and its modification. The following are included in the scope of educational psychology.

Human behavior: It studies human behavior in educational situations. Psychology is the study of behavior and education deals with the modification of behavior and hence, educational psychology pervades in whole field of education.

Growth and development: It studies growth and development of the child. How a child passes through various stages of growth and what are the characteristics of each stage are included in the study of educational psychology.

Learning process: It studies the law of learning. Learning is a major phenomenon in education. It studies how learning can take place most effectively and economically.

Heredity and environment: To what extent heredity and environment contribute toward the growth of the individual and how this knowledge can be used for bringing about the optimum development of the child, form a salient feature of the scope of educational psychology.

Personality: Educational psychology deals with the nature and development of the personality of an individual. In fact, education has been defined as an all-round development of the personality of an individual; personality development also implies a well-adjusted personality.

Individual difference: Every individual differs from another and it is one of the fundamental facts of human nature, which has been brought to light by educational psychology. This one fact has revolutionized the concept and process of education.

Intelligence and its measurement: The scope of educational psychology includes the study of the nature of intelligence, as well as its measurement. This is of great importance for a teacher or an educator.

Guidance and counseling: This is one of the most important fields or areas of study included in the field of educational psychology. Education is nothing, but providing guidance to the growing child. Thus, guidance forms an important aspect of educational psychology.

The following five areas were named by American Psychological Associations:

1. Human growth and development, including the effect of heredity and environment on various aspects of individual.
2. Learning: The nature of learning process, factors influencing the learning process, etc.
3. Personality and adjustment: It includes many subtopics such as mental health of the students and teachers character.
4. Measurement and evaluation statistics.
5. Techniques and methods of educational psychology.

Thus, educational psychology describes and explains the learning experience of an individual from birth to old age. Its subject matter is concerned with the conditions that affect learning.

IMPORTANCE

1. Educational psychology helps in the realization of educational aims.
2. It offers new viewpoints.
3. It ensures proper discipline in the proper manner.
4. It sets forth proper techniques and methods of teaching.
5. It keeps the educator informed about individual differences.
6. It helps in the understanding of group behavior.
7. It asks the teacher to teach according to the stages of development of the child.
8. It emphasizes the role of the learner.

AIMS AND OBJECTIVES

1. Developing proper attitudes in the teacher.
2. Assisting the teacher to set up appropriate educational situations.
3. Helping the teachers in teaching their pupils sympathetically and impartially.
4. Helping them in the organization of the subject matter.
5. Helping them to have a clear understanding of social relationships.
6. Assisting the teacher to understand their own job.
7. Making the teacher conversant with methods and techniques for the analysis of his/her and others behavior.

8. Organizing the proper guidance programs.
9. Guiding the administrators.
10. Helping them in planning out the proper evaluation techniques.
11. Furnishing the teacher with proper method.

GENERAL CATEGORIES

1. Learning is the most frequent topic in the field is by far.
2. Readiness of learning, which includes the phenomena of interest, aptitude and motivation.
3. Mental health and social adjustment, which focus on the noncognitive purposes of the school and correlates of intellectual learning.
4. Measurement and evaluation, which comprises the techniques for assessing the education growth of learners, diagnosing learning problems and clarifying the criteria to be used in an evaluation of the school.

CONCEPTS OF EDUCATION

1. Education modifies the behavior. It brings such changes in the behavior of a child, which is for their good. In the past, the education of a child meant the filling up of the child's mind with stuffed knowledge.
2. The modern education aims at the harmonious development of the personality of the child. The schools and the teachers are to create such situation, where the personality can be developed freely and fully.
3. Education is a social process; its main concern is the modification of behavior. Thus educational psychology studies the human behavior as it is influenced by the social process of education.
4. It also studies and investigates those processes that lead to the understanding of the way in which behavior is modified through education.
5. Education psychology constitutes the foundations of education. It provides an approach to educational problems and set of techniques for studying children, and problems that arise in their function.

Psychological Basis of Education

1. Psychology deals with response to any and every kind of situation, the life presents. Educational psychology deals with the behavior of the human being in educational situations.
2. To make an estimate of the value of educational psychology, it is necessary to understand the modern concept of education.
3. Education provides both experiences to the individual and their adjustment to the environment. It is also a process, which is individualistic as well as social in its nature.
4. The bringing of psychological basis in education has resulted in completely overhauling the outlook on education. Now, education is a much more pleasant process than what it was. Information and instructions are replaced by the words help and guidance. Love, sympathy and play are considered most important in the educational process.

VALUES OF EDUCATIONAL PSYCHOLOGY

1. The study of educational psychology should develop the student's interest in people, both children and adults and help him/her to understand them.
2. The study on educational psychology should have a favorable effect on the attitudes, behaviors and psychological understanding of students in both personal and professional relationship.
3. The study of educational psychology should enable the students, to use the body of knowledge that is derived from research studies in this field and that helps to explain the way in which learning occurs.
4. The study of educational psychology should improve the effectiveness of the prospective teacher's ability to learn.
5. The study of educational psychology should foster the student's appreciation and understanding of research on education.

Major Subdivisions of Educational Psychology

1. Psychology and education.
2. Human growth and development.
3. Learning.

4. Personality and adjustments.
5. Group psychology.
6. Measurement and evaluation.
7. Statistical and research methods.

ELEMENTS OF EDUCATIONAL PSYCHOLOGY

Learner

In educational process, the learner occupies the most important place. There can be no teaching without there being a learner. By the learner we mean the pupils, who individually or collectively comprise the classroom group.

The teaching in the classroom to a great extent depends on the personality's developmental stages and psychological problems of the students.

Learning Process

Learning process is the process by which people acquire changes in their behavior, improve performance, recognize their thinking or discover new ways of behaving and new concepts, and information.

This process may be directly observable as while the pupils learn writing, computing, talking, etc. or may be indirectly observable as in perceiving, thinking and remembering. The concern of the educational psychologist is with the way in which the learning process takes place.

Learning Situations

Learning situations refers to the environment in which the learner find himself/herself and in which the learning process takes place.

The teacher's attitude, classroom setting, emotional climate of the school and interest, community takes in the school affairs, may all form the part of the learning situations.

LIMITATIONS OF EDUCATIONAL PSYCHOLOGY

The application of educational psychology can be made in a limited manner keeping in view, the nature of teaching. In accordance with the nature of teaching, the experience, interest, attitude, etc. are as essential for a teacher as the knowledge of psychology.

The educational psychology is limited to the extent that the testing of facts or search of new facts is only helpful in arriving at a decision. They do not lead automatically to ultimate decisions or judgments. The educational psychology is bound by the boundaries of psychology.

CONCLUSION

Educational psychology is nothing, but one of the branches of applied psychology. It is an attempt to apply the knowledge of psychology to the field of education. It consists of the application of the psychological principles and techniques to human behavior in educational situations. In other words, educational psychology is the study of the experiences and behavior of the learner in relation to educational environment.

SUGGESTED READING

1. Aggarwal JC. Educational Research: An Introduction. New Delhi: Arya Book Depot; 1975.
2. Aggarwal JC. Essentials of Educational Technology. New Delhi: Vikas Publications; 1996.
3. Ausubel DP, Robinson FG. School Learning: An Introduction to Educational Psychology. New York: Holtt Rinehart and Winston Inc; 1969.
4. Best JW. Research in Education Englewood Cliffs. New Jersey: Prentice-Hall; 1970.
5. Dandapani S. Advanced Educational Psychology. New Delhi: Anmol Publications (P) Ltd; 2000.
6. Garrett HE. Statistics in Psychology and Education. Bombay: Vakils, Feffer and Simons Ltd; 1966.
7. Hilgard ER, Atkinson RL, Atkinson RC. Introduction to Psychology, 7th edition. New York: Harcourt Brace Jovanovich Inc; 1979.
8. Kasinath HM. Advance Educational Psychology. Gadag: Vidyanidhi Prakashan Muralidhar; 2000.
9. Koul L. Methodology of Educational Research. Vikas Publishing House (P) Ltd; 1984.
10. Richmond K. The Concept of Educational Technology. London: Kogan Page Ltd; 1970.

11. Sampath K, Panneerselvam A, Santhanam S. Introduction to Educational Technology. New Delhi: Sterling Publishers; 1981.
12. Seetharamu AS. Philosophies of Education. New Delhi: Ashish Publishing House; 1989.
13. Sodhi, Sandhu, Singh. Philosophies of Education. Ambala Cantt: The Indian Publication; 1989.
14. Srivastava SK. Tradition and Modernization Process and Change in India. Allahabad: Indian International Publication; 1976.
15. Tuckman Bruce W. Conducting Educational Research. New York: Harcourt Brace; 1972.

REVIEW QUESTIONS

1. Define educational psychology. Explain the scope and importance of educational psychology.
2. Explain the aims and objectives of educational psychology.
3. Define education. Explain the values of educational psychology.
4. Describe the elements of educational psychology.
5. Enumerate the limitations of educational psychology.

CHAPTER

16 Thinking and Reasoning

LEARNING OBJECTIVES

1. Definitions.
2. Nature of thinking.
3. Types of thinking.
4. Characteristics.
5. Tools of thinking.
6. Stages, elements.
7. Reasoning and creative thinking.
8. Problem solving.

INTRODUCTION

The primary basis of man's progress is thinking. Many problems can be solved with the help of thinking. Various processes of teaching are accomplished due to thinking only. It is possible to change the attitudes and thoughts of a person through thinking. Perception, memory, imagination and reason are included in thinking. Therefore, thinking is considered to be a complex process. Thinking is an incredibly complex process and a most difficult concept in psychology to define or explain. Thinking, the mental solution of problems, makes use of the symbols of objects instead of the objects. Thinking attempts the solution of problems by employing the trial and error method. There is a kind of flow in the activity of thinking; one problem leading to the thinking of another by reminding the person of that other problem.

NATURE OF THINKING

Thinking is the process of mentally solving the problems. It includes a flow of thoughts. Thoughts continue to come one after the other and this internal process continues till they are expressed. Here, attempts are made to solve the problems through trial and error method. If the person arises, its solution is sought through thinking or any new thought is evolved. Along with analysis, thinking also involves synthesis, foresight and hindsight. Here, one thinks about tangible objects through intangible signs and symbols, here thinking is a symbolic behavior.

The main form of thinking is reason and this is a process of mental research, healthy, saves time and behavior.

1. Thinking is essentially a cognitive activity.
2. It is always directed to achieve some end or purpose. In genuine thinking, we cannot let our thoughts wonder on without any definite end in mind; as happens in the case of daydreaming and imagination.
3. Thinking is described as a problem-solving behavior. From the beginning to the end, there is some problem around which the whole process of thinking revolves. But every problem-solving behavior is not thinking. It is only related to the inner cognitive behavior.
4. In thinking, there is mental exploration instead of motor exploration. One has to suspend immediately one's overt or motor activities, while engaging in thinking through some or other types of mental exploration.
5. Thinking is a symbolic activity. In thinking, there is a mental solution of the problem, which is carried out through some signs, symbols and mental images.
6. Thinking can shift very rapidly, covering an expanse of time and space, almost instantaneously.

DEFINITIONS OF THINKING

1. Thinking is the cognitive process that begins with the problem or work facing the person. It includes trial and error, but is affected by the readiness of person and ultimately it ends at the solution of problem or conclusion. —*Warren*
2. In strict psychological discussion, it is well to keep the thinking for an activity, which consists essentially of a connected flow of ideas, which are directed towards some end or purpose. —*Valentine*
3. Thinking is a mental activity in its cognitive aspect or mental activity with regard to psychological objects. —*Ross*

4. Thinking is behavior, which is often implicit and hidden, and in which symbols (images, ideas and concepts) are ordinarily employed. —*Garrett*
5. Thinking is an implicit problem-solving behavior. —*Mohsin*
6. Thinking is a problem-solving process in which we use the symbols in place of overt activity. —*Gilmer*
7. Thinking is the organization and reorganization of current learning in the present circumstances, with the help of learning and past experiences. —*Vinake*
8. Thinking is a perceptual relationship, which provides for the solution of the problem. —*Maier*
9. Thinking is a complex cognitive form of behavior, which occurs only at a relatively advanced stage of development, when simpler and more direct methods of dealing with environment have proved ineffective and simple memory is adequate to solve problem, thinking occurs. —*Whittaker*

TYPES OF THINKING

Imaginative Thinking

Here, thinking takes place without any basic sensory stimulus. Daydreaming and only being aware of future plans are major examples of imaginative thinking.

Creative Thinking

Creative thinking is related to creative activities; it is the basis of adopting new thoughts and attitudes in life, inventions, research and other creative activities. Creative thinking is chiefly aimed at creating something new. It is in search of new relationship and associations to describe and interpret the nature of things, events and situations. It is not bounded by any pre-established rules. Creative thinkers are great boons to the society, as they enrich the knowledge of mankind.

Positive Thinking

Here, the thoughts of person are of optimistic and positive point of view. This type of thinking identifies the good mental health.

Negative Thinking

Here, the person gives more importance to negative thoughts. This type of thinking is not good for health.

Perceptual or Concrete Thinking

Perceptual or concrete thinking is the simple form of thinking. The basis of this type of thinking is perception, i.e. interpretation of sensation according to one's experience. It is also named as concrete thinking, as it is carried over the perception of actual or concrete objects and events.

Conceptual or Abstract Thinking

Conceptual or abstract thinking does not require the perception of actual objects or events. It is also called abstract thinking, as it makes the use of concepts or abstract ideas. It is superior to perceptual thinking, as it economizes efforts in understanding and helps in discovery and invention. It is an abstract thinking, where one makes use of concepts, the generalized ideas and language. It economizes effects in understanding and problem solving.

Non-directed or Associative Thinking

In strict psychological sense, what we have discussed above in terms of the types of categories of thinking, constitutes real or genuine thinking. It is essentially a directed thinking, which pertains to reasoning and problem-solving procedure aimed at meeting specific goals.

Reflective Thinking

Reflective thinking is somewhat of a higher form of thinking. It can be distinguished from simple thinking in the following ways:

1. It aims at solving complex problems rather than simple problems.
2. It requires reorganization of all the relevant experiences and finding new ways of reacting to a situation or of removing an obstacle, instead of simple association of experiences or ideas.
3. Mental activity in reflective thinking does not undergo any mechanical trial and error type of effort. There is an insightful cognitive approach in reflective thinking.
4. It takes logic into account in which all the relevant facts are arranged in a logical order, in order to get to the solution of the problem in hand.

CHARACTERISTICS OF THINKING

A number of mental processes are included in thinking, which are as follows:

1. Thinking is affected by motives.
2. Thinking begins from general to specialty.
3. Analysis and synthesis have an important role in thinking.
4. Thought and language are very important in thinking.
5. Thinking begins with the beginning of problem.
6. Thinking can solve problem.
7. Brain remains active during thinking process.
8. Thinking enjoys challenges.
9. Thinking makes us able to suspend judgments.
10. Thinking challenges assumptions.
11. Thinking seeks problems as opportunities.

TOOLS OF THINKING

Images

The images, as mind pictures, are constant of personal experiences of objects, persons or scenes, once actually seen, heard or felt. These mind pictures symbolize the actual objects, experiences and activities. In thinking, we usually manipulate the images instead of actual objects, experiences and activities. The uses of images in thinking depend on no small measure upon the method of thinking, which the individual employs. Some people use other symbols in their thinking, instead of images.

Concepts

Concepts are the abstract forms of past experiences. Humanity is the quality of the human species, found equally in all human beings. A concept is a general idea that stands for a general class and represents the common property of all the objects or events of this general class. The concepts as a tool, economize our efforts in thinking. Concept is formed with the help of abstraction of mind. Concepts extend the limits of thinking to include both the past and the future. Reasoning cannot be done without concepts, which are both the past and the future.

Symbols and Signs

These represent and stand as substitutes for actual objects, experiences and activities. In this sense, they cannot be confined to words and mathematical numerals and terms. Traffic lights, railway signals, school bells, badges, songs, flags and slogans all stand for the symbolic expression. These symbols and signs stimulate and economize thinking.

Language

Language is the most efficient and developed vehicle used for carrying out the process of thinking. When one listens, reads or writes words, phrases or sentences, or observes gesture in any language, one is stimulated to think. Reading and writing of the written documents and literature, also helps in stimulating and promoting the thinking process.

Muscle Activities

Thinking in one way or the other shows evidence of the involvement of a slight incipient movement of groups of muscles. It can be easily noticed that there are slight muscular responses when we think of a word, resembling the movements used when we utter the word aloud. A high positive correlation has been found to exist between the thinking and muscular activities of an individual. The more we engage ourselves in thought, the greater is the general muscular tension and conversely as we proceed toward muscular relaxation, our thought processes gradually diminish.

Brain Function

Whatever may be the role of muscles, thinking is primarily a function of our brain. Our mind or brain is said to be the chief instrument or reservoir for carrying out the process of thinking. The mental picture of images can be stored, formed, reconstructed or put to some use only through the functioning of the brain.

STAGES OF THINKING

John Dewey says that there are distinct stages in thinking. They are awareness of the problem, defining it and evaluation of the same.

Awareness of the Problem

According to John Dewey, reason for thinking is confusion or doubt and hence, whenever we are aware or confronted with a problem we start thinking. Therefore, being aware of the existing problem is essential if we have to think. For instance, the student who is not aware that his/her behavior would lead to problem may not think before showing the behavior.

Defining the Difficulty

By having an awareness of the problem, one will be able to understand the kind of problem he/she has; this is important to find out the root cause of the problem.

Discovering the relationships and formulating the possible solutions to the problems is the third step. This helps in manipulating the information or as we have discussed in insight learning, this helps in perceptual reorganization assisting in problem solving.

Valuation

Valuation means testing the solution. This helps in taking the effective steps to solve a problem. Applying the solution is the last stage where we show the problem-solving behavior, i.e. the result of thinking.

ELEMENTS IN THINKING

Favorable Elements in Thinking

Interest and attention: Both interest and attention favor in thinking. Conclusive or authoritative thinking is extremely difficult if not impossible, when the subject is such as does not interest us. Attention too, is difficult in the absence of any interest. On the contrary, both attention and thinking are natural in a subject, which does interest us.

Strong motivation: It is needed in valid thinking, the latter being impossible in the absence of motivation. Organized and controlled thinking needs strong motivation. Thinking involves the solution of problems. The effort of the mind in thinking corresponds to the strength of motivation for the solution of problems. Motivation maintains enthusiasm and postpones fatigue.

Alertness and flexibility: These are also favor valid thinking, because they serve to keep external faults, from containing thinking. Alertness checks mistakes and fallacies from creeping into thinking. Flexibility keeps thinking free form conservation and blind beliefs. An alert person has new methods, ways and views and makes use of them in thinking, whenever necessary.

Time limit should not be rigid: When a solution to some problem is being sought, the time limit provided should not be too rigid because it so, then normal thinking is hampered and our mental facilities become invalid. Very inflexible and short-time limit cannot admit of valid thinking. Time limit for any interesting problem is superfluous because as it is every person exerts himself/herself to the maximum.

Wide range of wisdom: The wide range of wisdom is also a favorable factor in thinking. Thinking needs insight, which is constituted of hindsight and foresight. A proper development of the faculties of the mind is essential for these activities.

Incubation: Another factor, which favors thinking, is incubation. If the solution of some problem proves elusive despite strenuous and persistent effort, it is advisable to lay aside the problem and to involve oneself in some other activity. While one is engaged in this work, the mind ponders over the earlier problem and just as eggs are hatched by incubation, a solution is evolved through pondering in this manner.

Unfavorable Elements in Thinking

Emotion: It hinders thinking because strong emotion disturbs the mental equilibrium and thereby obstructs thinking. Even, if thinking is pursued in an emotional state, it will be extremely one-sided and biased. If the emotion is very faint, the speed of thinking will be augmented instead of being hindered. But, for correct thinking it is better to have control over the emotions.

Suggestion: It also obstructs thinking, because it makes it one-sided. Thinking moves along the path suggested. If for example, someone is told that he/she will not live that long, the person's level of thinking will be very badly affected, making him/her a pessimist. But it is not essential that suggestions should be invariably harmful to thinking, because healthy suggestions assist thinking.

Superstition: It is just as harmful as a prejudice. It contradicts reasoning; superstition is belief in something without any thinking or reasoning. Superstition is unreasoned belief. If for example, we superstitious believe some theory, opinion or person, we will always think in favor of him/her and never see his/her faults. The people who believe superstitious in a certain religion, believe mutually contradictory things, but never mentally reason them out.

Prejudice: It is like the two a fore side factor, has a detrimental effect on thinking, the only point of distinction being the extent of damage, which is more in this case than in the two cases discussed earlier. The word prejudice suggests the meaning namely some preconceived idea. If we are going to start thinking on some problems with an inclination in a particular direction, all our thinking will be colored by our bias and will not be impartial.

ASSESSMENT OF REASONING AND PROBLEM SOLVING

Wisconsin Card Sorting Test

Wisconsin Card Sorting Test (WCST) assesses abstract reasoning and flexibility in problem solving, stimulus cards of different color form and number are presented to patients to sort into groups, according to the principle established by the examiner, but unknown to the patient (e.g. to sort by color, ignoring form and number).

As the patient sorts the cards, he/she is told whether the responses are correct or incorrect and the number of trials required to achieve 10 consecutive correct responses is recorded. When the patient has mastered the task, the examiner changes the principle of sorting and the number of trials required to achieve correct sorting is recorded.

The procedure, repeated several times, measures the capacity for abstract thinking (i.e. the number of trials required to achieve a solution) and flexibility (perseverate error on successive sorting trials).

Persons with damage to the frontal lobes or caudate and some with schizophrenia give abnormal response.

Patients with cerebral disease are likely to lose the capacity to reason abstractly and to lack flexibility in problem solving or adopting to change situations.

REASONING

Reasoning plays a significant role in adjusting to one's environment. It not only controls one's abilities but also the total behavior and personality are affected by the proper or improper development of one's reasoning ability. Reasoning depicts a higher type of thinking, which is quite careful, systematic and organized in its functioning.

Reasoning is solving a problem by putting two or more elements of past experience together in a logical sequence to arrive at something new. Most human reasoning makes use of symbols—especially the verbal symbols. The process of reasoning follows some standard rules are rigid in nature and can be used as standards for reasoning. The rules are called logic. They prescribe what kind of implication statements can have and what kind of conclusion is permissible to draw from them.

Meaning of Reasoning

Reasoning is a form of thinking itself. When thinking process is guided by some logical principles, it is called reasoning. Good thinking and reasoning are clearly related. One facilitates the other. Reasoning is goal directed, as thinking is general. But in reasoning, the goal is imposed upon the process at every step. Every step weighs the advancement of the process, in terms of the accuracy, in the inaccuracy of the condition. When facts of data are put together according to the logical principles, reasoning is correct. Reasoning is mostly directed toward getting at certain definite conclusions and inferences. In this process, the facts are relevant to particular problems.

Definitions

1. Reasoning is a stepwise thinking with a purpose or goal in mind. —*Garrett*
2. Reasoning is the term applied to highly purposeful, controlled, selective thinking. —*Gates*
3. In reasoning, items (facts or principles) furnished by recall, present observation or both; are combined and examined to see what conclusion can be drawn from the combination. —*Woodworth*
4. Reasoning is the word used to describe the mental recognition of cause and effect relationships. It may be the prediction of an

event from an observed cause or the inference of a cause from an observed event. —*Skinner*

5. Reasoning is combining past experiences in order to solve a problem, which cannot be solved by mere reproduction of earlier solutions. —*Munn*

Characteristics of Reasoning

1. It is a genuine thinking and it involves a definite purpose or goal.
2. It is also an implicit act and involves problem-solving behavior.
3. Like thinking, here one makes use of one's previous knowledge and experiences.
4. Like thinking, there is a mental exploration instead of motor exploration in reasoning, as we try to explore mentally, the reason or cause of the event or happening.
5. Like thinking, reasoning is a highly symbolic function. The ability to interpret various symbols, development of concepts and linguistic ability helps much in reasoning.

Steps of Reasoning

1. Identification of the goal or purpose for which reasoning is to be directed.
2. The mental exploration or search for the various possibilities, cause and effect relationships or solutions for releasing the set goal or purposes based on previous learning or experiences and present observation or attempts.
3. Selection of the most appropriate possibility or solution by careful mental analysis of all the available alternatives.
4. Testing the validity of the selected possibility or solution, purely through mental exercise and thus, finally accept or reject it for actual solution of the problem.

Types of Reasoning

Inductive reasoning: In inductive reasoning, we usually follow the process of induction. Induction is a way of proving a statement or generalizing a rule or principle, by proving or showing that if a statement or a rule is true in one particular case, it will be true in all such cases, which appear in some serial order and thus, it may be applied generally to all such type of cases.

Deductive reasoning: It is just opposite to inductive reasoning. Here, one starts completely agreeing with some already discovered or pre-established, generalized fact or principle and tries to apply it to particular cases.

CREATIVE THINKING

At times, thinking leads to fertile results. Such thinking that brings about novel results is known as creative thinking. The creative thinkers like artists, writers or scientists try to create something new and non-existent in the world. In contrast with ordinary problems solving, creating solutions are new ones that other people have not thought of before. Creative thinking results in offering new and unique ways of conceptualizing the world around us. The word new is of importance in creative thinking. Usually, it appears that a creative thinker becomes aware of a new idea suddenly. The sudden appearance of new ideas is called insight. In fact, instead of being sudden such an insight is based on unconscious deliberations. All the discoveries or inventions of the scientists are instances of creative thinking.

Steps Involved in Creative Thinking

Preparation: In a way, all education is a preparation for creating thinking in general. But specific problems require special training and preparation in that particular field. The creative results in such thinking are mostly the results of insightful inspiration. But this inspiration is possible within the relevant field of training and experience. It cannot take place in a vacuum. Much emphasis is therefore, placed on training for creative thinking in the field of modern day educational psychology.

Incubation: The new ideas take some time to ripen or to get mature. They are to be hatched. The productive solution does not occur at the moment it is started. Often, the thinker has to struggle hard for the solution. Sometimes, he/she may even give up thinking about it in despair.

Illumination: When the solution occurs after the period of incubation, it occurs all of a sudden in the form of illuminating insight. Naturally, the thinker feels that something like inspiration is at work. He/she cannot explain it in terms of own attempts. He/she feels that the solution occurs by a sudden flash. But illumination can be well explained, taking the incubation period into account.

Verification: The solution of idea that results from illumination cannot be the final stage of creative thinking. The idea should well fit in the system of existing knowledge. Hence, evaluation of the solution is the essential stage following the solution. Especially, for the scientific invention, it is necessary to get the idea verified and see whatever it is correct and workable.

Revision: The final stage is that of revision, where the new solutions are further tested by applying them to other situations. Many thinkers find it necessary to get their ideas revised and modified before the results of their thinking are satisfactory.

PROBLEM SOLVING

Problem solving is an important characteristic of thinking that is a problem-solving behavior. It is always directed toward the solution of a problem. Whenever a need arises, man tries to satisfy it by some already established pattern of behavior. A problematic situation arises when this fixed pattern fails to satisfy the need. Man is constantly faced by some problems or the other, as his needs are numerous. Even when the needs necessary for his physical and social well-being are satisfied, he may still have a number of intellectual or spiritual needs, which has to get satisfied. Being thus constantly confronted with problems, man has to keep on thinking all the time. If he stops thinking, the problems due to the unsatisfied needs may affect his adjustment to life. He has to think in the most diverse possible manner.

Definitions

1. Problem-solving behavior occurs in novel or difficult situations in which a solution is not obtainable by the habitual methods of applying concepts and principles derived from past experience in very familiar situations. —*Woodward and Marquis*
2. Problem solving is a process of overcoming difficulties that appear to interfere with the attainment of a goal. It is a procedure of making adjustment in spite of interferences. —*Skinner*

Scientific Methods of Problem Solving

Problem Awareness

The first step in the problem-solving behavior of an individual concerns his/her awareness of the difficulty or problem that needs a solution. He/she must be confronted with some obstacle or interference in the path of the realization of needs or motives and consequently, he/she must be conscious of the felt difficulty or problem.

Problem Understanding

The difficulty or problem felt by the individual should be properly identified by a careful analysis. He/she should be clear about what exactly is the problem. The problem then should be pinpointed in terms of the specific goals and objectives.

Collection of the Relevant Information

The individual is required to collect all the relevant information about the problem through all possible sources in this step. He/she may consult experienced persons, read the available literature, revive his/her old experiences, think of possible solutions and put in all relevant efforts for widening the scope of knowledge concerning the problem in hand.

Formulation of Hypothesis or Hunch for Possible Solutions

In the light of the collected relevant information and nature of his/her problem, one may then engage in some serious cognitive activities to think of the various possibilities for the solution of one's problem.

Selection of a Proper Solution

Selection of a proper solution is an important step. All the possible solutions thought of in the previous step, are closely analyzed and evaluated in this step.

Gates and others (1946) have suggested the following activities in the evaluation of the assumed hypotheses or solution:

1. One should determine the conclusion that completely satisfies the demand of the problem.
2. One should find out whether the solution is consistent with other facts and principles, which have been well established.

3. One should make a deliberate search for negative instances, which might cast doubts on the conclusion.
4. Verification of the concluded solutions or hypothesis: The solution arrived at or conclusion drawn must be further verified by utilizing it in the solution of the various likewise problems. In case, the derived solution helps in solving these likewise problems and then only, one is free to agree with his findings regarding the solution of his problem.

An important step in problem solving is the direction or mental set. A wrong direction may interfere with the correct solution of the problem. A flexibility of mental set is often helpful in giving the proper direction to problem solving. The thinking, which is done in problem solving, is goal directed and is motivated by the need to reduce discrepancy between one state of affairs and another. The direction required for problem solving is given by the rules associated with the solutions of most of the problem. In everyday problems, these rules are supplied by our social experience. In some formal problems, they are the part of the problem itself.

Some of these rules, when followed correctly, guarantee a solution to a problem. In most problems, where such rules are not supplied, we fall back on our past experiences with problems, which are likely to lead a solution. The problem at hand is broken down in such smaller problems, each of which is a little closer to the end goal. However, there is no guarantee of correct solutions. Hence, thinking may be described as an implicit problem-solving behavior.

ATTRIBUTION

Social perception is the process through which one seeks to know and understand others. It is the most basic aspect of social life. We always try to understand others current or present feelings, moods, emotions, etc. The process through which we seek to determine the causes behind others behavior is known as attribution. In other words, attribute refers to our effects to understand the causes behind behavior and on some occasions, the causes behind our behavior. Attribute are influences that people draw about causes of events, others behavior and their own behavior. Attribution is necessary to understand our experiences. If we can attribute others behavior, it will help in making adjustments with others and to maintain self-image.

Theories of Attribution

Kelley's Covariation Model

Kelley's covariation model is based on assumption that people attribute behavior to factors that are present, when the behavior takes place and absent when it does not. According to Kelley, when people attempt to infer the cause of an actor's behavior, they usually consider three types of behavior:

1. Consensus: At first, we consider the extent to which an individual responds in the same manner to different stimuli or different situation.
2. Consistency: We consider constancy, the extent to which the individual reacts to the stimulus or event in the same way, on other occasions.
3. Distinctiveness: The extent to which the person reacts in the same manner for other different stimuli and events.

According to Kelley, low consistency favors an external attribution, but high consistency is compatible with either an internal or an external attribution.

James and Davis Correspondent Inference Theory

James and Davis correspondent inference theory describes how, with information about others behavior is used as a basis for inferring their stable traits. Hence, when we are making attributions about the people, we compare their action with alternative actions, evaluating the choices they have made. Informations about five factors is sought to make their inferences, which are as follows:

1. Whether the behavior considered is voluntary and freely chosen.
2. What is unexpected about the behavior (rare effects)?
3. Whether the behavior considered is socially desirable.
4. Whether the behavior considered impacts the person.
5. Whether the behavior considered is modifiable.

WAYS TO IMPROVE THINKING

Some of the ways to improve thinking are:

1. Keep yourself only with current project; clutters create confusion. Get organized and work with fresh canvas. On an average, we spend about 45 minutes a day looking for things.

2. Dedicate an hour of focus time to the most important task—multitasking is highly overrated and causes a loss of up to 40 percent efficiency. Get an hour of focused seclusion, to work on the most important task.
3. Stir up the visual sense and creative talents with exposure to the arts—go to a gallery, pick up an art book or spend time with nature.
4. Learn how to mind map: This is a best practice that allows you to visualize and map the projects and strategies. It is also a life-saving memory device that will help to remember more and organize thinking.
5. Give rest for thinking: When you have been working on something for more than an hour, you start losing concentration and focus. So stop, get up, walk around and go back to work.

ALTERATIONS IN THINKING

Psychosis

Psychosis is a major psychiatric disorder in which reality testing is not intact; behavior may violate gross social norm. It is just opposite to the nervous in which reality testing is intact and behavior may not violate social norms. Many psychiatric disorders such as schizophrenia, mania, depression, etc. come under psychosis. It includes various disturbances in thinking.

Delusion

Delusion is a false, persistent, irrational belief not shared by persons of some age, race, education standard, which cannot be altered by logical arguments.

Types of Delusion

The types of delusion and its description is show in Table 16.1.

Table 16.1: Types of delusion

Sl No	*Type*	*Description*
1.	Persecutory delusions	The individuals feel interfered, discriminates against threatened or mistreated, e.g. the patient says, my family members want to kill me

Contd...

Contd...

2.	Delusion of reference	The individual feels that others are talking about him/her, other's remarks/actions have special significance for him/her
3.	Delusions of influence/passivity	The individual believes that he/she is influenced and controlled by others, e.g. the cardiologist puts transmitter near heart that controls my feelings and thoughts
4.	Delusion of sin and guilt	The individual has a belief that he/she has committed unforgivable sin/some wickedness in past, leads to calamity to others; so, he/she is evil and worthless
5.	Hypochondriacal delusions	These are delusions of some bodily diseases
6.	Delusion of grandeur	The individual has an exaggerated feeling of importance, power, knowledge or identity

CONCLUSION

Thinking starts with a problem and concludes with its solution. This activity of thinking continues until the solution is found or till the person becomes fatigued by the effort. There cannot be any thinking in the absence of some problem. Problems in human life come in an incessant stream and they have to be solved by thinking. Thinking, the mental solution of problem, makes use of the symbols of objects, instead of the objects itself. Thinking attempts for the solution of problems by employing the trial and error method. There is a kind of flow in the activity of thinking, one problem leading to the thinking of another by reminding the person of some other problem. The instruments of thinking—images, imagination, signs, indications and such are also called internal activity. Thinking continues as an internal activity unless and until it takes the form of verbal thinking.

SUGGESTED READING

1. Bhatia, Craig. Elements of Psychology and Mental Hygiene for Nurses in India. Chennai: Orient Longman Ltd; 2000.
2. Clement I. Psychosocial Foundation of Nursing, 1st edition. New Delhi: Jaypee Brothers Medical Publishers (P) Ltd; 2010.
3. Denise F Polit, BP Hungler. Nursing Research Principles and Methods. Philadelphia: JB Lippincott Co; 1995.

4. Kaplan, Sadock. Synopsis of Psychiatry. Lippincott Williams and Wilkins; 1998.
5. Morgan, King. Introduction to Psychology. New Delhi: Tata McGraw-Hill Publishing Co Ltd; 1993.
6. Shaw ME. Group Dynamics. New York: McGraw-Hill; 1976.
7. Thompson RF. Introduction to Psychology. New Delhi: Haper and Row; 1975.

REVIEW QUESTIONS

1. Define thinking. Explain nature and types of thinking.
2. Explain the characteristics and tools of thinking.
3. Discuss the stages and elements of thinking.
4. Define reasoning. Explain the steps and types of reasoning.
5. Define creative thinking. Explain the steps of creative thinking.
6. Define problem solving. Explain the scientific methods of problem solving.
7. Discuss alterations in thinking.

CHAPTER 17 Aptitude

LEARNING OBJECTIVES

1. Definitions.
2. Meaning.
3. Measurement.
4. Values and uses.
5. Aptitude and nursing.

INTRODUCTION

The people differ from one another and within themselves in their performance in one or the other field of human activity such as leadership, music, art, mechanical work, teaching, etc. They usually come across the individuals who undergo similar circumstances, excel the other persons in acquiring certain specific jobs. Such persons are said to possess certain specific abilities or aptitudes, besides general intellectual abilities or intelligence, which help them in achieving success in some specific occupations or activities. Therefore, in a simple way, aptitude may be considered a special ability or specific capacity besides the general ability, which helps an individual to acquire a required degree of proficiency or achievement in a specific field.

MEANING AND CONCEPTS

An aptitude is the capacity of a person to achieve along special lines. It is a special tendency, bent, fitness or aptness due to a special neural or muscular organization possessed by an individual. Aptitudes make for special abilities and the achievements in special areas. Some of the well-known aptitudes are the mechanical, artistic, musical, numerical or nursing aptitudes. Aptitude is to be distinguished from person's ability. It shows that, although certain individuals do not possess certain ability, they can acquire it or have it, provide the opportunities that are available. Specific aptitudes can be assessed by means of specific aptitude tests. They can help in knowing people, who will be able to acquire a high degree of proficiency in fairly specific skills within minimum of training. The results of aptitude tests can be used for vocational guidance and adjustment.

An aptitude may be considered a special ability or specific capacity besides the general intellectual ability, which helps an individual to acquire degree of proficiency or achievement in a specific field.

An aptitude is the interaction of heredity and environment. Individuals born with certain potentialities and begin to learn immediately. Therefore, everything they learn enables them to learn still more.

It embraces any characteristics, which predisposes to learning including intelligence, achievements, personality, interests and special skills.

Intelligence is concerned with the general mental ability of an individual, but aptitude is related to specific abilities. Thus, the knowledge of intelligence of individuals predict their success in a number of situations involving mental function or activity.

Usually, interest and aptitude go hand in hand. A person must have aptitude for activity and an interest in a given activity to desirable success. But interest and aptitude both are not one and the same way.

Aptitude is measured by tests of general mental activity, which are used to facilitate prediction of scholastic success.

DEFINITIONS

1. Aptitude refers to those qualities characterizing a person's ways of behavior, which serves to indicate how well they can learn to meet and solve certain specified kinds of problems.

   —*Bingham*

2. Aptitude is a condition, a quality or a set of qualities in individuals, which is indicative of the probable extent to which they will be able to acquire under suitable training, some knowledge,

skill or composite of knowledge, understanding and skill, such as ability to contribute to art or music, mechanical ability, mathematical ability, to read and speak a foreign language.

—*Traxler*

3. An aptitude is a combination of characteristics indicative of an individual's capacity to acquire (with training) some specific knowledge, skill or set of organized responses, such as the ability to speak a language, to become a musician, to do mechanical work. —*Freeman*

MEASUREMENT OF APTITUDE

The term intelligence, ability and aptitude are often used interchangeably to refer the behavior that is used to predict future learning or performance. However, subtle differences exist between the terms (Table 17.1). Like intelligence tests, aptitude tests measure a student's overall performance across a broad range of mental capabilities. But aptitude tests also include items, which measure more specialized abilities such as verbal and numerical skills that predict scholastic performance in educational programs.

Table 17.1: Differences between intelligence and aptitude

Area	*Intelligence*	*Aptitude*
Ability	They exist usually to test the general mental ability of an individual	Aptitudes are concerned with specific abilities
Knowledge	By the knowledge of intelligence of an individual, we can predict the success in a number of situations involving mental function or activity	The knowledge of aptitudes acquaints us with those specific abilities and capacities of an individual, which give an indication of the ability or capacity to succeed in a special field or activity
Prediction	Predicting achievements of intelligence for general ability	Predicting achievement in some particular job, training, courses or specialized instruction, we need to know more about one's aptitudes (specific abilities)

Specific Nature of Aptitude Tests

1. Mechanical aptitude tests.
2. Musical aptitude tests.
3. Art judgment tests.

4. Professional aptitude tests, i.e. tests to measure the aptitudes for professionals like teaching, salesmanship, research work, etc.
5. Scholastic aptitude tests, i.e. tests to measure the aptitude for different course of institution.

Mechanical Aptitude Test

Some persons have a specific bent of mind for the tasks related to the use of mechanical abilities and thus, demonstrate their aptitude for all tasks and job that require the use of mechanical abilities. The term mechanical aptitude is not a single unitary function. It is a combination of sensory and motor capacities plus perception of spatial relations, the capacity to acquire information about mechanical matters and the capacity to comprehend mechanical relationships. Some of the well-known mechanical aptitude tests are:

1. Minnesota mechanical assembly test.
2. Minnesota spatial relation test.
3. The revised Minnesota paper form board (1948).
4. Stenquist mechanical aptitude tests (part I and III).
5. LJ O'Rourke's mechanical aptitude tests (part I and III).
6. SRA mechanical aptitude test.
7. Bennet tests of mechanical aptitude tests (Hindi) prepared by Manovigyan Shala, Allahabad. Usually, these tests contain the items of the following nature:
   a. Asking the subject to put together the parts of mechanical devices.
   b. Asking to replace cutouts of various shapes in their correct holes in the board.
   c. Requiring the ability to solve problems in geometric terms.
   d. Asking questions concerning the basic information about tools and their uses.
   e. Questions relating to comprehension of physical and mechanical principles.

Clerical Aptitude Tests

Clerical aptitude is also a composite function. According to Bingham, it involves several specific abilities as follows.

Perceptual ability: It is the ability to perceive words and numbers with speed and accuracy.

Intellectual ability: It is the ability to grasp the meaning of words and symbols.

Motor ability: It is the ability to use various types of machines and tools like typewriter, duplicator, cyclostyle machine, punching machine, etc.

Some of the popular clerical aptitude tests are as follows:

1. Detroit clerical aptitude examination.
2. Minnesota vocational test for clerical works.
3. The clerical ability test prepared by the Department of Psychology, University of Mysore, Mysore.
4. Clerical aptitude test battery (English and Hindi), Bureau of Education and Vocational Guidance, Patna (Bihar).
5. Test of clerical aptitude prepared by the Parsi Panchayat Guidance Bureau 209, Hornby Road, Bombay-1.

Sensory Aptitude

In sensory aptitude category, we can include all those aptitudes, which are related to the sensory capacities and abilities of the children. One may have aptitude in the task related to the use of sense of hearing; other may have aptitude in the task related to the use of the sense of sight, sense of smell, sense of taste or sense of touch. Here, depending upon their present ability concerning the particular sensory capacity, we can have an idea of their future success in the area or professions, where the use of such sensory ability or capacity is most demanded.

Musical Aptitude Tests

Musical aptitude tests have been devised for discovering musical talent. One of the important musical aptitude tests is discovered below:

Seashore measure of musical talent: It gives consideration to the following musical components:

1. Discrimination of pitch.
2. Discrimination of intensity of loudness.
3. Determination of time interval.
4. Discrimination of timbre.
5. Judgment of rhythm.
6. Tonal memory.

The instruction in these tests is of following nature: You will hear two tones, which differ in pitch. You are to judge, whether the second is higher or lower than the first. If the second is higher, record H; if lower, record L.

Aptitude for Graphic Art

Graphic art tests are devised to discover the talent for graphic art. The two important tests of this nature are:

1. The Meier art judgment test.
2. Horn art aptitude inventory.

In Meier art judgment test, there are 100 pairs of representational pictures in black and white. One member of each pair is an acknowledged art masterpiece, while the other is a slight distortion of the masterpiece. It is usually altered from the original, so as to violate some important principle of art. Tests are informed regarding, which aspect has been altered and are asked to choose from each pairs, the one that is better—more pleasing, more artistic and more satisfying.

Another important test of measuring aptitude for graphic art is the Horn art aptitude inventory. It requires the subject to produce sketches from given patterns to lines and figures. The created sketches of the subject are then evaluated according to the standard given by the author of this test.

Professional Aptitude

The aptitude related to the activities of various professions and occupations are included in this category. These aptitudes are able to predict the future success of an individual in the field or profession related to these aptitudes.

Tests for Scholastic and Professional Aptitudes

For helping in the proper selection of students for the study of specific courses of professions like engineering, medicine, law, business management, teaching, etc. The various specific aptitude tests have been designed. Some of these aptitude tests are:

1. Stanford scientific aptitude test by DL Zyve.
2. Science aptitude test (after higher secondary stage) NIE, Delhi.
3. Moss scholastic aptitude test for medical students.

4. Ferguson and Stoddard's law aptitude examination.
5. Tale legal aptitude test.
6. Pre-engineering ability test (Educational Testing Services, USA).
7. Minnesota engineering analogical test.
8. Coxe-Orleans prognosis test of teaching ability.
9. Teaching aptitude test by Jai Prakash and RP Shrivastav, University of Saugar (MP).
10. Shah's teaching aptitude test.
11. Teaching aptitude test by Moss FA and others, George Washington University Press.

Contemporary Trend in Aptitude Testing

Instead of utilizing specific aptitude tests for measuring specific aptitude in very specific field or area, the trend at present, has now been changed toward multiple aptitude tests battery to find the suitability of people for different professions, requiring different abilities on the basis of scores in the relevant aptitude tests in the battery. The examples of such tests are general aptitude test battery (GATB) and differential aptitude test (DAT).

General Aptitude Test Battery

General aptitude test battery developed by the Employment Service Bureau of the USA has 12 tests. Eight of which are paper-pencil tests as for name comparison, computation, vocabulary, arithmetic reasoning, form matching, test matching, three-dimensional spaces, etc. The other four require the use of simple equipment in the shape of moving pegs on boards, assembling and dissembling rivets and washers. From the scores obtained by the subject, the experimenter is able to draw inferences about the nine aptitude factors; intelligence, verbal aptitude and numerical aptitude, spatial aptitude, form perception, clerical perception, motor coordination, finger dexterity and manual dexterity. The GATB has proven to be one of the most successful multiple aptitude batteries particularly for the purposes of job classification.

Differential Aptitude Test

Developed by the USA Psychological Corporation. It has proved more successful in predicting academic success and found especially useful for providing educational and vocational guidance to secondary schoolchildren. The tests induced in the battery of DAT are as follows.

Verbal reasoning: It is a measure of ability to understand concepts framed in words. It is aimed at evaluation of the student's ability to abstract or generalize and to think constructively, rather than simple, fluency or vocabulary recognition. The word used in these items may come from history, geography, literature, science or any other content area.

Numerical ability: These items are designed to test understanding of numerical relationships and facility in handling numerical concepts. This test is a measure of the student's ability to reason with numbers, to manipulate numerical relationships and to deal intelligently with quantitative materials. Educationally, it is important for prediction in fields such as mathematics, physics, chemistry, engineering and other curricula in which quantitative thinking is essential. Various amounts of numerical ability are required in occupations such as laboratory assistant, book-keeper, statistical and shipping clerks, as well as in professions related to physical sciences.

Abstract reasoning: This test is intended as a verbal measure of the student's reasoning ability. It has many picture tests yielding ambiguous scores, because they require the student to discriminate between lines and areas, which differ, but slightly in size and shape. This test supplements the general intelligence aspects of the verbal and numerical tests.

Clerical speed and accuracy: This test is intended to measure speed of response in a simple perceptual task.

Perceptual ability: It is the ability to perceive words and numbers with speed and accuracy.

Intellectual ability: It is the ability to grasp the meaning of words and symbols.

Motor ability: It is the ability to use various types of machines and tools like typewriter, duplicator, cyclostyle machine, punching machine, etc.

Mechanical reasoning: This tries to test mechanical aptitude, which is a combination of sensory and motor capacities plus perception of spatial relations, the capacity to acquire information about mechanical matters and the capacity to comprehend mechanical relationships.

Space relations: It is the ability to visualize a constructed object from a picture of a pattern and an ability to imagine, how an object would appear if rotated in various ways for measurement of space perception. It means that these tests require mental manipulation of objects in three-dimensional spaces.

Language usage: This test has two sections.
Language usage-1: spelling.
Language usage-2: grammar.

VALUES OF APTITUDE TESTING

1. Aptitude tests are excellent predictors of future scholastic achievements.
2. They provide ways of comparing a child's performance with that of other children in the same situation.
3. They provide a profile of strengths and weaknesses.
4. They assess differences among individuals.
5. They have uncovered hidden talents in some children, thus improving their educational opportunities.
6. They are valuable tools for working with handicapped children.

USES OF APTITUDE TESTS

Instructional

Teacher can use aptitude test results to adopt their curricula to match the level of their students or to design assignments for students who differ orderly. Aptitude test scores can also help teachers form realistic expectations of students. Knowing something about the aptitude level of students in a given class can help a teacher to identify, which students are not learning as much as could be predicted on the basis of aptitude scores. For instance, if a whole class were performing less than would be predicted from aptitude test results, then curriculum, objectives, teaching methods or student characteristics might be investigated.

Administrative

Aptitude test scores can identify the general aptitude level of a high school. This can be helpful in determining, how much emphasis should be given to college preparatory programs. Aptitude tests can be used to identify students to be accelerated or given extra attention, for grouping and in predicting job training performance.

Guidance

The guidance counselors use aptitude tests to help parents develop realistic expectations for their child's school performance and to help the students to understand their own strengths and weaknesses. These tests are found to be very useful in helping the youngsters as well as youth in the selection of special courses of instruction, fields of activities and vocations.

Educational and Vocational

Aptitude tests can be safely used for the purpose of education and vocational selection. They help in making scientific selection of the candidates for various educational and professional courses as well as specialized jobs, as Munn puts it. The chief values of aptitude testing is, in fact that it enables to pick out from those who not yet have the ability to perform certain skills, those with a reasonable amount of training, will be most likely to acquire the skills in question and acquire them to a desirable level of proficiency.

APTITUDE AND NURSING

Aptitude is to be distinguished from present ability. A certain nurse may not at present have the ability to act as an operation theater nurse working with the surgeon, but she is clever and quick, able to think ahead and foresee what will be needed. She possesses a high degree of aptitude for theater work and has good chances with proper training to become a very successful operation theater nurse. Nursing is an arts and science, which requires high degree of aptitude for being a good bedside nurse. The nurse needs to foresee the need and progress of the patient. The aptitude differs from one area to another, based on their application of nursing.

CONCLUSION

Aptitude tests properly anticipate the future potentialities or capacities of an individual and thereby, help us in making selection of those individuals, who are best fitted for a particular profession and course of instruction or those who are likely to be more benefited by the preprofessional training or experiences. Aptitude testing when combined with the other information received through interest inventory, personality tests, intelligence tests and cumulative record, etc. can help to a greater extent, in avoiding the huge wastage of human, as well as material resources by placing the individuals to their proper places and lines of work.

SUGGESTED READING

1. Bennett GK, Seashore NG, Wesman AG. Differential Aptitude Tests. New York: Psychological Corporation; 1947.
2. Bingham WV. Aptitude and Aptitude Testing. New York: Harper and Brothers; 1937.
3. Brubaker J. Modern Philosophies of Education. New York: McGraw-Hill; 1939.
4. Crow LD, Crow A. An Introduction to Guidance. New Delhi: Eurasia Publishing House; 1962.
5. Freeman FS. Theory and Practice of Psychological Testing, 3rd Indian reprint. Bombay: Oxford and IBH; 1971.
6. Garrett HE, MR Schneck. Psychological Tests, Methods and Results. New York: Harper and Brothers; 1933.
7. Hull CL. Aptitude Testing. Yonkers. New York: World Books Co; 1928.
8. Stern W. Psychological Methods of Testing Intelligence. Baltimore: Warwick and York Inc; 1914.
9. Terman LM. Intelligence and its measurement: A symposium. Journal of Educational Psychology. 1921 Mar 12.
10. Wechsler D. The Measurement of Adult Intelligence, 3rd edition. Baltimore: Williams and Wilkins Co; 1944.

REVIEW QUESTIONS

1. Define aptitude. Explain the concept of aptitude.
2. Explain the various types of measurements of aptitude.
3. Discuss the values and uses of aptitude.
4. Describe the nurse's role in aptitude.

CHAPTER 18

Guidance and Counseling

LEARNING OBJECTIVES

1. Guidance: Definitions, principles, elements, characteristics, basic assumptions, purposes, need, types, steps involved.
2. Counseling: Definitions, meaning, characteristics, roles and rules, theories, educational guidance.

GUIDANCE SERVICE

The guidance is one of the major applications of psychology. It enables or assists the individual to solve educational, vocational and psychological problems. 'To guide' means a sort of help, assistance or suggestions for progress. In the field of psychology and education, the word 'guidance' is having a specific meaning. It refers to a process of helping the individual to discover himself/herself which means, the potentialities and propensities, capacities and capabilities, abilities and aptitudes, interests and natural endowments and to help him/her in achieving maximum advantage of the individual and state.

Concept of Guidance

1. Guidance refers to a process of assisting the individual to develop the body, mind, personality and character and to help the individual in achieving maximum educational, vocational and personal or psychological adjustments.
2. Guidance is regarded as a kind of specialized service provided to the individual to solve problems of crucial nature.

3. Guidance is regarded as any form of assistance given to child, who makes the best development of personality.
4. Guidance is not confined to a professional setting, since it is a continuous process starting from early childhood extending sometimes up to old age.
5. Guidance is the educational context, for example, assisting students to select courses of study appropriate to their needs and interests, achieve academic excellence to the best possible.
6. Guidance is not just providing direction; it is the imposition of one's view point on another, making decision for another individual, carrying burden of another's life, etc.

Definitions

1. 'Guidance' involves personal help given by someone, it is designed to assist a person to decide where he wants to go, what he wants to do or how he can best accomplish his purpose; it assists him to solve problems that arise in life. —*Jones (1951)*
2. Fundamental of all guidance is the help or assistance given by a competent person to an individual, so that the latter may direct his life by developing his point of view, make his own decision and carry out those decisions. —*Crow and crow*
3. The purpose of guidance is to help the student to make more favorable adjustments. —*Fowler*

Principles of Guidance

1. The debility of the individual is supreme.
2. Each individual is different from every other individual.
3. The primary concern of guidance is the individual in one's own social setting.
4. The attitudes and personal perceptions of the individual provide the basis for action.
5. The individual generally acts to enhance the perceived self.
6. The individual has the innate ability to learn and therefore, can be helped to make choices that will lead to self-direction and make the person consistent with reality.
7. The individual needs a continuous guidance process from childhood onwards.
8. Each individual may, at times, need the information and personalized assistance given by competent professional personnel.

Elements

1. Guidance focuses our attention on the individual and not on the problem.
2. Guidance helps to the discovery of abilities of an individual.
3. Guidance is based on interests, abilities, assets, needs and limitations of the individual.
4. Guidance gives rise to self-development and self-direction.
5. Guidance makes the individual to plan wisely for the present and future.
6. Guidance makes the individual to become adjusted in the new environment.
7. Guidance is helpful in achieving success and happiness.

Characteristics

1. The basis of guidance is individual differences, it is a known fact that no two individuals that are alike. Individuals are different in capacities, capabilities, potentialities, propensities, abilities, aptitude and variations within the individual.
2. Guidance is the basis of rigid code of ethics, it is important to follow a rigid code of ethics in programmed guidance.
3. The basis of guidance is on educational and vocational objectives, it means that realization of guidance in educational and vocational aims and objective.
4. Guidance is able to develop the insight of an individual; the counselor is helpful to the individual in such a way that the person gains insight to make own decisions and choices.
5. Guidance regards most of the individuals as average normal persons; it must be known to all the students that the services of guidance workers are available to all.
6. Guidance is slow, but a continuous process; individuals need considerable time to make suitable adjustments and are unable to make wise decisions, choices and adjustments in a day or so.
7. Guidance is universal, it is essential for all the pupils of all the stages. It is for those who seek it and also for those who do not seek it.
8. Guidance is planning, guidance personnel attempts to review the entire situation and gives plans for future in educational, vocational and social field.
9. Guidance is developmental as well as comprehensive; guidance is developmental because it is dealing with month-to-month, year-to-year and stage-to-stage.

10. Guidance is practical side of education; education sets the goal, while guidance makes the realization of that goal.
11. Guidance is mainly child-centered, guidance worker or counselor does not impose anything on individual, but he tries to find out the needs of the child and provides the child only with the suggestions.
12. Guidance is considered as an organized service and not incidental, i.e. it is a service, which is having a specific purpose.
13. Guidance is specialized and generalized service; many persons such as the teacher, parent, headmaster, counselor and career master play their specific role.

Basic Assumptions of Guidance

1. The differences between individuals in native is capacities, abilities and interests are quite significant.
2. Variations within the individual are quite significant.
3. Native abilities are not generally specialized.
4. Abilities and aptitudes do not depend upon race, color and sex.
5. There is need for assistance to certain crisis.
6. The school is in a strategic position to provide the needed assistance.
7. Guidance is progressive, self-directive, but not prescriptive.

Purposes of Guidance

Understanding the individual: The main purpose of guidance is to discover and understand capacities and potentialities of the individual and to make evaluation of the self, in relation to personal and social experience and to use the self more efficiently in everyday living.

Help the individual in making adjustments: Another aim of guidance is to assist the individual, so as to make satisfactory and maximum adjustments at home, in school, with teachers, to pupils and in society.

Develop personal abilities and potentialities: Another purpose of guidance is to help the individuals to develop their abilities, potentialities and points of view, to develop their body, mind, personality and character.

Improve school activities: The guidance program helps the school staff to solve problems and improve all the activities of the school.

Coordinating home, school and society: Erickson has correctly said that one of the important purposes of guidance has been coordinating home, school and community, which influences the child.

Need for Guidance

Educational need: Guidance must be given to the students to select subjects of counsel, to select books, hobbies and cocurricular activities, to develop study habits, to organize time and work, to concentrate on studies, to build social relationship and to make satisfactory progress and adjustments in school.

Psychological need: Guidance is required from psychological and social point of view. Youth of 20th century is subjected to much great emotional strain at home and in the community. The number of problems in delinquent children, backward children and maladjusted children has been increasing in schools.

Vocational need: The vocational guidance is essential for helping the individual to know himself, for knowing the world of work, adequate information about jobs, skills and opportunities for making a right choice in the vocation, according to the abilities, interest and aptitudes and to obtain suitable jobs in their chosen fields.

Social need: Society is becoming complex, been started changes have occurring in the entire structure of the economic, social and political system.

Types of Guidance

1. Educational guidance.
2. Vocational guidance.
3. Religious guidance.
4. Guidance for home relationship.
5. Guidance for citizenship.
6. Guidance for leisure and recreation.
7. Guidance for personal well-being.
8. Guidance in right doing.
9. Guidance in thoughtfulness and cooperation.
10. Guidance in wholesome and cultural action.

INDIVIDUAL GUIDANCE SERVICE

Individual guidance service is some type of help, which is provided to individual to understand and develop the potentialities, make the best use of the potentialities and solve problems. Individual problems are concerned with physical health problems, home, school and leisure time problems, sex problems, other emotional and psychological problems and vocational problems.

Stages of Individual Guidance Service

At Elementary Stage

1. The childhood period refers to the period of growth and development.
2. During this stage, the basic foundations of physical, intellectual, emotional, social and other type of personality development are laid.
3. It is considered to be the most impressionable period of life, when the character traits, attitudes, values and habits get developed.
4. Some of the tasks or purposes of individual guidance service at this stage are to make a right start in the school, to build good physique and to make emotional adjustments.

At Secondary Stage

Secondary stage is regarded as the most critical stage of individual's development because it is the stage of stress and strain, storm and strife, heightened emotionality and hypersuggestibility, anxieties and worries, conflicts and frustrations. The main aims of individual guidance at this stage are as follows:

1. To make the individual to solve problems concerning physical health.
2. To make the individual to solve problems concerning sex, emotional and mental health.
3. To guide the individual in making family adjustments.
4. To advise the individual in making social adjustments including adjustment at school.
5. To guide the individual in making suitable progress in the school.

At College Stage

The main purposes, aims or functions of individual's guidance at college stage are as follows:

1. Guidance is essential, to help the individual in solving all types of emotional problems, sex problems and other personal problems.
2. Guidance is needed, to help the individual in making adjustment with new environment.
3. Guidance is also needed, to help the individual in developing healthy ideas and building a new philosophy of life.
4. Guidance is essential, to help them in participating in social activities.
5. Guidance is also essential, to help the individual in making suitable educational progress.
6. Guidance helps the individual in getting suitable job.

Need for Individual Guidance Service

Problems concerning physical health: The advice and treatment of an expert may be required by an individual for curing physical ailment and building up the physique.

Family problems: There are many family problems such as the strained relationship between child and parents, husband and wife, brothers and sisters, constant quarrels between the father and mother, presence of stepfather or stepmother in the house, etc. Jealousy among various siblings in the family may contribute another factor in home environment, which may become a potent cause of maladjustments.

Utilization of leisure time: In order to utilize the leisure time profitably, individual might require guidance. He/she might need to be guided in sports, games and hobbies.

Personal problems: Sometimes, the main cause of maladjustments are personality problems such as bullying, teasing, frightened, anxiety, nail biting, thumb sucking, grinding of teeth and inferiority complex. These difficulties require competent guidance.

School problems: The individual may be unable to make progress in various academic, physical, social and recreational activities of school and thus, require guidance.

Vocational problems: The individual might require guidance for selecting the occupation, adequate training for a particular occupation or the change of an occupation.

Religious problems: The individual might be having certain religious doubts or wrong philosophy of life for which he/she might require guidance.

Marital problems: Happy man is one who has got the good life partner. For carrying out the right choice of a partner, the person might require guidance.

Sex problems: Sometimes, individuals have sex problems due to menstruation, nightmares, excessive sex curiosity, heterosexual interests and activities. In order to help the individual in solving sex problems and in leading a healthy sexual life, individual guidance becomes essential.

Old age problems: Old age brings its own problems. At this age, various organs of the body loses their strength and the various senses like eyesight, hearing and smell, etc. will start growing feeble day by day. Such an age group requires guidance regarding proper utilization of time and for keeping the body in strength.

Steps Involved in Individual Guidance Service

Collection of Facts

1. Post (display) of all physical details such as age, sex, physical health and defects like defect in eyesight, hearing and defect in nose, throat, etc. are to be noted.
2. Family details such as family background, size, education, income of parents, order of birth in the family and other members in the family, discipline in the home, mutual relations between different members of the family are to be noted.
3. Details regarding attitude towards school, classmates, teachers, subjects, cocurricular activities, achievements in examinations, sports and cocurricular activities. Failure and promotions, positions and distinction in the class and main difficulties in school or college subjects are to be noted.
4. The details concerning vocational choices, special skills, vocational interests and ambitions, jobs held in the past, satisfied or dissatisfied during the job, reasons of dissatisfaction, relation with the employer, etc. are to be noted.

5. The details of social development such as individual's relation with parents, brothers and sisters, other relatives, playmates, class fellows, teachers, friends, neighbors, etc. are to be noted.
6. Then, the details concerning mental abilities such as intelligence, aptitudes and other mental abilities should be collected with the help of various tests and examinations intended for the purpose are to be noted.
7. Finally, the details concerning other qualities of personality like individual's emotional maturity, interests, motives, ambitions and ideals are to be noted.

Sources

Parents: They can provide quite useful information about the child. This information can be obtained by inviting parents to school on special occasions or contacting them at their homes.

Teacher: They are also able to provide much information about the student. This information has been based on observation, individual records, marks secured in examinations, interview and home visits.

Students: The primary source of student's (individual's) data is being studied by themselves and by other individuals in the school. Their friends and companions can also provide much useful information about them.

Guidance worker: A guidance worker can obtain information about students from many sources. He/she may able to collect this information from family doctors, social workers and members of the community.

Diagnosis of the Problem

1. After collecting relevant information concerning individual, the guidance worker would like to analyze the information, so as to find out the ways and means of solving the problem.
2. This process involving the analysis of information and efforts to find out ways and means of solving the problem is called diagnosis of the problem.
3. The guidance worker is unable to impart individual guidance to the individual without proper diagnosis of the problem.

Prognosis

1. It involves visualizing the extent to which the guidance workers will be successful in solving a person's problem.
2. Guidance workers visualize the result to the guidance, which he/she offers to the individual so as to solve the problems.
3. For example, by observing a person's past performance in mathematics and by measuring his mental abilities, it is possible to make some tentative estimate of what he will achieve after the guidance is rendered.

Therapy

1. Here the guidance worker offers a satisfactory solution of the problem. He will make the individual gain an inspiration for the problem.
2. Various techniques used in therapy include suggestion sublimation through substitution, rational persuasion, re-education, play therapy, change in environment, psychoanalysis, group therapy, occupational therapy and non-directive therapy.

Follow-up Action

After providing guidance, it becomes essential to know that up to what extent the problem is solved. Hence, follow-up becomes essential. Individual guidance is more or less incomplete without follow-up. The following methods find use in follow-up study:

1. Card file method: In this method, details of interview such as name age, sex and address of the interviewer, purpose of interview and details of the problems have been indicated.
2. Questionnaire method: Guidance workers give questionnaire to counselee. In the questionnaire, those items are included, which deals with various aspects of the progress of problems concerning, which the advice was provided.
3. Contact through letters: In this method, counselee is contacted through letters, which can be used even to provide further guidance to the person.

COUNSELING

We have quite often heard the term counseling used in newspaper in the context of counseling for engineering, demission, computer-related admissions and so on. Counseling forms the heart of all guidance programs. We know that proper functioning of the heart is essential for a human; similarly the success or failure of the guidance programmed could be determined by counseling service.

Meaning of Counseling

1. Counseling refers to a progress in which the people are made to approach at an individual level. The person gets help in educational, vocational or psychological field only at problem points.
2. In counseling, the subject matter would be pupil's needs, abilities, aims, aspirations, plans, decisions, actions and limitations.
3. Counseling may be referred to a sort of specialized, personalized and individualized service, which makes effective use of information gathered about any individual.
4. This information provides self-insight, self-analysis and self-direction. This self-direction helps individual to make maximum educational, vocational and psychological adjustments.

Definitions

1. Counseling is a process involving an interaction between a counselor and a client in a private setting, with the purpose of helping the client to change his behavior, so that satisfactory resolutions of needs may be obtained. —*Pepinsky (1954)*
2. Counseling or assisting an individual in the solution of his problems. The interview has an important place in guidance, but is only one-stage in the whole process of counseling. —*Crow and Crow*
3. Basically counseling involves understanding and working with the individual to discover his unique needs, motivations and potentialities and to help him appreciate them. —*Bernard and Fullmer*

Characteristics of Counseling

1. Counseling is based on person-to-person relations.
2. It involves two individuals; one seeking help and the other, a professionally trained who can help the first.
3. The main aim is to help the counselor to discover and solve his personal problems independently.

4. In order to help and assist properly, the counselor must establish a relationship of mutual respect, cooperation and friendliness between the two individuals.
5. The counselor will try to discover the problems of the client and helps him/her to set up goals and guide him/her through difficulties and problems.
6. The main emphasis in the role of counseling process is laid on the counselor's self-direction and self-acceptance.
7. Counseling is democratic. The counselor sets up a democratic pattern and allows the councelee to do freely whatever he/she likes, while with the consultant and not under the consultant.

Rules and Roles of Counseling

Remedial Role

1. It entails working with individuals or groups, to assist them in remedying problems of one kind or another.
2. As noted by Kagan et al (1988) remedial interventions may include personal or social counseling or psychotherapy for an individual or couples (e.g. marital counseling).
3. Crisis intervention and various therapeutic services for students requiring assistance with unresolved life events are additional examples of work at the remedial level.

Preventive Role

1. It is one in which the counseling psychologist seeks to anticipate, circumvent and if possible, forestall difficulties that may arise in the future.
2. Preventive interventions may focus on what are called psycho-educational programs aiming to forestall the development of problems or events.
3. Examples include drug prevention/awareness programs, suicide prevention programs for high-risk individuals and psychological adoption of orphan children, which gives them a feeling of belongingness.

Educational and Developmental Role

1. The purpose, which is to help individuals to plan, obtain and derive maximum benefits from the kind of experiences that will enable them to discover and develop their potentialities.

2. Examples of this would include various workshops or seminars. Another example might be a study skill class, the college students are aimed at making the good students even more effective.
3. The key features of the developmental role are that when performing it, one is going beyond prevention and is involved in enhancement.

Goals of Counseling

1. Facilitating behavioral change.
2. Enhancing coping skills.
3. Promoting decision-making.
4. Improving relationships.
5. Facilitating client potential.

Comparison of Counseling with Other Terms

1. Guidance and counseling: These are not synonyms. Counseling forms a part of guidance. Not all of it.
2. Counseling and interview: Interview is a part of counseling; it is only a technique, which is used in the process of counseling.
3. Counseling and advising: Counseling does not give advice; a wise counselor ever provides advice until it becomes absolutely essential.
4. Counseling and teaching: Counseling does not mean teaching. Teaching is related to academic and instinctual problems, whereas counseling is related to social and emotional problems.
5. Counseling and psychotherapy: Counseling is not considered as psychotherapy, although it is used by psychotherapist as one of the techniques of treatment. Counselor does work in educational setting, while psychotherapist works in medical setting.

Theories of Counseling

Directive Counseling

EG Williamson is the leading architect of this school of thought.

1. It also called prescriptive or counselor-centered counseling.
2. It is considered to be problem-centered and pedocentered.
3. It is the counselor, who prepares plans and sees through the process.

Assumptions

1. All the efforts should be done to tackle the problem of the counselee.
2. As counselor is more competent than the counselee; it means that the former plays a more active role than the client.
3. Counseling is more or less an intellectual rather than emotional process and hence an intellectual aspect is assigned more weightage than emotional aspects.

Steps of directive counseling

1. Analysis: Collection of data is carried out from a variety of sources by using a variety of tools and techniques.
2. Synthesis: Summarizing and organizing the data are to be carried out so as to reveal the client's assets, liabilities, adjustments and maladjustments.
3. Diagnosis: At this stage, an attempt should be made to find out the root cause of the problem exhibited by the client.
4. Prognosis: At this stage, the future development of the client's problems should be predicted.
5. Treatment: It includes establishing report, advice or plan programs.
6. Follow-up: Here the counselor makes an attempt to help the client with new problem or with recurrences of the original problem and ascertains the effectiveness of counseling provided to the client.

Advantages of directive counseling

1. It is more economical in time.
2. Emphasis is mainly laid on the problem, but not on the individual.
3. Directive counseling lays more emphasis on the intellectual rather than the emotional aspects of personality of the individual, but not at the emotional level.
4. The directive counseling methods used have been direct, persuasive and explanatory.

Limitations of directive counseling

1. The counselee would never become independent of the counselor.
2. Directive counseling is unable to keep the counselee away from making mistakes in future.

Non-directive Counseling

Carl Rogers is the chief architect of this school of thought.

1. It is also known as permissive counseling or client-centered counseling.
2. In this type of counseling, the client is the one who forms the pivot or the center. It is the counselee who plays the main role; the counselor remains mostly passive.
3. It is the counselee who actively participates in the process, gets insight into own problems by using the counselor and takes decisions to take an action.

Assumption of non-directive counseling

1. Independence and integration of the client becomes more important than the client.
2. Emotional aspects have been more significant than intellectual aspects.
3. Creating an atmosphere in which the client can work out the understanding is being more important than cultivating self-understanding in the client.
4. Counseling results in a voluntary choice of goals and a conscious selection of courses of action.

Steps of non-directive counseling

1. The client is able to recognize the need of counseling and come for help; help is sought and not given.
2. The counselor is able to define the situation and creates congenital atmosphere.
3. Attitude of the counselor should be friendly with sympathy and affection. He should be interested in the problem of child and should encourage free expression of feeling regarding the problem of individual.
4. The counselor makes an attempt to understand the feelings of the individual.
5. The counselor accepts as well as recognizes the positive and negative feelings.
6. The counselor will pay attention to negative self-feelings of the client or child and changes him/her from negative self-feelings to positive self-feelings, from emotional release to gradual insight.
7. The counselor makes the client to translate the insight to action.
8. A decreased need for help is desired and the client is the one who decides to the contact.

9. Positive steps toward the solution of the problem situation begin to start.

Advantages of non-directive counseling

1. It is slow, but sure process, which makes the individual capable of making adjustments.
2. No tests are used in it and therefore, avoid all that is laborious and difficult.
3. It is able to remove the emotional block and makes the individual to bring the repressed thoughts in conscious level, thereby reducing the tension.

Limitations of non-directive counseling

1. It is quite slow and time-consuming process. In school, it is not feasible, as counselor has to attend many students.
2. The child, the client or the student is unable to make the decisions himself/herself. Hence, we fail to rely upon his/her resources, judgment and wisdom.
3. There are many individuals who may lead from stage to stage. The counselor's passive attitude might be able to irritate the counselee so much that he/she might hesitate to express the feelings.

Eclectic Counseling

Eclectic counseling may be defined as the synthesis and combinations of directive and non-directive counseling.

In this counseling, the counselor has been neither too active as in directive counseling nor too passive as in non-directive counseling.

In elective counseling, first of all the counselor considers the personality and needs of the counselee and then selects the directive or non-directive technique that would serve the purpose for the best. Throne is the chief architect of eclectic counseling.

Steps of eclectic counseling

1. To diagnose the cause.
2. To analyze the problem.
3. To prepare a tentative plan for modifying factors.
4. To secure effective conditions for counseling.
5. To interview and stimulate the client to develop own resources and to assume its responsibility for trying new models of adjustments.

6. To do proper handling of any related problems, which may be able to contribute to adjustments.

Generalizations

1. Generally, passive methods should be used whenever possible.
2. Passive techniques are preferred in the early stages, if the client is telling his/her story. This allows release of emotional stress.
3. Active methods are to be used with specific indication.
4. Complicated methods should not be tried until simpler methods have been failed.
5. All counseling should be client-centered.
6. Every child should be given an opportunity to resolve his/her problems indirectly.
7. Directive methods are generally involved in situational maladjustment, where a solution cannot be achieved without involving cooperation of other persons.
8. Some degree of directiveness will be inevitable in all counseling even in reaching the decision to use passive methods.

Limitations of eclectic counseling

1. Eclectics are not possible, because it is not possible to merge directive and non-directive concepts together.
2. According to some writers, eclectics are vague, superficial and opportunistic.

Basic Principles of Counseling

1. Acceptance: The client must be accepted as a whole person; as a human being.
2. Respect for the individual: Importance is attached to respect for individual.
3. Permissiveness: All schools of counseling would accept relative permissiveness in counseling relationship.
4. Learning: All schools of counseling should accept the learning element in counseling.
5. Thinking in rather than for the client: It is another basic principle of counseling.

Functions or Duties of Counselor

1. Programs of guidance and its organization—these include vocational information service, self-inventory service, personal

data collection service, counseling service, vocational preparatory service, placement and employment service, follow-up or adjustment service.
2. Orientation implies a sort of preparation, which includes collecting data about sources of jobs, disseminating information to pupils and planning activities.
3. Data collection should be done about the individual, administering the test and analyzing the same.
4. Interviews and individual counseling should be held.
5. Contacts should be made outside agencies like parents, guidance bureaus and employment exchanges.
6. Placement and follow-up work should be done.

Characteristics or Qualifications of Counselor

Personality Traits

1. Breadth of interest: A counselor must be interested in various types of people, jobs and organization.
2. Cooperation: A counselor should cooperate with all the staff in a cheerful manner.
3. Refinement: A counselor should not be overconfident, but should be modest and humble toward the pupils.
4. Magnetism: A counselor should create confidence in others and put others at ease.
5. Considerateness: A counselor should understand the difficulties of a teacher, exhibit human understanding and possess real love for fellow men.

Training and Preparation

Good education, which includes knowledge of humanities like sociology, psychology, economics, history, geography, etc.

1. To know principles of guidance.
2. To know objectives, curriculum and methods of secondary schools.
3. To know vocational activities.
4. To know methods of imparting occupational information.
5. To know psychological tests in guidance services.
6. To know about organization of guidance services.

Experiences

1. Competence as a leader in guidance program.
2. Competence as a counselor.
3. Competence in interpreting and using information.
4. Competence in placement and follow-up services.
5. Competence in using community resources.
6. Competence in evaluating the counseling service itself.

EDUCATIONAL GUIDANCE

Guidance services are meant to help students to make proper adjustments with the environment in which they are living and also make the best possible contributions commensurate with one's strengths and limitations. Educational guidance refers to guidance to students in all aspects of education.

The emphasis is on providing assistance to students to perform satisfactory in their academic work, choose the appropriate course of study, overcome learning difficulties, foster creativity, improve levels of motivation and utilize institutional resources such as library, laboratory, etc. optimally.

Definitions

1. The educational guidance deals with assistance given to pupils in their choices and adjustments with relation to schools, curriculum, courses and school life. —*Jones*
2. Educational guidance refers to a process, which is concerned with bringing about an individual pupil, which has distinctive characteristics on one hand and differing group of opportunities and requirements on the other, a favorable setting for the individual's development or education. —*Myer*

Objectives

1. To monitor academic program of students.
2. To identify special learners such as academically backward, gifted and creative.
3. To assist students in further education.
4. To provide assistance to special learners by catering to their educational needs.

5. To diagnose the learning difficulties of students in different subjects.
6. To help students in their adjustments to curriculum and co-curricular demands of the educational programs.
7. To provide career information.

Need of Educational Guidance

1. *Wastage and stagnation:* There occurs a lot of wastage and stagnation in education. The number of failures in the examination is responsible for much wastage to the nation.
2. *Diversified curriculum:* The curriculum is being diversified in the higher secondary and multipurpose schools. Therefore, the need for guidance in the selection of subjects of studies is becoming an utmost necessity.
3. *Decision for further education:* Educational guidance is needed in order to help the pupil to make the best use of their potentialities and resources.
4. *Preparation for future vocation:* An urgent need is required for preparing and helping the pupils for further vocation, while keeping in view their potentialities, interests and aptitudes and the demands of the society.

For a balanced life, simple vocational education is not sufficient, children must be educated to live and help together.

Purposes of Educational Guidance

1. *Wise selection of the curriculum:* It is known that the pupil's success in the field of education depends upon the wise selection of curriculum. Hence, an important purpose of education assists in selecting a curriculum in accordance with their abilities, aptitudes and interests.
2. *Improvement in methods of study:* Another aim of educational guidance is to improve the methods of study. The methods of study include such factors as mode of reading, mode of taking notes, methods of memorizing and summarizing.
3. *Providing special methods of education to backward students:* Guidance is mainly given to evolve special methods of education for pupils who usually fail in examinations, show signs of delinquency, indiscipline or run away from classes. The methods of education for backward children are evolved by keeping in view,

the causes of backwardness including special schools, specialists with special curriculum and special methods of teaching.
4. *Making special arrangements for gifted students:* Another specific aim of educational guidance is to arrange special educational programs for the gifted students.
5. *Taking into account, the failures in examination*: A large number of failures at various examinations is responsible for much wastage and stagnation. Many students lose their mental equilibrium as a result of failure.
6. Educational guidance is to help the students to secure information concerning the possibility and desirability of further schooling.
7. Educational guidance is to help them to know the requirements for entrance into the school of their choice.
8. Educational guidance is to help the students to find the purpose and functions of different types of schools.
9. Educational guidance is to guide them in selection of vocations.

Stages of Educational Guidance

At Elementary Stage

1. To help pupils to develop good habits, right attitudes and basic skills.
2. To help pupils to make a good beginning.
3. To help pupils to plan intelligently.
4. To help pupils to obtain the best out of their education.

At Secondary Stage

1. Helping the child to know himself.
2. Helping the child to understand the environment.
3. Helping the child to make the right choice of subjects.
4. Helping the child to know about the college education.

At College Stage

1. Providing library facilities for broadening the mental horizon of the students.
2. Providing special guidance for certain subjects and preparation for examination.
3. Providing special guidance for selection of books and reference books.

4. Guiding the individual to learn how to read books, make notes, summarize and organize the materials, and make use of quotations.

Factors Involved in Educational Guidance

1. Secondary schools become less selective.
2. Emphasis upon individual difference.
3. Growing complexity of the world of work.
4. Expansion of the school programs.
5. The concept of the child growth and development.
6. Beneficial effects of group testing.
7. Influences of social and economical conditions.

Basic Principles of Educational Guidance

1. Guidance should be provided to all.
2. Standardized tests should be employed.
3. Selection of curriculum should be done.
4. Remedy should be given in the beginning.
5. Relevant information has to be obtained.
6. Follow-up study must be there.
7. Relationship between school and parents should be set up.

VOCATIONAL GUIDANCE

In this scientific and technological age, one of the most important aspects of man's life is vocation. Therefore, one has to choose vocation for himself/herself. One of the main aims of education is to give maximum help in one's professional life. If vocational aim of education is not fulfilled, then education becomes worthless.

Vocational guidance is fundamentally, an effort for conserving the priceless native capacities of youth and the costly training provided for youth in the school. It conserves, this richness of all human resources by the individual to invest and use them, which will bring greatest satisfaction and success to himself and greatest benefit to society.

Definitions

1. Vocational guidance, as assistance, given to an individual in solving problems related to occupational choices and progress

with due regard, for the individual's characteristics and their relation to occupational opportunity.

—International Labor Organization

2. Vocational guidance is the process of assisting the individual to choose an occupation, prepare for it and enter upon and progressing with it. *—Vocational Guidance Association*

Need of Vocational Guidance

1. To increase the number of occupations.
2. Vocational guidance is to maintain the health.
3. To promote personal and social values.
4. To discover and utilize the human potentialities.
5. To meet the needs of an individual and complex nature of the society.
6. To promote financial growth of an individual and society.

Special Aims of Vocational Guidance

1. To assist the student to acquire such knowledge of the characteristics and functions, the duties and rewards of the group of occupations.
2. To enable the student to find what general and specific abilities, skills, etc. are required for the group of occupations.
3. To give opportunity for experiences in school that will give much information about conditions of work and will assist the individual to discover his/her own abilities, help in the development of wider interests.
4. To help the individual develop, the point of view that all honest labor is worth and that the most important bases for choice of an occupation.
5. To assist the individual to acquire a technique of analysis of occupation information and to develop the habit of analyzing such information, before making a final choice.
6. To assist the student to secure such information about himself/herself, his/her abilities (general and specific), interests and powers, as this may be needed for wise choice.
7. To assist economically handicapped children, who are above the compulsory attendance age to secure through public or private funds, scholarships or other financial assistance.
8. To assist the student to secure knowledge of the facilities offered by various educational institutions for vocational training and

the requirements for admission to them, the length of training offered and the cost of attendance.

9. To keep the worker to adjust himself/herself to the occupation in which he/she is engaged; to assist to understand relationship with other workers in own related occupation and to society as a whole.
10. To enable the student to secure reliable information about the danger of alluring shortcuts to fortune.

Characteristics of Vocational Guidance

1. It helps the child to develop potentialities to the optimum level.
2. It is a process, which helps the person to impart occupational information, broadening the occupational horizon and including his/her interests in vocational self-help.
3. It is a process, which helps individual to select an occupation for life, to prepare for it and to be place against a suitable job. Also progress in the job is to be watched.
4. It is a process, which helps the person to develop and accept an integrated and correct picture of himself/herself and role in the economy of the society to which he/she belongs.
5. It is a process, which helps the individual to evaluate his/her role in terms of reality or practicability.
6. It is a process, which helps the individual to achieve the vocational goal. The process of achieving the vocational goal should be useful to society.
7. It is a process, which helps the individual to make adjustments in relation to occupation or job.

Stages of Vocational Guidance

At Elementary Stage

1. It is in this period where habits, skills and attitudes develop.
2. For developing the basic skills and attitudes.
3. For developing the habit of doing the work in a neat and systematic manner.
4. For developing good interpersonal relationships.

At Secondary Stage

1. To help pupils to appraise or to know their vocational assets and liabilities.

2. To make pupils to be familiar with various occupations and their requirements.
3. To help pupils to make a right choice.
4. To help pupils to prepare themselves for entering into the occupations of their choices.
5. To help pupils to get suitable jobs in their chosen field.
6. To help pupils to think seriously, whether to go to college or not.

At College Stage

1. To help pupil for making a comprehensive study of the cancer, which they would like to pursue.
2. To help pupils to relate their studies to vocations that is open to them.
3. To help pupils for acquainting themselves with different avenues of work.
4. To help pupils to acquainting themselves with avenues for higher studies and various programs for financial assistance, scholarships, stipends, grants, fellowship, etc.
5. To help pupils to make contacts that would help in putting their plan into successful operation.

SUGGESTED READING

1. Anthikad Jacob. Psychology for Graduate Nurses, 4th edition. New Delhi: Jaypee Brothers Medical Publishers (P) Ltd; 2007.
2. Bhatia BD, Craig Margaretta. Elements of Psychology and Mental Hygiene for Nurses in India. Chennai: Orient Longman; 2005.
3. Das G. Educational Psychology. New Delhi: Kind Books.
4. Gross Richard, Kinnison Nancy. Psychology for Nurses and Allied Health Professionals. London: Hodder Arnold; 2007.
5. Hilgard RE, Atkinson CR, Atkinson LR. Introduction to Psychology, 6th edition. New Delhi: Oxford and IBH Publishing Co Pvt Ltd; 1975.
6. Hurlock B Elizabeth. Developmental Psychology. A Lifespan Approach, 5th edition. New Delhi: Tata McGraw-Hill Edition; 2002.
7. Khan MA. Psychology for Nurses. New Delhi: Academa Publishers; 2004.
8. Kuppuswamy B. An Introduction to Social Psychology. Bombay: Media Promoters and Publishers (P) Ltd; 1994.

9. Mangal SK. Advanced Educational Psychology, 6th edition. New Delhi: Prentice Hall of India (P) Ltd; 2007.
10. Mangal SK. General Psychology. New Delhi: Sterling Publishers (P) Ltd; 2006.
11. Matlin W Margaret. Psychology, 3rd edition. Philadelphia Harcourt Brace College Publishers; 1999.
12. Morgan T Clifford, King A Richard, Weisz R John. Introduction to Psychology, 7th edition. New Delhi: Tata McGraw-Hill Publishing Company Ltd; 2004.
13. Myers G David. Social Psychology, 6th edition. Boston: McGraw-Hill College; 1991.
14. Nagaraja Rao, Begum Shamshad B, Sudarshan CY. MCQs in Psychology for Nursing and Allied Sciences. New Delhi: Jaypee Brothers Medical Publishers (P) Ltd; 2006.
15. Ramnath Sharma. Psychology and Mental Hygiene for Nurses. Meerut: Kedarnath Ramnath and Co.
16. Robert S Feldman. Understanding Psychology, 6th edition. New Delhi: Tata McGraw-Hill Edition; 2004.
17. Sinclair C Helen, Fawcett N Josephine. Altschul's Psychology for Nurses, 7th edition. London: Bailliere Tindall; 1991.
18. Skinner E Charles. Educational Psychology, 4th Edition. New Delhi: Prentice-hall of India (P) Ltd; 1996.
19. Taylor E Shelley. Health Psychology, 6th edition. New York: Tata McGraw-Hill Edition; 2006.

REVIEW QUESTIONS

1. Define guidance. Explain principles and elements of guidance.
2. Explain characteristics and basic assumption of guidance.
3. Discuss the need and purpose of guidance.
4. Enumerate the various types of guidance services.
5. Define counseling. Explain the meaning and characteristics of counseling.
6. Discuss the various theories of counseling in detail.
7. Define education guidance. Explain the needs and objectives.
8. Define vocational guidance. Explain the needs and special aims.

CHAPTER 19

Mental Illness

LEARNING OBJECTIVES

1. Definition.
2. Characteristics.
3. Common signs and symptoms.
4. Concepts of normal and abnormal behaviors.
5. Burdens of mental disorders.
6. Misconceptions about mental illnesses.
7. Mental health team.

DEFINITION

Mental and behavioral disorders are understood as clinically significant conditions characterized by alterations in thinking, mood (emotions) or behavior associated with personal distress and/or impaired functioning [World Health Organization (WHO) 2001].

CHARACTERISTICS

1. Changes in one's thinking, memory, perception, feeling and judgment resulting in changes in talk and behavior, which appear to be deviant from previous personality or from the norms of community.
2. These changes in behavior cause distress and suffering to the individual or others or both.
3. Changes and the consequent distress cause disturbance in day-to-day activities, work and relationship with others (social and vocational dysfunction).

FEATURES

The features of mental illness are classified under four headings:

1. Disturbances in bodily functions.
2. Disturbances in mental functions.
3. Changes in individual and social activities.
4. Somatic complaints.

Disturbances in Bodily Functions

Sleep: Disturbed sleep throughout the night, no sleep at all, difficulty in falling asleep or waking up in the middle of night and failing to fall asleep again. In addition, the individual may experience lethargy and lack of freshness in the morning.

Appetite and food intake: Increased or decreased appetite, weight loss or weight gain, nausea, vomiting.

Bowel and bladder movement: Diarrhea or constipation, increased micturition, bedwetting.

Sexual desire and activity: Decreased interest in sex, premature ejaculation, impotence or lack of sexual satisfaction. In some conditions, there can be excessive sexual desire or lack of social inhibitions.

Disturbances in Mental Functions

Behavior: The patient may exhibit overactivity, restlessness, irritability, may be abusive to others for trivial or no reasons at all or the patient may become dull, withdrawn and not respond to external or internal cues. At times the patient may behave in a bizarre way, which the family members may find irritating. Sometimes the patient's behavior can be dangerous to self or others.

Speech: Patient talks excessively and unnecessarily or talks very little or stays mute. The talk becomes irrelevant and un-understandable (incoherent).

Thought: Patient expresses peculiar and wrong beliefs, which others do not share.

Emotions: Patient may exhibit excessive emotions like happiness, anger, fear or sadness. Sometimes, emotions can be inappropriate to situations. He/she may laugh to self or weep without any reason.

Perception: The patient may perceive without any stimulus. There can be misinterpretation of perception. For example, a mentally ill person can see things or hear sounds or feel objects, which do not exist or which others do not see. This is known as hallucinations. A patient, who is hallucinating is seen talking to self, laughing or weeping to self, wandering in the streets and behaving in a manner, which others may find abnormal.

Attention and concentration: Patient may have decreased attention and concentration; may get distracted easily or have selective inattention.

Memory: Patient may lose the memory and start forgetting important matters.

Intelligence and judgment: In some mental illnesses, intelligence and the ability to take decisions deteriorate. Patient loses reasoning skills and abilities, may not be able to perform simple arithmetic or commit mistakes in routine work.

Level of consciousness: In some mental illnesses due to possible brain damage there may be changes in the level of consciousness. Patient fails to identify his/her relatives. He/she can be disoriented to time and place, and may remain confused or become unconscious.

Changes in Individual and Social Activities

Patients may neglect their bodily needs and personal hygiene. They may also lose social sense. They behave in an inappropriate manner in social situations and embarrass others. They behave strangely with their family members, friends, colleagues and others. They may insult, abuse/assault them.

Somatic Complaints

Patient may complain of aches and pains in different parts of the body, fatigue, weakness, involuntary movements, etc.

COMMON SIGNS AND SYMPTOMS OF MENTAL ILLNESS

Disturbances in Motor Behavior

Motor retardation, stupor, stereotypes, negativism, ambitendency, waxy flexibility, echopraxia, restlessness, agitation and excitement.

Disorders of thought, language, communication, pressure of speech, poverty of speech, dysarthria, flight of ideas, circumstantialities, loosening of association, tangentiality, incoherence, perseveration, neologism, clang association, thought block, thought insertion, thought broadcasting, echolalia, delusions, obsessions and phobias.

Disorders of perception—illusions, hallucinations, depersonalization, derealization.

Disorders of emotion—blunt affect, labile affect, elated mood, euphoria, ecstasy, dysphoric mood, depression, anhedonia.

Disturbances of consciousness: Clouding of consciousness, delirium and coma.

Disturbances in attention: Distractibility, selective inattention.

Disturbances in orientation: Disorientation of time, place or person.

Disturbances of memory: Amnesia, confabulation.

Impaired Judgment

Disturbances in Biological Function

Persistent deviations in temperature, pulse and respiration, nausea, vomiting, headache, loss of appetite, increased appetite, loss of weight, pain, fatigue, weight gain, insomnia, hypersomnia and sexual dysfunction.

CONCEPTS OF NORMAL AND ABNORMAL BEHAVIORS

Psychiatry as evident from the above is concerned with abnormal behavior in its broadest sense, but defining the concepts of normal and abnormal behaviors such has been found to be difficult. These concepts are much under the influence of sociocultural factors.

Several models have been put forward in order to explain the concepts of normal and abnormal behaviors. Some of them are given below.

Medical Model

Medical model considers organic pathology as the definite cause for mental disorder. According to this model, abnormal people are the ones who have disturbances in thought, perception and psychomotor activities. The normal are the ones, who are free from these disturbances.

Statistical Model

Statistical model involves the analysis of responses on a test or a questionnaire or observations of some particular behavioral variables. The degree of deviation from the standard norms arrived at statistically, characterizes the degree of abnormality.

Statistically normal mental health falls within two standard deviations (SDs) of the normal distribution curve.

Sociocultural Model

The beliefs, norms, taboos and values of a society have to be accepted and adopted by individuals. Breaking any of these would be considered as abnormal. Normalcy is defined in context with social norms prescribed by the culture. Thus, cultural background has to be taken into account when distinguishing between normal and abnormal behavior.

Behavior Model

Behavior that is adaptive is normal, maladaptive is abnormal. Abnormal behavior is a set of faulty behaviors acquired through learning.

Problems of Mental Disorders

1. Self-care limitations or impaired functioning related to mental illness.
2. Significant deficits in biological, emotional and cognitive functioning.
3. Disability, life process changes.
4. Emotional problems such as anxiety, anger, sadness, loneliness and grief.
5. Physical symptoms that occur along with altered psychological functioning.
6. Alteration in thinking, perceiving, communicating and decision-making.
7. Difficulties in relating to others.
8. Patient's behavior may be dangerous to self or others.
9. Adverse effects on the well-being of the individual, family and community.
10. Financial, marital, family, academic and occupational problems.

BURDENS OF MENTAL DISORDERS

Mental disorders are common, affecting more than 25 percent of all people at some time during their lives. They are also universal, affecting people in all countries and societies, individuals of all ages, women and men, the rich and the poor from urban and rural environments. They have an economic impact on societies and on the quality of life of individuals and families. Some of them are:

1. Mental disorders at any point of time are present in about 10 percent of the adult population. Around 20 percent of all patients seen by primary healthcare professionals have one or more mental disorders.
2. During the last 2 decades many epidemiological studies have been conducted in India, which show that mental disorders prevail in 18 to 207 per 1,000, with median 65.4 per 1,000 at any given time. About 2.3 percent of the population suffers from seriously incapacitating mental disorders or epilepsy. A large number of adult patients 10.4% to 53.0% coming to the general outpatient department are diagnosed as mentally ill.
3. It is estimated that in 2000, mental disorders accounted for 12 percent of the total disability adjusted life years (DALYs) the year lost due to all diseases and injuries. Common disorders, which usually cause severe disability, include depressive disorder, substance use disorders, schizophrenia, epilepsy, Alzheimer's disease, mental retardation and disorders of childhood and adolescence.
4. More than 450 million people today suffer from mental and behavioral disorders. Within the next 20 years depression will have the dubious distinction of becoming the second biggest cause for global burden of disease (GBD).
5. Worldwide 70 million people suffer from alcohol dependence, 50 million from epilepsy, 24 million from schizophrenia and another 20 million people attempt suicide every year.
6. Global burden of disease, 2000 estimates show that mental and neurological conditions account for 30.8 percent of all years lived with disability (YLD). Depression causes the largest amount of disability, accounting for almost 12 percent of all disabilities. Six neuropsychiatry conditions figured in the top 20 causes of disability worldwide, which include:
   - Unipolar depressive disorders
   - Alcohol use disorders

- Schizophrenia
- Bipolar affective disorders
- Alzheimer's and other dementias
- Migraine.

7. Mental illnesses cause massive disruption in the lives of individuals, families and communities. Individuals suffer the distressing symptoms of disorders. They also suffer because they are unable to participate in work and leisure activities often as a result of discrimination. They worry about not being able to show their responsibilities toward their family and friends, and are fearful of being a burden to others. Mental illnesses are common to all countries and cause immense suffering. People with these disorders are often subjected to social isolation, poor quality of life and increased mortality. These disorders are thus the cause of staggering economic and social costs.
8. It is estimated that one in four families has at least one member currently suffering from mental illness. These families are required not only to provide physical and emotional support but also to bear the negative impact of stigma and discrimination present in all parts of the world.
9. Families in which one member is suffering from a mental disorder make a number of adjustments and compromises that prevent other members of the family from achieving their full potential in work, social relationships and leisure. These are the human aspects of the burden of mental disorders that are difficult to assess and quantify.
10. The impact of mental disorders in communities is large and manifold. There is the cost of providing care, the loss of productivity and certain legal problems associated with some mental disorders.

MISCONCEPTIONS ABOUT MENTAL ILLNESS

Beliefs about mental illness have been characterized by superstition, ignorance and fear. Although, time and advances in scientific understanding of mental illness have dispelled many false ideas, there remain a number of popular misconceptions. Some of them are:

Mental illness: It is caused by supernatural power and is the result of a curse or possession by evil spirit. Many people do not consider mental illness as an illness, but possession by evil spirits or curse that has befallen on the patient or family because of past sins or misdeeds in previous life.

Mentally ill people show bizarre behavior: Patients in mental hospitals and clinics are often pictures as a weird lot, who spend their time in exhibiting useless bizarre behavior like twisting of hands, etc.

Mentally ill people are dangerous: People, who have or had a mental illness, are viewed with suspicion and as dangerous persons.

Mental illness is something to be ashamed of: This idea arouses an unsympathetic, cruel attitude toward mentally ill person. This is the reason why many people hide mental illness in the family.

Mental illness is not curable: People object to have normal relationship with mentally ill people or to give them employment even after being cured or even to accept them as neighbors.

Mental illness is contagious: The fear that it is contagious is the main false notion, which leads people to view suspiciously or object to marital relations with a person belonging to the household of the mentally ill.

Mental illness is hereditary: It is not a rule that children of mentally ill patients should become mentally ill.

Marriage can cure mental illness: A mentally ill person can get worse, if he/she gets married when he/she is ill, as marriage can become an additional stress. A patient, who has recovered can get married and live a normal life like any other person.

Mental hospitals: These are the places where only dangerous mentally ill individuals are treated and restraint is a major form of treatment. People hesitate to take their relatives to mental hospitals for treatment because of fear. Further, as a former patient of a mental hospital, he/she as well as his/her family members is often isolated. Therefore, people seek help from mental hospitals only as a last resort.

GENERAL ATTITUDE TOWARD THE MENTALLY ILL PATIENTS

1. In general, the community responds to the mentally ill through denial, isolation and rejection. There is also a lack of

understanding of mental illness as any other illness and a lack of tendency to reject both the patients and those who treat them.
2. Mentally ill patients are viewed as people with no capacity for understanding.
3. People feel mental illness cannot be cured and even if the patient gets better, complete physical rest is considered essential.
4. The mentally ill are by and large perceived as aggressive, violent and dangerous.

An individual's values and personal beliefs affect his/her attitude about mental illness, the mentally ill and treatment of mental illness. There still exists a stigma surrounding individuals, who need or use psychiatric mental health services. The need continues for public education to modify or alter misconceptions about mental illness and people with mental disorders.

MENTAL HEALTH TEAM

Multidisciplinary approach refers to collaboration between members of different disciplines, who provide specific services to the patient.

The multidisciplinary team includes:
1. A psychiatrist.
2. A psychiatric nurse.
3. A clinical psychologist.
4. A psychiatric social worker.
5. An occupational therapist or activity therapist.
6. A pharmacist and a dietitian.
7. A counselor.

Psychiatrist

Psychiatrist is a medical doctor with special training in psychiatry. He/she is accountable for the medical diagnosis and treatment of patient. Other important functions are:
1. Admitting patient into acute care setting.
2. Prescribing and monitoring psychopharmacologic agents.
3. Administering electroconvulsive therapy.
4. Conducting individual and family therapy.
5. Participating in interdisciplinary team meetings.
6. Owing to their legal power to prescribe and to write orders, psychiatrists often function as leaders of the team.

Psychiatric Nurse

Psychiatric nurse is a registered nurse with specialized training in the care and treatment of psychiatric patients; he/she may have a Diploma, MSc, MPhil or PhD in psychiatric nursing. He/she is accountable for the biopsychosocial nursing care of patients and their milieu. Other functions include:

1. Administering and monitoring medications.
2. Assisting in numerous psychiatric and physical treatments.
3. Participating in interdisciplinary team meetings.
4. Teach patients and families.
5. Take responsibility for patient's records.
6. Act as patient's advocate.
7. Significant interaction between patients and others.

Clinical Psychologist

Clinical psychologist should have a Masters Degree in psychology or PhD in clinical psychology with specialized training in mental health settings. He/she is accountable for psychological assessments, testing and treatments. He/she offers direct services such as individual, family or marital therapies.

Psychiatric Social Worker

Psychiatric social worker should have a Masters Degree in social work or PhD degree with specialized training in mental health settings. He/she is accountable for family case work and community placement of patients. He/she conducts group therapy sessions, emphasizes intervention with the patient in social environment in which he/she will live.

Occupational Therapist or Activity Therapist

An occupational therapist or activity therapist is accountable for recreational, occupational and activity programs. He/she assists the patients to gain skills that help them to cope more effectively to gain or retain employment, to use leisure time.

Counselor

A counselor provides basic supportive counseling and assists in psychoeducational and recreational activities.

SUGGESTED READING

1. Anthikad Jacob. Psychology for Graduate Nurses, 4th edition. New Delhi: Jaypee Brothers Medical Publishers (P) Ltd; 2007.
2. Bhatia BD, Craig Margaretta. Elements of Psychology and Mental Hygiene for Nurses in India. Chennai: Orient Longman; 2005.
3. Gabor D. First contact body language. How to Start a Conversation and Make Friends, Revised edition. New York: Rockefeller Center: Fireside Publications; 2001.
4. Grant. Child Development in India, 3rd edition. New Delhi: Ashish Publishing House; 1992. p. 21.
5. Morgan CT. A Brief Introduction to Psychology. New Delhi: Tata McGraw-Hill; 1975.
6. Morgan CT, King RA. Introduction to Psychology, 6th edition. New Delhi: Tata McGraw-Hill; 1982.
7. Munn, Norman L. Introduction to Psychology. New Delhi: Oxford and IBH; 1973.
8. Robinson DN. An Intellectual History of Psychology. New York: Macmillan; 1976.
9. Santrock JW. Child Development, 7th edition. Sydney: Brown and Benchmark Publishers; 1996.
10. Tendon BN. Management of severely malnourished children by village workers through ICDS in India. Journal of Trop Pediatri. 1984 Oct;30(5):274.

REVIEW QUESTIONS

1. Define mental illness. Explain the characteristics, and common signs and symptoms of mental illness.
2. Discuss the concepts of normal and abnormal behaviors.
3. Enumerate the burdens of mental disorders.
4. Explain the misconceptions about mental illness.
5. Describe mental health team in detail.

CHAPTER

20

Assessment of Knowledge, Skills, Attitude and Evaluation

LEARNING OBJECTIVES

1. Definitions.
2. Evaluation in nursing.
3. Steps in evaluation.
4. Principles of evaluation.
5. Purpose and scope of evaluation.
6. Personality tests.
7. Rating scale.
8. Checklist.
9. Anecdotal records.
10. Objective structured practical examination.

INTRODUCTION

Evaluation includes a variety of procedures. A vast variety of evaluation procedures is available for measuring the results of teaching and learning. Evaluation procedures can be classified as qualitative and quantitative techniques. It can also be classified in terms of aspects of behavior to be evaluated and in term of evaluative method used.

DEFINITIONS

1. Evaluation is a relatively new technical term introduced to designate a more comprehensive concept of measurement. It is implied in conventional tests and examination.

   —*Wringhtone*

2. Evaluation is essential in the never-ending cycle of formulating goals, measuring progress toward them and determining the new goals, which emerge as a result of new warnings.

   —*Clara M Brown*

3. Evaluation in education is a process of judging the effectiveness of educational experiences through careful appraisal.

   —*LE Heidgerken*

4. Evaluation is a process used to determine what has happened during a given activity or in an institution.

   —*John W Best*

Evaluation requires many skills that are of equal importance with the other elements of the instructional process. A complete evaluation program for a teacher of nursing would encompass evaluation of the following:

a. Educational objectives.
b. Teaching and learning procedures.
c. Student's progress.
d. Outcomes.

EVALUATION IN NURSING

The very essence of nursing requires the nurses to evaluate constantly the patient's nursing needs, as well as his/her own activities in meeting these needs, guiding the patient to evaluate his/her own health needs, determining how well he/she is meeting them and planning with him/her to maintain an optimal level of health.

All of this requires continuous evaluation. The nurses must evaluate the results of the interventions they perform for the patients. By evaluating the condition of patients, they can provide better care to their patients.

General Evaluation Plan

1. Evaluation in education is a systematic process, which enables to measure the extent to which the student has achieved the educational objectives.
2. This plan should include a list of learning outcomes and the techniques to be used in evaluating the outcomes.
3. It must be planned jointly by teachers and others including students involved in teaching and learning process.
4. It should be a group activity.

Steps in Construction of Test

Groulund summarized the preliminary steps in construction of test as follows:

1. Objectives and specific learning outcomes must be identified and defined in terms of desired changes in pupil behavior.
2. Subject matter contents must be outlined.
3. A table of specification, which related to the subject matter content, should be developed.
4. Specific test questions are constructed in accordance with the table of specification.

STEPS IN EVALUATION

According to LE Heidgerken:

1. Starting objectives.
2. Defining changing in behavior expected as outcomes.
3. Listing and briefing describing situations that give opportunity for the expression of the behaviors described.
4. Developing appropriate and systematic means of electing kinds of behavior implied in the objectives to be evaluated.
5. Receding on ways of recording and summarizing (scores, rating or describing) behavior as the basic of evidence collected.
6. Checking validity, reliability and difficulty of the measures used.
7. Establishing conditions that permit the students to give the best performance.
8. Assigning scores on the basis of the above step.
9. Developing methods of interpretation.

Criteria for Selecting Evaluation Tools or Devices

Major criteria used in selecting and developing evaluation tools are:

1. Sample of objectives.
2. Sampling of the content.
3. Checking validity, reliability, practicability and usefulness.

Evaluation Methodology

There is certain methodology for evaluation. The educational spiral illustrated by Gilbert is given below. It has four steps. They are:

1. Defining objectives.
2. Planning evaluation system.
3. Preparing.
4. Implementing evaluation.

The processes are repeated giving feedback and re-examining the objectives and making necessary changes in the education system (programs). Evaluation is continuous process and the results are used for the educational spiral—Gilbert.

PRINCIPLES OF EVALUATION

1. The objectives of evaluation must be stated clearly, before evaluation is made.
2. Evaluation techniques should be selected in terms of the purposes to be served.
3. Comprehensive evaluation requires a variety of evaluation techniques.
4. Proper use of evaluation technique requires awareness of their limitation, as well as on their strength.
5. Evaluation is a means to an end and not an end itself. Evaluation procedures would be related in terms of the decisions to be made.
6. Evaluation procedures must contribute to improved decisions of instruction, guidance and administrative nature.
7. Since, evaluation involves getting evidence about the behaviors that are desired as educational objectives, an appropriate method of evaluation is required.
8. Evaluation assures that it is possible to estimate the typical reaction of the students by getting evidence about a sample of the reaction (behavior).

PURPOSES OF EVALUATION

1. Evaluation procedures help the students to know the desired behaviors to be achieved and what the desired behaviors to be achieved and what they should learn.
2. It helps the students to identify their difficulties and problems in learning and know the progress they make.
3. To guide the teacher and students in selecting of future learning.

4. To provide guidance and counseling to the students related to learning.
5. To provide judgment as to the appropriateness and feasibility of determined objectives.
6. To provide the teacher with clues to the effectiveness of the course plan, teaching method and effectiveness of learning experience provided.
7. To decide promotion and placement, etc.
8. To report the parents, the achievement of the students.
9. To diagnose each student's strength and weakness and suggest remedial measures.
10. To motivate and encourage students to learn.
11. To determine the level of knowledge and understanding of students at various levels.
12. To gather information needed for administrative purpose, such as selecting students for honors course. Placement of students for advanced standing programs and meeting graduation requirements. Evaluation helps the administration to determine effectiveness of curriculum, its strength and weakness to interpret to the public, the goals and accomplishments of the school.

SCOPE OF EVALUATION AND ASSESSMENT

1. Value judgment.
2. Effectiveness of appraisal or method of instruction.
3. Provide baseline for guidance and counseling.
4. Placement and promotion in jobs.
5. Ascertaining the extent to which the educational objectives have been attained.
6. Development of attitudes, interests, capabilities, creativity, originality, knowledge and skills, etc.
7. Development of tools and techniques.
8. Development of curriculum and its revision.
9. Interpretation of results.

CHARACTERISTICS OF EVALUATION PROCEDURE

Essential Characteristics

1. *Validity:* It is the extent to which the test used really measures, what it is intended to measure.

2. *Reliability:* It is the term used to indicate the consistency with which a test measures, what it is designed to measure.
3. *Objectivity:* This is the extent to which independent and competent examiners agree on what constitutes a good answer for each of the item of measuring instruments.
4. *Usability:* This implies such factors as the time taken to conduct the test, the cost of using it and practicability for everyday use.

Other Characteristics

1. *Relevance:* It is the degree to which the centers established for selecting questions, so that they confirm to the aims of the measuring instrument.
2. *Equilibrium:* Achievement of correct proportion or balance among questions allotted to each of the objectives of a course and representatives of the sample of the tasks included in the test.
3. *Discrimination:* This refers to the quality of each element of measuring instruments, which makes it possible to distinguish between good and poor student in relation to a given variable.

EVALUATION TOOLS

Evaluation tools are divided into three domains:
1. Intellectual skills.
2. Communication skills.
3. Practical skills.

Intellectual Skills

The test and scales that have met the criteria of testing are known as intellectual skills.

Characteristics of Standardized Tests

According to Thorndike:
1. A fixed set of test items, designed to measure clearly designed sample of behaviors.
2. Specific direction for administering and scoring the test.
3. Standard content and procedures.

Types of Standardized Test

They are of five types:
1. Achievement tests.
2. Aptitude tests.

3. Personality tests.
4. Intelligence test.
5. Prognostic test.

Intelligence Tests

Meaning of Intelligence

Binet describes intelligence as:

1. The tendency of thought to take and maintain a definite direction.
2. The capacity to make adaptation for the purpose of attaining a desired end.
3. The power of self-criticism.

Measurement of Intelligence

Intelligence is measured through a complicated process. It involves a comparison and establishment of a relationship between chronological age (CA) and mental age (MA). This relationship is expressed by the term intelligence quotient (IQ). When the MA is divided by the CA and the quotient is multiplied by 100, the result is IQ.

$$IQ = \frac{MA}{CA} \times 100$$

Classification of Intelligence Tests

Intelligence tests may be classified under three categories, such as:

1. *Individual tests:* These tests are administered to one individual at a time. These cover age group from 2 to 18 years. These are:
   a. The Binet-Simon tests.
   b. Revised tests by Terman.
   c. Mental and scholastic tests of Burt.
2. *Group tests:* These are administered to a group of people. Group tests had birth in America—when the intelligence of the recruits who joined the army in the First World War was to be calculated. These are:
   a. The army alpha and beta test.
   b. Terman's group tests.
   c. Otis self-administrative tests.
3. *Performance tests:* These tests are administered to the illiterate person. These tests generally involve the construction of certain

patterns or solving problems in terms of concrete material. Some of the famous tests are:

a. Koh's block design test.
b. The cube construction tests.
c. The pass along tests.

4. *Aptitude test:* According to Traxler, aptitude is a present condition, which is indicative of an individual's potentials for the future.

Hahn and Macheam, aptitude is correctly referred to as latent potentialities, undeveloped capacities to acquire abilities and skills; and to demonstrate achievements.

Measurement of Scholastic Aptitude

1. *School marks and scholastic aptitude:* This is the traditional method of measuring aptitude.
2. *Occupation of parents and scholastic aptitude:* McNemur tested the IQ of children's following different occupations. He found that children of professional peoples, engineers, doctors, lawyers, etc. got higher IQ at all age levels than children of clinical, skilled trade and retail business people. The lowest IQ was of the children of day laborers. This study indicated a positive relationship between the intelligence of the child and the occupational status of the father.
3. *Teacher's observation and scholastic aptitude:* The following points may be observed:
   a. Rapidity in comprehending material of study.
   b. Rapidity and accuracy in reading.
   c. Ability in attaching new problems.
   d. Large vocabulary.
   e. Eagerness to answer questions.
   f. Deficiency in one or more skills (a negative criterion).

Scholastic Aptitude Test

The Yale educational aptitude test: The battery contains test designed to measure a person's relative aptitude or ability in the following areas:

1. Verbal facility.
2. Linguistic ability.
3. Verbal reasoning.
4. Quantitative reasoning.

5. Mathematical aptitude.
6. Spatial visualizing.
7. Mechanical ingenuity.

Based on these aptitude tests, students are admitted to courses like social sciences, pure sciences, and mathematical and applied sciences.

Mechanical Aptitude Tests

Mechanical aptitude tests are designed to measure fundamental aptitude of tool usage, space visualization and shop arithmetic in the area of mechanical ability. In general, there are two types of mechanical aptitude tests which are given below.

1. Performance test in which the subject is expected to do something with special equipment.
2. Paper-and-pencil test in which the response is given on paper.

Personality Tests

Warren and Carmichael defined personality as, "the entire organization of a human being at any stage of development."

McDougall defines personality, a synthetic unity of all mental features and functions in their intimate interplay.

Characteristics of Personality

1. Personality is self-consciousness. We do not attribute personality to animals.
2. Personality is through social. Its development and growth takes place only in social environment.
3. Personality is continuous, adjusting itself to environments.
4. Personality is always striving for certain ends.
5. Personality functions as unified whole.

Usually, the following methods are employed to assess personality:

a. Questionnaires.
b. Observational method.
c. Case history method.
d. Interview method.
e. The rating scales.
f. Projective techniques.
g. Autobiography method.
h. Personal inventories.

Methods of Studying Personality

1. Clinical.
2. Psychometric.
3. Experimental.

Clinical methods: It is one of the oldest methods of studying personality. A psychologist collects the information from the person himself/herself.

Clinical methods include:

1. Projective techniques.
2. Interview technique.
3. Motor technique.
4. Situational tests of personality.

Characteristics of clinical method:

1. These are observer-dependent.
2. These are primarily qualitative.
3. Data collected can be analyzed in various ways.
4. The reliability and validity are not very high.

Psychometric methods: do not require the presence of the observer. The responses are self-recorded and are qualitative assessment. These are relatively easy to administer.

Whereas, most of the clinical methods give a global and complex picture of personality, the psychometric methods tell us only something about specific traits. Questionnaires and tests of personality come under this category.

Experimental method: It has helped in contributing to the theory of personality and perception. The controlled conditions in the laboratory, have made it possible to study the person under conditions of stress in the laboratory leading to greater understanding of factors leading to disorganization and breakdown.

Achievement Tests

Practical uses of achievement tests are detailed below.

Administrator's Use

1. Tests help to evaluate the extent to which the objectives of education are being achieved.
2. Tests help to classify school objectives.

3. Tests discover the types of learning experiences that will achieve these objectives with the best possible results.
4. To evaluate, revise and improve the curriculum in the light of these results.
5. To discover background children, who need help and to plan for remedial instructions for such students.
6. To select talented pupils for special classes and courses.
7. To decide proper classification of students.
8. To get a better understanding of the needs and abilities of pupils.
9. To select students for the award of special merits or scholarships.
10. To group pupils in a class, students are grouped in such a way that individual differences are as slight as possible.
11. To help the parents in recognizing the strengths and weaknesses of their children, so that they direct their energies on suitable goals only and do not put heavy demands on them.
12. To determine the efficiency of one school with the others.
13. To determine the general level of achievement of a class and thus, to judge the teaching efficiency of the teacher. The level of achievement of a class may be judged based on the achievement of the class in the beginning and at the end of the school years.

Teacher's Role

1. The teacher will come to know the general range of abilities of students in the class.
2. In the light of above, he/she will select appropriate materials of instruction, so that all individuals benefit from instruction to the maximum.
3. The teacher will determine and diagnose the weakness of the students in various subjects.
4. The teacher will spot out brilliant and backward children.
5. The teacher will determine the progress of the group in a particular subject over a period of time.
6. By studying the results of the student on achievement tests and intelligence tests, the teacher will determine, whether or not the students are working at their maximum capacity.

Classification of Achievement Tests

1. Oral tests.
2. Written tests (standardized tests).
3. Essay tests.
4. Objective tests.

Achievement tests can be classified according to functions it serves.

1. *Mastery tests:* It measures the knowledge, skill and other learning outcomes that all pupils must acquire.
2. *Survey tests:* It gives individual student's score and is compared with the general achievement score.
3. *Diagnostic tests:* These are constructed, so that parts scores and individual items response reveal specific disabilities and deficiencies of achievement. It helps in identification of specific disabilities.

Standardized Written Test

Tests and scales that have met the criteria of testing are known as standardized tests.

Written tests are of two types. They are:

1. Standardized tests.
2. Teacher made test.
   a. Free response type includes:
      i. Essay type.
      ii. Short answer.
   b. Fixed response type:
      i. Very short answer.
      ii. Objective type.
         - Yes or no, true or false type
         - Multiple choice type
         - Matching type
         - Rearrangement type.

Communication Skill

1. Direct observation.
2. Indirect observation.

Observation Techniques

Observational techniques are systematic methods of recording the observations of students for the purposes of evaluation. Anecdotal records, checklists, rating scales and sociometric techniques are included in this category.

RATING SCALE

Rating scale is a device for systematically recording observer's judgments, concerning the degree to which a quality or trait is present and require indication of how much or how little that characteristic is indent (Groulund).

Types

1. *Numerical rating scale:* It is, where the rather checks or circles a number to indicate the degree to which a characteristic is present. For example, indicate the degree to which pupil contribute to class discussion. The number represents the following values:
   a. Outstanding.
   b. Above average.
   c. Average.
   d. Below average.
   e. Poor.
2. *Graphical rating scale:* Direction place an X anywhere along the horizontal line. To what extent does the pupil participate in class discussion?
   a. Never.
   b. Seldom.
   c. Occasionally.
   d. Frequently.
   e. Always.
3. *Descriptive graphic scale:* Place an X anywhere along the horizontal line, add a comment to clarify the rating.
   a. Never participate or participate as much as or participate more than any person.
   b. Quite, passive other group members comments.
4. *Rating method:* In this method, the pupils being rated are ranked in the order in which the rater estimates those possess the characteristics being judged.

Definition of Rating

Rating is a term applied to expression of opinion or judgment regarding some situation. Opinions are usually expressed on a scale of values.

Principles of Effective Rating (Groulund)

1. Only these learning outcomes, which can be evaluated and stated, clearly should be checked by rating scale.
2. The characteristics evaluated should be directly observable.
3. The characteristics and points on the scale should be clearly defined.
4. Raters should omit rating, where they feel unqualified to judge.
5. Rating from several observers should be combined, wherever possible.

Qualities of Rating Scale

1. Clarity.
2. Reliance.
3. Precision.
4. Variety.
5. Objectivity.
6. Uniqueness.

The sociometric techniques are a method for evaluating the social relationship existing in a group.

a. Each group member is asked to indicate those individuals, they would prefer to work with for some group work or situation or choose as leader with some particular qualities.
b. The number of choices each person receive as an index of this social acceptance and analysis of sociometric results provides, information concerning leadership potential, social adjustment and personality characteristics.
c. Sociometric procedures are especially useful in emulating personality triads.

Advantages and Disadvantages

Advantages

- Easy to administer
- Easy to score
- Can be used for a large group of students
- Wide range of applications
- Clarity of feedback to students.

Disadvantage

Misuse can result in a consequent decrease in objectivity.

CHECKLIST

Checklist is a prepared list of statements relating to behavior traits, performance in some area or practical work or a product of some performance list or an artwork.

Steps of Checklist (Groulund)

1. Identify and describe clearly each of the specific desired actions in the performance.
2. Add to the list those actions, which represent common error, if they are limited in number and can be clearly identified.
3. Arrange the desired actions and likely errors in the appropriate order in which they are expected to occur.
4. Provide a simple procedure for numbering the actions in sequence or checking each action as it occurs.

Advantages

- Easy to evaluate
- Easy for scoring
- Better content validity.

Disadvantages

- Takes a lot of time
- Observer must be trained
- Individual checklist is needed for each candidate.

ANECDOTAL RECORDS

Anecdotal records are factual description of the meaningful incidents and events, which the teacher has observed in the lives of pupils.

1. Anecdotal records attempt to describe those episodes—most typical of student's behavior, in the area of personal or social adjustment. The report may be negative, positive or outstanding performance of behavior.
2. The incidents record shortly after it happens.
3. It is made in practical area/clinical area, where the student's actual behavior is observed.

Advantages

- Supplements and validates of other structured instruments
- Provision of insight into total behavior incidents
- Use of formative feedback
- Economical and easy to develop
- It provides a description of actual behavior in a natural situation.

Disadvantages

- Anecdotal records are carelessly recorded; the purpose will not be fulfilled
- Subjectivity
- Lack of standardization
- Difficulty in scoring
- Time-consuming
- Limited applications
- The amount of time required is more in maintaining an adequate system of records
- Not objective in nature.

SELF-REPORT TECHNIQUES

Information from individuals is taken by interview or questionnaire regarding, how one feels about certain situations and activities the individual is interested in most and personal problems of great common to the individuals. Interview involves a face-to-face relationship between the interviewers and interviewee. Information is elicited by direct questioning, which may be structured or unstructured.

SCHOLASTIC ACHIEVEMENT TEST

Academic Achievement

1. Written test.
2. Oral test.
3. Practical tests.
4. Daily work.
5. Achievement in skill.

WRITTEN TEST (CLASSROOM TEST)

Written test is the most common types of evaluation device used by teachers because of the case in developing, administering and scoring test. But it cannot measure all the learning outcomes expected from the students, it measures mostly the knowledge or intellectual domain only.

Classroom tests are playing central role in the evaluation of pupil progress. The purposes of constructing classroom test are to develop available instrument for evaluating pupil's achievements.

Principles of Classroom Tests—Groulund (1971)

1. The test construction procedures must take into the account, the use to be served by the test.
2. The type of the test 'inter' used should be determined by the specific learning outcomes to be measured. For example, knowledge, inputs, principles.
3. Test 'inter' should be based on a representative sample of the course content and the specific learning outcomes to be measured.
4. The 'inter' should be proper level of difficulty.
5. The 'inter' should be as constructed that extraneous factor do not prevent the pupil from responding.
6. Test 'inter' should be so constructed that the pupil obtains the correct answer, only if he/she has obtained the desired learning outcomes.
7. The test should be so constructed that it contributes to improved teaching and learning process.

Steps of Constructing of a Classroom Test

1. Identifying and defining the objectives in terms of desired changes in behavior and to specify the learning outcomes as the first step in evaluation.
2. Outlining the content of subject matter.
3. Making a table of specification, which relates the objectives to the content of subject matter.
4. The construction of specific test questions in accordance with the specification.

Common Defects of Written Examination

1. *Triviality:* It is essential for each question to be important and useful.
2. *Error:* In phrasing the questions, especially multiple choice questions.
3. *Basis:* Examiners preference for an answer, when other option or correct answer is available.
4. *Complicated instruments:* Make it difficult to understand them especially when, language other than mother tongue is used.
5. *Ambiguity:* Use of language, which may lead to spend more time in trying to understand the question than in answering it. It is said to be an ambiguous question. This leads the student to give relevant answer to the question asked.
6. *Complicity:* Expecting students to answer very difficult questions, which can be answered by the best student.
7. *Obsolescence:* Forcing the student to answer in terms of the outmoded ideas of the examiners, a bias often aggravated by the traditional teaching methods.

Grading of Answer Papers

There are two methods of grading answer paper:

1. Absolute grading.
2. Relative grading.

Absolute Grading

Absolute grading is the system of assigning grades by which the student get the marks for the answers, depending on how well he has met the requirements of the model answer and is expressed in percentage.

Relative Grading

Relative grading tells the student, how the answers rated in relation to other students doing the same test, by indicating whether or not is average, above average or below average.

Marking System of Evaluation

1. In marking system, the answer papers are assessed and given a number as 0 to 100 scales and the percentage of marks obtained by the students is clearly marked.

2. The position of conciliate in the class or in the university examination can be decided exactly in the marking system and top rankers easily identified.

Grading System of Evaluation

1. In grading system, the student is evaluated on the five or seven scale pattern and gives a grade, e.g. O, A+, A–, B+, B– and C, etc.
2. The grade is given according to a criteria decided by faculty of the school as between 90 and 100, O outstanding; 81 to 100, A+, very good and so on.

Types of Classroom Tests

There are two general types of classroom tests:
1. Objective type.
2. Essay type.

OBJECTIVE TYPE TEST

Advantages

1. The objective type questions are highly structured and require students to select the correct answer from limited number of alternatives.
2. The student must demonstrate the specific knowledge, understanding or skill called the item.
3. This contributes to objective scoring, which is quick, easy and accurate.
4. It covers large content area and can include minute details of the subjects.
5. More reliable because these are free from personal opinion in scoring.
6. These are an effective means of testing because they save time and yield more reliable, valid, fair and important results.
7. It can be scored easily by using machines or computers.

Disadvantages

1. Student cannot present the answer in their own way.
2. These are inappropriate for measuring the ability to select, organize and explain ideas.
3. More time is required to prepare good objective type questions.

Types

1. *Supply type:* Students are required to supply the answers.
2. *Selection types:* Students are required to select the answers from the given number of alternatives.

Classification of objective type test is given in the Table 20.1.

Table 20.1: Classification of objective type tests

Sl No	*Supply type*	*Selection type*
1.	Short answer	True or false (alternative response type)
2.	Completion type	Matching type Multiple choice Interpretive items (complex achievement)

Supply Type

Short answer type: Examples are given below:

1. Who is the Father of our Nation? (Mahatma Gandhi).
2. Who was the first Prime Minister of India? (Pandit Jawaharlal Nehru).

Completion type: For example: The formula for ordinary common salt is ________ (NaCl).

Selection Type

True or false (alternative response items): For example: State whether following statement is true or false.

Water boils at 120°C—these items are statements, which the learner has to decide are true or false, right or wrong, correct or incorrect, yes or no, fact or opinion, agree or disagree and the like. In each case, there are only two possible answers by Groulund.

Uses

1. To measure ability to identify the correctness of statements of facts, definition of terms, etc.
2. To measure the students ability to distinguish principles.

Limitations

True or false method is limited to the more elementary learning outcomes in the knowledge area.

Matching type: Matching exercises consists of two parallel columns with each word, number or symbol being matched to a word, sentence or phrase in the other column. The items in the column for which a match is sought are called premises and the item in column from which the selection is made is called responses (Groulund).

Steps for constructing matching items

1. Keep the test item to be matched and place the shorter response on the right.
2. Make the list brief to maintain homogeneity. It will also help the students to read the longer premise time and rapidly go through the list of responses doing the test quickly.
3. Place all the items for one matching question in the same page.
4. When writing matching items, the number of choices should always exceed the number of statements, so that guessing is reduced.
5. The students have to identify the pairs of items that are to be associated, matched on the basis implicated (Table 20.2).

Advantage

These questions are easy to construct.

Disadvantage/limitation

Matching items are limited to the measurement of actual information based on simple associations, ability to identify relationship between two things and promote memorization.

Table 20.2: Example for matching type

Sl No	*Column A*	*Column B*
1.	Seen in yellow fruits and vegetables like papaya, carrots	Vitamin A
2.	Fish and cod liver oil are the sources	Vitamin A, D
3.	Citrus fruits are rich sources in this vitamin	Vitamin C
4.	Found in parboiled rice	Vitamin B
5.	Helps in clotting of blood	Vitamin B_{12}

Multiple choice questions: It consist of a problem and a list of suggested solutions. The problem may be stated in the form of a question or an incomplete statement called stem of the item. Each question has three parts; the key, which is the correct response or alternative and distractors or incorrect responses. There should be at least three options given to reduce the chances of guessing. The question may ask for only one correct answer or the best answer.

Example

1. Stem—the vitamin necessary for healing wound is ____________
   a. Distractors (incorrect response).
   b. Vitamin A.
   c. Vitamin B.
   d. Vitamin C (correct response).
   e. Vitamin D.
   f. Key (correct response).

Advantages

1. High quality and feasibility.
2. It can measure effectively the learning outcomes.
3. The objective test is more reliable.
4. Free from ambiguity and vagueness.
5. Saves time of teachers as computers can correct them.
6. There can be several question bank and used from time-to-time.

Limitations

1. The work process is time consuming to construct multiple choice questions (MCQs).
2. Test of higher levels of intellectual functioning is difficult to form.
3. MCQs are limited to learning outcomes at the verbal level, but it cannot determine how the pupils will perform in an actual situation.
4. It is inappropriate for measuring the ability to organize and present ideas.
5. It takes some experience in setting proper MCQs.
6. It is difficult to find sufficient number of incorrect, but possible distractors.

Interpretive items: It consists of a series of objective items, written materials, tables, charts, graphs, maps and pictures. Students are presented with a common set of data and asked to identify relationship in the data to recognize valid conclusions, to appraise assumptions and inferences. Interpretive exercises measure complex achievements (Groulund).

Uses

Useful for assessing the higher levels of cognitive domain to apply principles and to recognize assumptions and inferences.

Appraising the Test

After the objective test has record, it is describable to appraise the effectiveness of the test items. The effectiveness of each item can be determined by analyzing the pupil's response to the item. This item analysis data provides for the general improvement of classroom instruction, since it provides insight into instructional weakness and clues to their improvement.

Item Analysis Procedure

Item analysis, the teacher has to rank. The paper in order from the highest to the lowest score. Divide the paper, approximately, one third in three groups, the top scores 1/3 according to rank and the low scores 1/3 for each test item, tabulate the number of pupils on the upper and lower groups who selected each alternative.

Estimate the difficulty of each item, which is the percentage of pupils who got the item right. Estimate the discriminating power of each item. This is the difference between the number of pupils in the upper and lower groups, who got item right. Evaluate the effectiveness of the directors in each item. Effectiveness of the distracters can be obtained by impacting the item analysis data.

ESSAY TYPE TESTS

Essay type of examination may be one of the oldest type of examination and mostly used in India even today. Essay type questions permit the pupil to respond by selecting, organizing and presenting the facts he considers appropriate. Essay type examinations are of two types based on the freedom of response allowed to the pupil.

1. The extend response type, e.g. describe the role of evaluation in relation to the curriculum goals.
2. Restricted response type, e.g. discuss the advantage and disadvantage of essay and objective type examination.

Principles for Preparing Essay Type Test

1. Do not give too many lengthy questions.
2. Avoid phrases, e.g. discuss briefly.
3. Questions should be well structured with specific purposes or topic at a time.

4. Word should be simple, clear unambiguous and carefully selected.
5. Do not allow too many choices.
6. According to the level of student's difficulty and complexity, items has to be selected.

Scoring Problem

1. For every question set out the elements, which according to you should appear in the answer by point scoring system?
2. Score the answers of all the students for one question, before going on to the scoring of another question.
3. When two or more teachers correct the same test, they should agree on the scoring procedures before they test the answer script.
4. The time allowed and the marks allotted will act as guide to the students to answer the questions.

Advantages

1. Provide candidate with opportunity to demonstrate knowledge and ability to recognize ideas and express them effectively.
2. Can measure understanding, thinking, skills and other complete learning outcomes.
3. Preparation of question is relatively easy.
4. Freedom of responses in own words influence fulfilling and writing skill to influence the score guessing is minimized.
5. Encourage pupil to concentrate on larger units of subject matter with special emphasis on the ability to organize, integrate and express idea effectively.
6. Test the ability to communicate in writing depth of knowledge and understanding.
7. The student can be free to communicate, his/her ability for independent thinking.
8. The student can demonstrate the ability to organize ideas and express them effectively in a logical and coherent fashion.

Disadvantages

1. Low content validity.
2. Lacks objectivity.
3. Provides little useful feedback.

4. Scoring difficulty.
5. Inefficient for measuring knowledge of facts.
6. Only few questions could be used in a test, therefore, sampling of content is limited.
7. Subjective scoring, which is slow, difficult and inconsistent.
8. Low marker reliability.
9. Marking is time consuming.
10. Ambiguous and unclear for students to understand.
11. Writing ability of student affects marking.
12. Student fatigue.

ORAL EXAMINATIONS

1. Oral examination has been traditionally used along with practical examinations and in professional courses in the clinical area.
2. This type of examinations consists of a dialogue with the examiners, who asks questions to the student, usually in an actual or simulated situations.
3. It is better that oral examination is evaluated by two examiners to make it reliable or objective.
4. A predetermined evaluation term could be used by the examiner. Time limit must be traced for each student.
5. Viva voce (viva) examination must be done with care after a practical examination.

Advantages

1. Oral examinations provide direct personal contact with the examinee.
2. Provide opportunity for clarifying answers and doubts.
3. Require the candidate to formulate his/her own answers.
4. It provides flexibility in moving from strong points to weak points.

EXAMINATIONS

1. Examinations are most commonly used evaluating method in the education system of our country.
2. Examinations are given the highest priority.
3. Teachers, students, parents, the university and board all give more importance to examination.

4. The standards and place of a rehired in relate, depends on the percentage and number of students passed in the trial examination.
5. This type of emphasis on examination makes the students nervous and scared of examinations.
6. They try to memorize the answer without understanding and even engage in malpractice during the examinations.
7. These types of examinations prevent critical thinking and reasoning power in the students.
8. It is highly important that the examinations are objective as possible as fair to the students.
9. They should be comprehensive, but brief, precise and clear.
10. The examination must be to take the factor of practicability into account.
11. It must be easy for administration, scoring and interpretation of the results.

Disadvantages

1. Lack of standardization.
2. Make student nervous and afraid of examinations.
3. Provide favoritism or abuse of the situations.
4. Lack of objectivity and reproducibility of results.
5. Unsuitable environment to conduct the examinations.
6. It is costly because of professional time. Only few students can be examined in a day.

PRACTICAL EXAMINATION

Practical examinations are integral part of nursing examinations. The aim of practical examination is to evaluate the nursing competence or practical skills. Practical examination is essentially a combination of test methods like rating scales, checklists, etc. An oral examination also accompanies the practical test in order to supplement the information obtained through it. The students proceed through a series of 'steps' and undertake a variety of practical tasks like assessing the patient, formulating nursing diagnosis according to priority, planning the care, implementing the care and evaluating the care. Marking sheets, checklists and rating scales are prepared in advance to improve the reliability of scoring. All students are thus evaluated on the same criteria by the same examiners.

Practical skill can be evaluated by two methods:

1. Direct observation: For example, clinical area, practical tests by the use of evaluation format.
2. Indirect observation: For example, carrying out the projects.

PERFORMANCE APPRAISAL IN NURSING

Introduction

Performance appraisal or merit rating is one of the oldest and most universal practices of management. The approach resulted in an appraisal system in which the employee's merits like initiative, dependability and personality were compared with others and ranked or rated. The trend nowadays is in the direction of attempting to measure, what man does (performance appraisal) rather than what he is (merit rating). Appraisal can be made by one or more supervisors or by subordinate or by peers. There can be even a system of self-appraisal in which the employee can evaluate his/her own performance and potentials.

Definitions

1. Performance appraisal refers to all the formal procedures used in the working organizations to evaluate the personalities and contribution of group members.
2. Performance appraisal is a periodic formal evaluation of how well-personnel have performed their duties during specific period.
3. Performance appraisal (also called merit rating or efficiency or service rating) is the process of reviewing an individual's performance and progress in job and assessing his/her potentials.

Purposes of Appraisal

1. Appraisal can serve as a basis for job change or promotion. By establishing, whether the nurse can contribute still more in a different or higher job, it helps in suitable promotion and placement.
2. By identifying the strengths and weakness of an employee, it serves as a guide for formulating a suitable training and development program to improve the quality of performance in present work.

3. It serves as a feedback to the employee. By letting the employee know, how well he is doing or where he/she stands with his/her superior, it tells him/her what he/she can do to improve his/her present performance and go up in the management hierarchy.
4. It serves as an important incentive to all the employees, who are by the existence of an appraisal system assured of the management's continued interest in them and of their continuous possibility to develop. The employees realize that not only they are being continuously observed but that they have not been forgotten.
5. The existence of regular appraisal system tends to make the supervisors and executive more observant of their subordinates because they will be expected periodically to fill out rating forms and would be called upon to justify their estimates. Their knowledge results in improved supervision.
6. Performance appraisal often provides the rational foundation for payment of piecework, wages, bonuses, etc. The estimates of the relative contributions of employees of their characteristics help to determine the rewards and privileges.
7. Performance appraisal serves as a mean for the evaluation of the effectiveness of devices for the selection and classification of workers. Alternatively, knowledge of the characteristics of the supervisors and the inferior workers can be helpful in selection and placement of workers.
8. Permanent performance appraisal records of employees help the management to give up sole reliance upon personal knowledge of supervisors, who may be shifted.

Judgmental Purposes

1. Purpose of determining salary standards and salary increase and/or awarding merit increases then it is carried for judgmental purposes.
2. Selecting qualified individuals for promotion transfers, denoting or terminating employees, due to unsatisfactory performance.
3. Performance evaluation that are not done for judgmental purposes carry the highest states.

Developmental Purposes

Performance appraisal may predominantly educate and involve coaching the employee to gain professionally through working within the organizational goals.

1. Identifying talents in the organization.
2. Determining training and development needs of individuals or groups.
3. To improve interpersonal relationship among groups.
4. Establish standards of performance and gaining acceptance of those standards.
5. Provides employee recognition.
6. Discover employee aspiration.
7. Reconcile with goals of the organization.
8. To provide team building.
9. To give employee feedback.

Principles of Performance Evaluation

1. Evaluation must contain content that is relevant to individuals being evaluated in a particular setting.
2. Criteria that are used to evaluate performance should be stated and standards should be specified, whenever possible.
3. Performance evaluation should be able to discriminate between excellent, good and poor performance.
4. Any performance evaluation must be practical or in measurement terminology. It must have utility.

Tactics of Performance Evaluation

Irancerich, Donnelly and Gibson identified five possible parties, who could evaluate or rate another person.

1. Supervisor.
2. Peers.
3. Rates.
4. Subordinates of the vertex.
5. Raters outside the organizational environment.

In most of the cases, employees should be rated by their immediate supervisors.

When Should Evaluations Occur?

1. Most organizations evaluate older or tenured employees about once or twice a year.
2. New employees are evaluated about 6 weeks to 2 months after being hired and employees at various stages of development may be evaluated more or less often than twice a year, depending on the objectives set during the previous evaluation.

3. Progressive discipline procedure is an example of evaluation done often every 2 weeks.

An evaluation should contain a progress note at the bottom that is written by the evaluator. It should designate when the evaluation will occur and the objectives for the period of time until the date.

Essentials of a Good Appraisal System

1. *Appraisal system must be easily understandable:* If the system is too complex or too time consuming, it may be anchored to the ground by its own dead weight of complicated from which nobody, but the expert understands.
2. *It must have the support of all line people who administer it:* If the line people think it is too theoretical, too ambitious and too unrealistic or that it has been foisted on them by ivory towered, staff consultants who have no comprehension of the demands on the time of line operators, they will resent it. A similar goodwill and understanding must exist between the rater and the rates.
3. *The system should fit the organization's operations and structure:* A system that may work extremely well at a company, those activities are compact. Similarly, where the operations are interdependent and interlinked, performance data pertaining to any one individual cannot be regard as sufficiently discrete or reliable for appraising the performance.
4. *The system should be both valid and reliable:* The validity of rating is the degree to which they are truly indicative of the intrinsic merit of employees. The reliability of rating is the consistency with which the ratings are made either by different raters or by on rater at different times.
5. The system should have built in incentives that is awarded should follow satisfactory performance.
6. *The system should be periodically evaluated to be sure that is continuing to meet its goals:* Not only there is a danger that subjective criteria may become more salient than the objective standards originally established, there is the further danger that the system may become rigid in a tangle of rules and procedure, many of which are no longer useful.

Criteria of Performance Appraisal

Criteria may be classified into two main categories: Objective criteria and subjective criteria. Amount of quality of production, work sample tests, length of service, amount of training necessary, absenteeism, accidents, etc. are all examples of objective criteria. Rating of employee's job proficiency by their supervisors, peers and subordinates, extent of upward communication of ideas, degree of knowledge about corporate goals, contribution to sociocultural values, etc. are all examples of subjective criteria. Since, all subjective criteria depends upon human judgment and opinion; these are subject to certain kinds of errors likely to be found in the rating process.

Performance Appraisal Methods

Rating Method

Rating means the judgment of one person by another. Rating is, in essence, direct observation. Rating is a team applied to expression of opinion or judgment regarding some situation, object or character. Opinions are usually expressed on a scale or values. Rating techniques are devices by which such judgments may be quantified. The oldest and simplest method of performance appraisal is to compare one man with all other men and place him in a simple rank order. In this way, ordering is done from best to worst of all individuals comprising the group.

Rating Scale Method

As the name implies, these methods provide some kind of a scale for measuring absolute differences between individuals. The scales used are generally of two types.

Discrete: Where two or more categories are provided, representing discrete amounts of ability or degrees of the characteristics, the rater can tick mark the category, which feels best, describes the person being rated. Thus, for example, the characteristic job knowledge may be divided into five categories on a discrete scale. Exceptionally good, above average, average, below average and poor.

Continuous (or graphic): Where just above the category notation as uninterrupted line is provided. There are four kinds of standards used in rating scale namely, numerical or alphabetical, descriptive-adjective, man-to-man and behavior sample.

Checklist Method

Sometimes, the method used for performance appraisal is a list consisting of a number of statements about the worker and his/her behavior. Each statement on this list is assigned a value depending upon its importance. The method has advantages of requiring only a reporting of facts from the rater. Since, the values assigned to different statements do not appear on list, the rater does not know, how highly he/she has rated a given individual. He/she also does not have to distinguish among various categories for each of the several traits considered for each of the several employees working under him/her.

Forced-choice Method

A forced-choice rating form consists of a number of statements, which desired an individual being rated. These statements are grouped in 2s, 3s and 4s. Sometimes, the groups on the rating form are made of favorable statements only, sometimes all above unfavorable statements only and sometimes, they have both favorable and unfavorable statements in equal number. When all groups on the rating form contain favorable statements only, the rater must check one statement in each group, which he/she believes best characterizes the individual being rated. When all groups are made of unfavorable statements, the rater must check one statement in each group, which he/she believes is the least descriptive of the individual being rated. When each group has two favorable and two unfavorable statements, the rater makes two checks in each group, one for the statement, which best describes the individual and one for the statement, which is least descriptive.

Field Review

Under field review method, appraisal of worker is done by the personal officer by collecting oral rating about them from the supervisor at the place of work. The personal officer later writes his notes and initiates the supervisor to make additions or corrections. This method is not widely used because supervisors generally resent what they consider the staff interference.

Critical Incident Technique

In critical incident technique method, the first step is to draw up for each job a list of critical job requirements, i.e. those requirements, which are vital for success or failure on the job. The concept of a critical incident differs from that of an anecdote. Fivers and Gosnell define a critical incident as one that makes a significant difference in the outcome of an activity. It may be the positive factors that contribute toward the cusses of the behavior or it may be the negative factors that interfere with the completion of the assignment.

Confidential Report

A confidential report by the immediate supervisor is still a major determinant of the subordinate promotion or transfer. The format and pattern of this varies with each organization.

Performance Appraisal Tool

The type of appraisal tool used is not so important as how it is utilized. A formal written tool may have specific guidelines or a more open-ended format. General topics may be addressed in an anecdotal or incident type format. The tool or evaluation form should facilitate accurate appraisal of the individual's performance, as well as provide an opportunity to stimulate personal goals of the individual and goals of the organization. There are two primary categories of performance appraisal tools: structured and fixed.

Structured (Traditional) Tool

The forced distribution scale is a norm-referenced tool that prevents the evaluator from rating all individuals in the same manner. The evaluator is provided with a schematic diagram and asked to rate the individual. According to all individuals, the manager evaluates. The evaluator has indicated that the individuals rated are in the top 10 percent of employee, but is not the best employee. This scale also provides the employee with a brief visual picture of how this evaluator has ranked performance in reference to others. This type of scale can undetermine group cohesion and communication effectiveness by its very nature of rank ordering individual performance.

Flexible (Collaborative) Tool

The evaluation focus can also be conducted with a collaborative approach. One method that has been used for many years is management by objectives (MBO). The MBO method is similar, but more rigid in structure. An MBO approach requires that the employee establish clear and measurable objectives at the beginning of each rating period. These objectives are then addressed individually and in writing by both the employees and the manager during the performance appraisal interview. The approach can be simplified, if it is performance based and outcome or results oriented. Then, in effect, the employee has created a performance contact, as well having defined goals for future professional performance.

Performance Appraisal in Clinical Nursing Practice

The term clinical practice is familiar to individuals involved in nursing, but perception of this term varies considerably. To some, it implies a series or an aggregate of tasks and to others, the term implies a process. Clinical practice may be viewed as the way or the medium through which a professional practitioner ministers to his/her client. The clinical practice may be conceptualized, as the way the nurse utilizes a particular consultation of abilities to meet the health needs of the client.

Performance appraisal implies systematic or formal evaluation of the individual with respect to the performance on the job and potential for development. It is the rational and continuous process of evaluating the performance of employees on a particular job in terms of the job required. Performance appraisal should be differentiated from job evaluation. Job evaluation involves the determination of worth of different jobs, while performance appraisal is concerned with the measurement of the worth of individuals to the organization. In job evaluation, the focus is on the job, while under performance appraisal the emphasis is on the performance and potentials of an employee.

Conclusion

Systematic and objective appraisal of the performance of managers is an important element in staffing. The livelihood and career prospectus of employees depend largely on their appraisals. In case of small enterprises, employee's performance may be evaluated by the supervisors or foreman. But in modern large scale enterprises, formal systems of performance appraisal are required for a rational judgment of individual employee's efficiency, performance and capacity.

OBJECTIVE STRUCTURED PRACTICAL EXAMINATION (OSPE)

Testing, measurement and evaluation play an important role in all educational institutions, including nursing educational institutions. Evaluation tool have far reaching consequences for students in their success or failure, consequently educators have the responsibility for development of testing devices or procedures that fairly evaluates student's achievements and yields accurate results. The traditional system of practical examination in nursing education consists of either assigning a procedure to a student or a patient for identifying the needs on a priority basis for giving care. This depends upon student's ability and availability of the patient for a particular procedure. In spite of the innovations in the mode of evaluation of student's performance, the importance of conventional system of practical examination cannot be denied.

What is OSPE?

Objective structured practical examination is a new pattern of practical examination. In OSPE, each component of clinical competence is tested uniformly and objectively for all the students who are taking up a practical examination at a given place.

Through OSPE, one gets a reasonable idea of the extent of achievement of each student in every practical skill related to a particular discipline. It can be used for formative and summative evaluation.

How to Organize an OSPE?

In order to organize an OSPE, one has to spell out the objectives of practical experiences in a given discipline, related to a particular subject such as practical examination in medical, surgical and nursing, each student is suppose to do the following:

1. *Demonstrate practical skills:* This may be done by assessing a student:
   a. To monitor and record oral temperature.
   b. To convert 39°C to F.
   c. To attach a heart monitor to a patient.
   d. To test urine for sugar.
   e. To start an intravenous (IV) drip on a patient.

2. *Make correct and accurate observations:* This may be done by assigning a student:
   a. To interpret type of fever from the given graph.
   b. To identify the type of arrhythmia from the electrocardiograph (ECG) provided.
   c. To differentiate between normal and abnormal ECG.

These questions may not require the examiners to observe the student in action. These questions can be answered on a paper, which can be collected later for evaluation.

3. *Analysis and interpret data:* This is one of the important skill components to be judged for the continuity of patient care. The nurse has to perform this task, where he/she may come across normal and abnormal data in relation to patient's investigation reports. The student is asked to interpret the data given below:
   a. Hemogram: Normal or abnormal.
   b. Liver function test reports.
   c. Renal function test reports.
   d. Laboratory reports.
4. *Identify patient's problems:* In order to organize the work, nurse has to identify the patient's problems and set priority, so as to clear the immediate needs of the patient, such as to identify the following problems:
   a. Dyspnea on the basis of observations.
   b. Rigor following blood transfusion.
   c. Coning following lumbar puncture.
   d. Cerebrospinal fluid (CSF) rhinorrhea following head injury.
5. *Plan of alternative nursing interventions in a given situation:* In order to provide the need based on the care, the nurse plan's alternative nursing interventions, as in case of airway obstruction, the student nurse is expected to do the following:
   a. Keep the patient in side-lying position.
   b. Do oropharyngeal suction.
   c. Check and record vital signs.
   d. Starts oxygen inhalation, if required.
   e. Keep the things ready for endotracheal intubation.
   f. Assist the doctor in intubating the patient.

In order to assess certain practical skills, the OSPE is organized in the form of several stations through which the candidate rotate till complete one full round (Table 20.3).

Table 20.3: Types of stations

Sl No	*Stations*	*Question*	*Method of scoring*
1.	Procedure station	Check and record blood pressure (BP)	Observed and scored by the examiner A using checklist
2.	Question station	List five factors, which help in maintaining BP	Answer on a sheet provided
3.	Procedure station	Take oral temperature and record it	Observed and scored by the examiner B
4.	Question station	Convert 39°C to F by using the formula	Answer a sheet provided
5.	Procedure station	Test the urine albumin and record it	Observed and scored by the examiner C
6.	Question station	List five causes of albuminuria	Answer on a sheet provided

How to Score Students in OSPE?

1. For each specific skill, a checklist is prepared by breaking the skill being tested into essential steps and scores is assigned to each step, which is proportional to the importance of the steps related to a particular procedure.
2. The objectivity in assessment is achieved by getting each component tested at one particular station by the same examiner and to rotate through all the students.
3. The time allowed is same for all the stations, 3 to 5 minutes is the length of time allocated to each station.

Advantages

1. The OSPE helps us to observe and assess student for different professional and technical skills in a real life situation.
2. It enables us to have an overall view of the student's performance.

Disadvantages

1. The OSPE is subjective, as the student's score depends on the whims, fancies and mood of the examiner.
2. It is time consuming and there is a lack of standardized conditions in bedside, which affects student's score.
3. Realizing the magnitude of the problem prevailing in assessment of students.

Student's Instructions Regarding OSPE

1. Write your roll number in bold figures and display it on your white coat, so that the examiner can identify the candidate.
2. Students are asked to report at a particular time, all of them are collected in a room or hall and explained the procedure of examination.
3. Students may be given instructions that they will rotate around station (numbered 1–6), spending 3 minutes at each station.

SUGGESTED READING

1. Aggarwal JC. Education Vocational Guidance and Counseling, 8th edition. New Delhi: Doaba House; 1998. pp. 257-71.
2. Basavanthappa BT. Nursing Education, 1st edition. New Delhi: Jaypee Brothers Medical Publishers (P) Ltd; 2011.
3. Flippo Edwin B. Principles of Personnel Management. New York: McGraw-Hill; 1975.
4. George K Aleyamma. Principles of Curriculum Development and Evaluation. Namakkal District, Tamil Nadu: Vivekananda Press; 2002. pp. 120-90.
5. Gupta CB. Principles and Practice of Management, 4th edition. New Delhi: National Publishing House. pp. 316-30.
6. Heidgerken E Loretta. Teaching and Learning in Schools of Nursing: Principles and Methods, 3rd edition. New Delhi: Konark Publishers Pvt Ltd; 1994. pp. 629-68.
7. John W Best, James V Kahn. Research in Education, 7th edition. New Delhi: Prentice-Hall of India Pvt Ltd; 2002. pp. 25-6, 106-7.
8. Lancaster Jeanette. Nursing Issues in Leading and Managing Change. St Louis: Mosby Publications; 1999. pp. 496-502.

REVIEW QUESTIONS

1. Define evaluation. Explain steps, principles and purpose of evaluation.
2. Discuss the evaluation tools in detail.
3. Explain personality test, achievement test and standardized test.
4. Define rating scale. Explain the steps of rating scale.
5. Explain anecdotal record, objective type of tests and multiple choice questions.
6. Short notes:
   a. Practical examination.
   b. Performance appraisal in nursing.
   c. Objective structured practical examination.

CHAPTER
21

Social Psychology

LEARNING OBJECTIVES

1. Definitions.
2. Principles.
3. Scope of social psychology.
4. Development of social psychology in education.

INTRODUCTION

Social psychology is one of the latest extensions of the great movement of scientific thought, which achieved its most striking results in the investigation of physical phenomena. The advances of natural science were the indispensable conditions for a study of psychology. In the study of man, psychology occupies a unique and commanding position. We may say that what physics is to the natural sciences, psychology is to the sciences of man. All activities in society—economic, political, artistic have their center in individuals, in their strings, needs and understanding. The individual is the point of intersection of nearly all that is of consequence in the social sphere. For purpose of convenience, we may divide our interest and concentrate on a particular phase of social process.

With the increasing variety of courses offered in psychology and education, it is inevitable that social psychology will trespass upon related fields. In spite of possible overlapping, it has been decided that social psychology is an independent discipline that is required today, because of several transformations, with the growth of mass industrialization, the concentration of great populations in cities and spread of rapid communication have altered the human situation in definite ways.

MEANING AND NATURE

Psychology and sociology, each often claims the whole domain of human behavior as its individual bailiwick. The history of these two disciplines reveals basic differences in their approaches to the understanding of human behavior. These differences have been generally, the result of varying approaches to the types of problems posed for different levels of behavior analyzed by the two disciplines. One has emphasized one level of obstruction and the other, another. Some differences have stemmed from differing definitions in describing the significant problems. For example, in the early psychology, psychologists tended to emphasize the physiological basis of behavior and minimized social and cultural experience, while sociology tends to minimize the physical basis; and emphasized social processes and conditions.

DEFINITIONS

Our glance at representative topics of social psychology, its ground rules and the converging trends in the present state of its development was preparation for definition of social psychology. The definition of any class of objects or events requires specification of what it is and what it is not. This is not an easy matter in our complex subject matter.

Major generalizations are implied in defining a discipline, such as the claim that we know its scope and how to go about studying its problems. There has been disagreement on these matters, since the first two books appeared under the label of *'Social Psychology'* in 1908. One was written by the psychologist William McDougall and the other by the sociologist Ross EA. Since then, several textbooks on social psychology have appeared.

The definition of social psychology offered here is suggested by three converging trends in contemporary social psychology that were noted above, namely:

1. Increased adherence to the ground rules of the scientific approach and utilization of scientific methods and techniques.
2. Awareness of the need for checks to guard against ethnocentric conclusions.
3. Conception of behavior within its appropriate frame of reference as a product of interacting influences coming both from the individual and social surroundings.

Social psychology is, "the scientific study of the experience and behavior of the individual in relation to social stimulus situations."

Let us take the terms in the definition one by one as an orientation to the principal theoretical issues in social psychology and its relation to the social sciences.

PRINCIPLES

Scientific Study

Specifying that social psychology is a scientific study, underscores the task of adhering closely to the ground rules of science and their ramifications in the actual operations of research. Policy makers, religious leaders, novelists and commentators on the social scene cannot be held accountable for adhering to the ground rules of communicability and reproducibility of methods that permit verification, but social psychologists can be. In this book, the scientific ground rules, their associated methods and the techniques are presented on the whole, through the summaries of significant research studies that exemplify their use.

Of the Individual

The phase of the individual specifies that the unit of analysis in social psychology is the individual. Because the field is social psychology and not psychological sociology, its concepts refer to the individual's perception.

The individual is the unit of analysis for social psychology whether the investigator happens to be stationed in a university's department of psychology or sociology (the field's twin parents). Social psychologists today do not use concepts such as 'group mind'. A group cannot perceive, feel or think. The designation 'social' in the label refers to the fact that a particular task is to study the individual's behavior in relation to those aspects of surroundings that are interpersonal or sociocultural. When the individual has traffic first with these aspects of the environment, they are external to his/her, i.e. on the stimulus side of the familiar stimulus-organism-response (S-O-R) scheme for analysis.

Experience and Behavior

Experience is a general term that refers to the awareness of the individual and not just to past experiences as conveyed in expressions such as 'my experience has shown that'. What a person perceives feels, learns or remembers in a word, the experience—is inferred from his/her behavior, i.e. the deeds and words as well as subtle expressions and movements. For this reason, some psychologists refer to all psychological phenomena as behavior. The terms consciousness, mind and 'awareness' were for a time almost banished from academic psychology.

In Relation to

In any definition, the choice of words is important. The importance of these particular words reflects controversies during the earlier development of social psychology. The phase 'determined by' was deliberately avoided in our definition. The individual is not merely a passive recipient, a tabula rasa, reflecting the imprints of the environment, whether social or not. Anything that impinges on the individual from the social world around his/her is processed, motives, desires, attitudes and ideas enter into processing. The processing reflects selectivity in what he/she reacts to and whom transacts with, the processing is also affected by what he/she confronts. Hence, experience and behavior that count for the individual and in the social process is always a joint product of influences in the social environment and those from within him/her, whatever may be at a given time with all of past learning, enduring and momentary motives and viewpoints toward, the issue at hand.

Social life is the natural habit of the human individual. It is not alien to the nature. Therefore, how an individual learns the requirements and values of the group and culture, how he/she responds to pressures from them and the molding of his/her behavior within these requirements are not the sole problems of social psychology.

Social Stimulus Situations

The final phase in the definition of social psychology is social stimulus situations. The phase seems self-explanatory. To show that it is not, we shall consider more seriously, what constitutes a social situation for the individual at a given time. This analysis will enable us to indicate the scope and variety of social stimuli that an individual may encounter in the surroundings.

RELATIONSHIP BETWEEN SOCIAL PSYCHOLOGY AND EDUCATION

"Social psychology is an attempt to understand and explain how the thought, feeling and behavior of individuals are influenced by the actual, implied or imagined presence of others." —*Allport FH*

There is an increasing complexity in social life and also personal life of an individual in the society, because of explosion of population, explosion of knowledge and industrialization. This has greater impact on the education field. Because of this, the educationists, administrators, parents, teachers and the persons involved in the educational activities are confronting many problems in the execution of educational programs in spite of their knowledge of psychology and sociology. This might have happened because psychology deals with individual behavior as a separate entity apart from the society, whereas sociology deals with society group behavior without emphasizing the individual. It is from this angle, it is very significant to deal with social psychology in relation to education, because social psychology studies the behavior of the individual in a social context.

Social psychology begins with the individual and looks at political, social and cultural systems through the eyes of the individual, whereas political science, sociology and cultural anthropology begin as the larger systems and look at the individual through the eyes of this system in all.

SCOPE OF SOCIAL PSYCHOLOGY

The scope of social psychology is not restricted to a particular field. It is inclusive of many of the aspects as its subject matter for the study. This idea becomes more clearer by Krech and Crutchfield saying that social psychology is concerned with every aspect of the individual's behavior in the society. Therefore, we can define social psychology as the science of behavior of the individual in the society.

Newcomb's (1900) contention is that interaction constitutes subject matter of social psychology. Therefore, we can say that it encompasses all types of interaction processes for its study.

The subject matter of social psychology is composed of two psychologically important aspects of the individual. One is directly observable, the overt behavior—what the individual does and the second one is not directly observable but determines behavior—psychological dynamics, what the individual experiences. The first is referred to as the phenotypic self and the second as genotypic self.

It deals with mass communication and the social structure, intergroup attitudes, interpersonal attraction, interpersonal perception, social power, prejudice and stereotypes, group norms and social control, social roles, leadership, group productivity and satisfaction, self and personality, social motivation, social interaction, socialization, affiliation, social organization, attitudes, etc. which are social, psychological approaches to the problem of human nature.

SCOPE OF EDUCATION

Once again, it is difficult to explain the scope of education, because it is an open system and a very comprehensive discipline. In the real sense of the term, it is a process, which goes on from birth to death, encompassing each and every aspect of human life.

Pestalozzis conception of education is that "it reforms and elevates society. It involves a natural and harmonious development of all the faculties of the individual; it requires an active cooperation between home and school."

Therefore, we can say that education is joint endeavor of home, school and society to bring about a desirable behavioral change among children, so that they become contributing citizens of the society.

Education as a discipline is concerned biological, physical, mental, intellectual, emotional, cultural and spiritual development of the individual.

Scope of education is very broader, because it stretches its hands toward different directions as vocational education, technical education, adult education, non-formal education, guidance and with social, counseling, etc. Its scope ranges from teaching three R's (reading, writing and arithmetic), through development of values, attitudes, etc. to the all-round development and self-realization of the individual.

By observing the scope of social psychology and of education we can say that both of them concentrate, emphasize and deal with the individual for his/her harmonious development and in turn make the society a place suitable for human existence. As such it is very significant to study the relationship between social psychology and education.

Social psychology deals with the behavior of the individual in a 'social context'. School is a miniature 'society', where deliberately planned educational programs are executed. Therefore, education and social psychology are inter-related.

Formulation of social objectives for education, incorporation of social objectives into curricular or design of classroom, social process as a means of achieving social goals, etc. require helping from social psychologists to educationists.

Educators often face a series of social problems such as prejudice, pupil's dislike of school and conflicts among students and also among staff members that can be solved easily with the help of social psychology.

Education refers to school-related behavior and related variables. Education is fundamentally an interpersonal process, carried out through the interdependent cooperation of two roles—educator and learner, requires for its elucidation precisely the kinds of analytical tools and data provided by social psychology.

The knowledge of social psychology provides the knowledge about individual and group differences, which provide a basis for developing alternative educational treatment of different individuals or groups that would benefit all, more than teaching everyone the same way would.

Schools are complex social environments, where in addition to learning, social interaction takes place. Therefore, social psychology, which focuses its attention and discusses elaborately on 'social interaction' helps the education field, particularly school program to a large extent. In the same way, education also helps in social interaction, understanding the group norms, which leads to minimizing group conflicts, developing right types of attitudes, inculcation of values, better interpersonal relationship, etc.

Therefore, in conclusion, educational problems provide sophisticated and complex issues to challenge social psychologists to utilize the best available theory and methods and to challenge the field to develop new approaches. In a parallel way, the social psychological perspective is important for educators and significantly improves educational practice.

From the above discussion, we can see how intimately social psychology and education are related. Discussing this, Radsick and

High, shall argue that educational psychology must be fundamentally not cognition or a developmental/personality psychology, but a social psychology.

Though this much of intimate relationship is there between social psychology and education, educational issues were ignored by social psychologists; previously say up to 1954–1955. Only after this period, the educational issues drew attention of social psychologists and led to the development of social psychology of education. If is from this points of view, we shall discuss largely the development of social psychology of education.

DEVELOPMENT OF SOCIAL PSYCHOLOGY OF EDUCATION

There were many reports and textbooks, containing laboratory experiments, mainly in psychology and educational psychology, up to 1935. Among them, very few of them contained about social factors. For example, Thorndike's 1914 edition of his book contained a chapter *The Social Instincts.* Pressay's (1933) text included a chapter *Social Psychology of Childhood and Adolescence.* Erdrich and Carroll (1935) text included *Measurement of Personality Attitudes and Interests in Learning and Instructions.*

In 1941, Trow complained that, most of the educational psychologists were limiting their investigation to the psychology of the individual, neglecting the social aspects of individual behavior.

In 1954, Geizhals complained in his book '*The Handbook of Social Psychology*' that usually, textbooks contain chapters on the social psychology of industry and politics. Social psychologists have tended to ignore educational issues.

From the views of the above two authors, we can observe that though there was a change in the attention from educational psychology to social psychology emphasizing on the social aspects of the individuals behavior, there was very little or no attention of social psychologists toward the educational issues. At the same time, it reveals that initiation and awareness about the necessity of knowledge of social psychology to the educational field. Because of this, there was initiation to the development of social psychology of education. Some of the more successful texts by Ritchie (1981), Jander (1957) and

Perkins (1969), contained some of the aspects of educational issues viewed from the social psychological perspective.

Though the work started in social psychology of education, since 1959 to bridge the gap between social psychology and education, the work was geared up in 1970s and then social psychology of education became a subdiscipline finding clearly its scope.

Social psychology for education merely uses social psychological principles to explain educational problems. Here, mostly the researches are carried out in laboratory settings (not in educational settings).

In contrast, the social psychology of education defines its scope according to a problem focus on educational issues. The topics in social psychology of education are those social psychological issues that concern the social functioning of individuals and groups in educational systems, i.e. the topics of social psychology of education does not necessarily correspond to the standard topics of social psychology. Here, researches are carried out on the education setting itself.

CONCLUSION

The scope of social psychology and education are vast and inclusive of many of the aspects. They are intimately related to a larger extent. The knowledge of social psychology helps to a greater extent in solving the educational problems. This intimate relationship of mutual contribution led to the development of a new discipline, namely 'social psychology of education'. This deals mainly with the educational issues from the social psychology perspective, which helps in achieving educational goals.

SUGGESTED READING

1. Abram Kardiner. The Psychological Frontiers of Society. New York: Columbia University Press; 1945.
2. Allport FH. Social Psychology. Boston: Houghton Mifflin; 1924.
3. Allport GW, Kramer BM. Some roots of prejudice. J Gen Psychol. 1946;22:9-39.
4. Allport GW. Personality: A Psychological Interpretation. New York: Holt; 1937.

5. Allport GW. The Nature of Prejudice Reading. Massachusetts: Addison Wesley Publishing Company; 1954.
6. Argyris C. Interpersonal Competence and Organizational Effectiveness. Homewood, IL: Irwin-Dorsey Press; 1962.
7. Argyris C. Personality and Organization. New York: Harper; 1957.
8. Lindesmith AR, Strauss AL. Readings in Social Psychology. New York: Holt, Rinehart and Winston; 1969.

REVIEW QUESTIONS

1. Define social psychology. Explain the concepts of social psychology.
2. Explain the principles of social psychology.
3. Discuss the relationship between social psychology and education.
4. Describe the scope of social psychology.
5. Enumerate the development of social psychology in education.

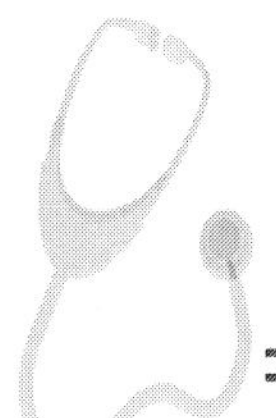

Previous Years University Questions (2011–2006)

POST BASIC BSc NURSING QUESTION PAPERS

PSYCHOLOGY-2011-QP-FEB-FIRST YEAR

Long Essays

1. Define intelligence. Explain the classification of intelligence test.
2. What is the nature and causes of individual differences?
3. Explain the laws of learning and their application in education.

Short Essays

4. Methods of memorizing.
5. Tools to improve memory.
6. Determinants of attention.
7. Types of thinking.
8. Type-cum-trait theory of personality.
9. Self-actualization theory.
10. Emotional states.
11. Define attitude and explain the nature of attitude.
12. Characteristics of a mentally healthy person.

Short Answers

13. Teacher's qualities.
14. Forgetting.
15. Behavior.
16. Extrovert.
17. Motives.
18. Conflict.

19. Id, ego, super ego.
20. Mnemonics.
21. Reasoning.
22. Abstract thinking.

PSYCHOLOGY-2010-QP-CODE: 1701

Long Essays

1. Define psychology. Discuss the methods used in psychology to study behavior.
2. Correlate the influence of hereditary and environment on the development of an individual.
3. How frustration and conflict causes stress? Discuss the role of a nurse in stress management.

Short Essays

4. Discuss the uses of psychology in the field of nursing.
5. Discuss the factors influencing creativity.
6. Examine the development of attributes.
7. Define perception. What are the errors in perception?
8. Describe the types of attention.
9. Explain the role of emotion in causing illness.
10. What do you mean by sensory disorder? How these disorders affect personality?
11. a. Explain the role of autonomic nervous system in emotion.
    b. Define mental retardation. Enumerate different types of mental retardation.
    c. What is thinking? Briefly discuss the types of thinking.

Short Answers

12. Physiological motives.
13. Mental age.
14. Problem-solving methods.
15. Individual differences in behavior.
16. Twins.
17. Concepts.
18. Memory.
19. Fluctuation of attention.
20. Insightful learning.
21. List of laws of learning.

PSYCHOLOGY-2009-QP-CODE: 1743

Long Essays

1. Discuss the role of hereditary and environment in the development of human behavior.
2. Define forgetting. Explain theories of forgetting.
3. Define problem solving. Explain scientific steps involved in problem solving.

Short Essays

4. Bring out the differences between biological and social motives.
5. Discuss the perceptual disturbances.
6. Explain factors influencing perception.
7. Discuss Erikson's theory of personality.
8. Describe operant conditioning by Skinner.
9. What is forgetting? How it can be minimized?
10. Theories of intelligence.
11. Define creative thinking. Discuss stages of creative thinking.
12. Importance of individual differences in the field of nursing.

Short Answers

13. Structuralism.
14. What is contributed by environment?
15. Meaning of attitude.
16. Steps of evaluation.
17. Measurement of emotions.
18. Social motives.
19. Conflicts.
20. Eysenck's theory of personality.
21. Measurement of memory.
22. Questionnaire method.

PSYCHOLOGY-2008-QP-CODE: 1701

Long Essays

1. Define psychology. Critically evaluate the different methods used in the study of psychology.
2. Define perception. Discuss the factors influencing perception. Explain extrasensory perception.

3. What is intelligence? Discuss the types of intelligence and various tests used to measure intelligence quotient (IQ).

Short Essays

4. Scope of educational psychology.
5. Define conflicts. How is it related to emotions?
6. Explain the varieties of attention. What is degree of attention?
7. Define personality and discuss the psychosocial factors that influence the development of personality.
8. Describe Skinner's instrumental conditioning in learning.
9. Explain the psychoanalytic theory of personality.
10. What is memory? Explain long-term memory and short-term memory.
11. Define frustration. Explain the sources of frustration.
12. What are the essential features for a teacher to be effective?

Short Answers

13. Stress.
14. Drive and needs.
15. Motivational cycle.
16. Id.
17. Creative thinking.
18. Individual differences.
19. Attitudes.
20. Concepts.
21. Social motives.
22. Regression.

PSYCHOLOGY-2007-QP-CODE: 1701

Long Essays

1. Define psychology and explain the scope of psychology in nursing profession.
2. What is motivation? Enumerate the theories of motivation.
3. Define personality and explain the methods used to assess the personality.

Short Essays

4. Determinants of attention.
5. James-Lange and Cannon-Bard theories of emotion.
6. Methods of educational psychology.
7. Narrate the importance of personality in nursing.
8. Explain biological motives.
9. Principles of hereditary.
10. Trial and error method of learning.
11. Define intelligence. Explain different types of intelligence tests.
12. Explain meaning and nature of thinking.
13. Define forgetting and explain the causes of forgetting.

Short Answers

14. Reasoning.
15. Integrated responses.
16. Extrasensory perception.
17. Span of attention.
18. Extinction.
19. Steps in problem solving.
20. Attitude change.
21. Evaluation.
22. Personal motives.
23. Reinforcement.

PSYCHOLOGY-2006-QP-CODE: 1701

Please refer 2010 Question Paper.

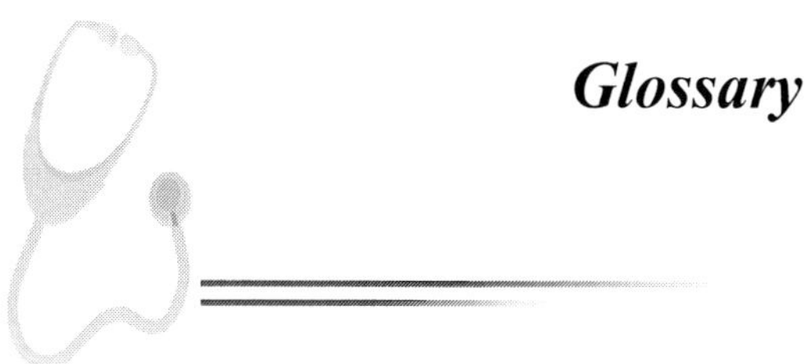

Glossary

A

1. *Absolute threshold:* The smallest quantity of physical energy that can be reliably detected by an observer.
2. *Abstract or general intelligence:* It is the ability to respond to words, numbers, letters, etc. This type of intelligence is acquired by the study of books and related literature. Mostly good teachers, lawyers, doctors, philosophers, etc. have this type of intelligence.
3. *Abstract reasoning test:* This test is intended as a verbal measure of the student's reasoning and yielding ability. It has many picture test yielding ambiguous scores, because they require the student to discriminate between lines or areas, which differ slightly in size and shape. This test supplements the general intelligence aspects of the verbal and numerical tests.
4. *Accommodation:* In Piaget's theory, the process of modifying existing cognitive structures in response to experience and new information.
5. *Acculturation:* The process by which members of minority groups comes to identify with and feel part of the mainstream culture.
6. *Achievement testing:* An achievement test is a systematic procedure for measuring a representative sample of learning tasks. Although, the emphasis is usually on measuring a set of intended learning outcomes, as defined by the instructional objectives, it should not be implied that the testing will be limited.

7. *Action potential:* A brief change in electrical voltage that occurs between the inside and the outside of an axon when a neuron is stimulated; it serves to produce an electrical impulse.
8. *Activation-synthesis theory:* The theory that dreaming results from the cortical synthesis and interpretation of neural signals triggered by activity in the lower part of the brain.
9. *Acute illness:* Illness characterized by symptoms that are of relatively short duration, are usually severe and affect the functioning of the clients in all dimensions.
10. *Adaptation:* Process by which changes occur in any of a person's dimensions in response to stress.
11. *Adjustment:* It is defined as an interaction between a person and his/her environment by which he/she adapts and depends upon his/her personal characteristics and circumstances of a situation producing a more harmonious relationship between him/her and the environment.
12. *Adrenal hormones:* These that are produced by the adrenal glands and that are involved in emotion and stress.
13. *Aggression:* A general term applying to behavior aimed at hurting other people, also applies to feelings of anger or hostility. Aggression functions as a motive, often in response to threats, insults or frustrations.
14. *Agoraphobia:* A set of phobias, often set off by a panic attack, involving the basic fear of being away from a safe place or person.
15. *Alarm reaction:* The first stage of the general adaptation syndrome consists of prompt responses of the body, many of them mediated by the sympathetic system, which prepare the organism to cope with stressors.
16. *Algorithm:* A problem-solving strategy guaranteed to produce a solution, even if the user does not know how it works.
17. *Alternative hypothesis:* An assertion that the independent variable in a study will have a certain predictable effect on the dependent variable; also called experimental or research hypothesis.
18. *Amygdala:* A brain structure involved in the arousal and regulation of emotion and the initial emotional response to sensory information.
19. *Analytical intelligence:* It is academic problem-solving skills, based on combined operations of execution, performance and knowledge. These three operations will enable to encode

stimuli, hold information in short-term memory, make calculations, perform mental calculations, mentally compare different stimuli and retrieve information from long-term memory.

20. *Anorexia nervosa:* An eating disorder, characterized by fear of being fat, a distorted body image, radically reduced consumption of food sand emaciation.
21. *Antidepressant drugs:* These are used primarily in the treatment of mood disorders, especially depression and anxiety.
22. *Antipsychotic drugs:* These are used primarily in the treatment of schizophrenia and other psychotic disorders.
23. *Antisocial personality disorder (APD):* It is characterized by antisocial behavior such as lying, stealing, manipulating others and sometimes violences and a lack of guilt, shame, and empathy (sometimes, called psychopathy or sociopathy).
24. *Applied psychology:* The study of psychological issues that have direct practical significance; also, the application of psychological findings.
25. *Appreciation learning:* While conceptual learning is on the affective side, a child from the very beginning utilizes his/her inborn trait of esthetic sensibility and acquires concepts colored by appreciation.
26. *Aptitude:* It is a combination of characteristics, indicative of an individual's capacity to acquire (with training) some specific knowledge, skill or set of organized responses such as the ability to speak a language, to become a musician, to do mechanical work, etc.
27. *Archetypes:* Universal, symbolic images that appear in myths, art, stories and dreams; to Jungians, they reflect the collective unconscious.
28. *Arithmetic mean:* An average that is calculated by adding up a set of quantities and dividing the sum by the total number of quantities in the set.
29. *Assimilation:* In Piaget's theory, the process of absorbing new information into existing cognitive structures. In Piaget's theory of cognitive development, the modification of one's environment, so that it fits into already developed ways of thinking and behavior.
30. *Associated areas:* Regions of the cerebral context involved in such complex physiological functions as the understanding and production of language, thinking and imagery.

31. *Associative learning:* Conceptional learning is helped by associative learning in amazing a wealth of knowledge. New concepts are tagged with the past concept through association.
32. *Attitude:* Attitude is the evaluation expressed in terms such as liking or disliking, pro or anti, favoring or not favoring and positive or negative. They are the feeling tone aroused by any attitude object. Attitude is thought to guide behavior. For example, if a person shows unfavorable attitude toward smoking, he/she will show negative attitude towards smokers.
33. *Attitude relevance:* Because the world abounds with attitude issues, each of us can be concerned only with a limited number of issues, those which are of special importance to us. It has been suggested recently that, relevant attitudes are better guide to subsequent behavior than irrelevant attitudes, i.e. for any given attitude issue, the link or correlation between attitude and behavior should be much stronger for those individuals for whom the attitude is relevant than for those individuals for whom it is not. This effect has been demonstrated for experimentally induced relevance.
34. *Attitudinal learning:* Attitudes are generalized dispositions for certain particular concepts, things, persons or activities. A child develops an attitude of affection toward his/her mother, an attitude of reverence toward the teacher and an attitude of belongingness toward the family. His/her attitude toward play is most favorable. All this he/she learns and adopts gradually.
35. *Attribution theory:* The theory that people are motivated to explain their own and other's behavior by attributing causes of that behavior to a situation or disposition.
36. *Autonomic nervous system:* The subdivision of the peripheral nervous system that regulates the internal organs and glands.
37. *Availability heuristic:* The tendency to judge the probability of a type of event by how easy it is to think of examples or instances.
38. *Avoidance goals:* They framed in terms of avoiding unpleasant experiences such as trying not to look foolish in public.
39. *Axon:* A neuron's extending fiber that conducts impulses away from the cell body and transmits them to other neurons.

B

1. *Basic concepts:* The concepts that have a moderate number of instances and that are easier to acquire than those having few or many instances.
2. *Basic psychology:* The study of psychological issues in order to seek knowledge for its own sake rather than for its practical application.
3. *Behavior modification:* The application of conditioning techniques to teach new responses or to reduce or eliminate maladaptive or problematic behavior.
4. *Behavior therapy:* A form of therapy that applies principles and techniques of classical and operant conditioning to help people change self-defeating or problematic behaviors.
5. *Behavioral genetics:* An interdisciplinary field of study concerned with the genetic bases of individual differences in behavior and personality.
6. *Behavioral records:* In behavior therapy, a method of keeping careful data on the frequency and consequences of the behavior to be changed.
7. *Behaviorism:* An approach to psychology that emphasizes the study of observable behavior and the role of the environment as a determinant of behavior. The view that human and animal behavior can be understood predicted and controlled without recourse to explanations involving mental states.
8. *Behaviorology:* It is an independently organized discipline featuring the natural science of behavior. Behaviorologists study the functional relations between behavior and its independent variables in the behavior-determining environment. Behaviorological accounts are based on the behavioral capacity of the species, the personal history of the behaving organism and the current physical and social environment in which behavior occurs. Behaviorologists discover the natural laws governing behavior.
9. *Binocular cues:* Visual cues to depth or distance, requiring two eyes.
10. *Biological perspective:* A psychological approach that emphasizes bodily events and changes associated with actions, feelings and thoughts.

11. *Biological rhythm:* A periodic, more or less regular fluctuation in a biological system; may or may not have psychological implications.
12. *Bipolar disorder:* A mood disorder in which episodes of both depression and mania (excessive euphoria) occur.
13. *Borderline personality disorder:* A disorder characterized by intense, but unstable relationships, a fear of abandonment by others, an unrealistic self-image and emotional volatility.
14. *Brain stems:* The part of the brain at the top of the spinal cord, consisting of the medulla and the pons.
15. *Brightness:* Lightness or luminance; the dimension of visual experience related to the amount of light emitted from or reflected by an object.
16. *Bulimia:* An eating disorder characterized by episodes of excessive eating (binging) followed by forced vomiting or use of laxatives (purging).

C

1. *Case study:* A detailed description of a particular individual being studied or treated.
2. *Cell body:* The part of the neuron containing the nucleus surrounded by cytoplasm but not incorporating the axon and dendrites.
3. *Central nervous system (CNS):* The portion of the nervous system consisting of the brain and spinal cord.
4. *Cerebellum:* A brain structure that regulates movement and balance and that is involved in the learning of certain kinds of simple responses.
5. *Cerebral cortex:* A collection of several thin layers of cells covering the cerebrum; it is largely responsible for higher mental functions. Cortex is Latin for 'bark' or 'rind'.
6. *Cerebral hemispheres:* The two halves of the cerebrum.
7. *Cerebrum:* The largest brain structure, consisting of the upper part of the brain; divided into two hemispheres, it is in charge of most sensory, motor and cognitive processes. Cerebrum is the Latin word for 'brain'.
8. *Childhood (infantile) amnesia:* The inability to remember events and experiences that occurred during the first 2 or 3 years of life.

9. *Chromosomes:* Within every cell, rod-shaped structures that carry the genes.
10. *Chunk:* A meaningful unit of information; it may be composed of smaller units.
11. *Circadian rhythm:* A biological rhythm with a period (from peak to peak or trough to trough) of about 24 hours; from the Latin *circa,* 'about', and *dies,* 'a day'.
12. *Clairvoyance:* It is the ability to gain information about an object, person, location or physical event through means other than the known human senses.
13. *Classical conditioning:* The process by which a previously neutral stimulus acquires the capacity to elicit a response through association with a stimulus that already elicits a similar or related response.
14. *Clerical aptitude:* It is also a composite function. It involves several specific abilities like perceptual ability, intellectual ability and motor ability.
15. *Client-centered (non-directive) therapy:* A humanist approach to therapy devised by Carl Rogers, which emphasizes the therapist's empathy with the client, the therapist's ability to see the world as the client does and the use of unconditional positive regard.
16. *Cloning:* It is a technique of producing one or more individuals, plants or animals or human beings: who are genetically identical to the original plant or animal or man. In short, it is the duplication process or carbon copy process.
17. *Clouding:* The consciousness is a very mild form of altered mental status in which the patient has inattention and reduced wakefulness.
18. *Cochlea:* A snail-shaped, fluid-filled organ in the inner ear, containing the organ of Corti, where the receptors for hearing are located.
19. *Coefficient of correlation:* A measure of correlation that ranges in value from –1.00 to +1.00.
20. *Cognitive dissonance:* A state of tension that occurs when a person simultaneously holds two cognitions that are psychologically inconsistent or when a person's belief is incongruent with his/her behavior. When two contradictory feelings: belief or behavior exists, it creates a state of tension and the person tries to reduce tension by changing the feelings, beliefs or

behaviors. For example, if a nurse student studies hard for a test, he/she expects to do well. But if he/she studies hard and fails, dissonance is aroused.

21. *Cognitive ethology:* The study of cognitive processes in non-human animals.
22. *Cognitive perspective:* A psychological approach that emphasizes mental processes in perception, memory, language, problem solving and other areas of behavior.
23. *Cognitive schema:* An integrated mental network of knowledge, beliefs and expectations concerning a particular topic or aspect of the world.
24. *Cognitive therapy:* A form of therapy designed to identify and change irrational, unproductive ways of thinking and hence, to reduce negative emotions and their behavioral consequences; it is often combined with behavioral techniques.
25. *Collective unconscious:* In Jungian theory, the universal memories and experiences of humankind, represented in the symbols, stories and images (archetypes) that occur across all cultures.
26. *Collectivist cultures:* The cultures in which the self is regarded as embedded in relationships and harmony with one's group is prized above individual goals and wishes.
27. *Commitment:* It is the extent to which he/she feels reluctant to give up his/her initial position (attitude). Greater the strength of commitment to their own attitude, it is harder for the individual to change his/her attitude.
28. *Competitive evaluation:* All evaluation systems can be grouped into two categories: those that force a student to compete with other students (no referenced) and those that do not require interstudent competition, but instead are based on a set of standards of mastery criterion reference. Traditionally, schools have required competition among students and many teachers believe that competition among students is necessary for motivating. Many also believe that competition is needed to prepare students for adulthood in a competitive world, especially for getting ahead in their future employment.
29. *Concept:* A mental category that groups objects, relations, activities, abstractions or qualities having common properties. A concept is a symbol that stands for common properties of things. Concepts enable us to divide things into classes. Objects with common features are grouped under the same class. For

example, we use the concept of flowers to refer to jasmine, lotus, etc. with the concept of 'soft'; we sort out objects into soft and hard. The concepts as a tool, economize our efforts in thinking. For example, when we listen to the word 'elephant', we are at once reminded not only about the nature and qualities of the elephants as a class but also our particular experiences and understanding about them emerges from our consciousness, which stimulates our present thinking.

30. *Conceptual learning:* As concrete thinking leads to abstract thinking, perceptual learning is followed by conceptual learning. A concept is a general idea, universal in character. A child sees a particular cow and forms some ideas of a cow, with some particular characteristics. Here the ideation is on the basis of one particular cow. This is the particular percept, but when the child sees a number of cows, with some common characteristics, he/she locates certain general qualities in all the cows and on the basis of these he/she forms a conception of 'cow'. This is on the basis of percept, which is made general.
31. *Conceptual or abstract thinking:* Like perceptual thinking, it does not require the perception of actual objects or events. It is an abstract thinking, where one makes use of concepts, the generalized ideas and language. It is regarded as a superior type of thinking to perceptual thinking, as it economizes efforts in understanding and problem solving.
32. *Concrete intelligence:* It is related to concrete materials. This type of intelligence is applicable when the individual is handling concrete objects or machines. The person uses this intelligence in the operation of tools and instruments. For example, engineers, mechanics generally have this type of intelligence.
33. *Conditioned response (CR):* The classical-conditioning term for a response that is elicited by a conditioned stimulus; it occurs after the conditioned stimulus, is associated with an unconditioned stimulus.
34. *Conditioned stimulus (CS):* The classical-conditioning term for an initially neutral stimulus that comes to elicit a conditioned response after being associated with an unconditioned stimulus.
35. *Conditioning:* A basic kind of learning that involves associations between environmental stimuli and the organism's responses. It is a form of learning in which a reflex or some aspect of behavior is brought under the control of a stimulus; we will

define conditioning in terms of the procedures used to bring it about. These procedures, with examples, are described below. Although conditioning has been investigated in humans and animals, with generally similar findings, the majority of experiments on conditioning have employed animal subjects, in which learning prior to the experiment can be more easily controlled.

36. *Cones:* Visual receptors involved in color vision.
37. *Confabulation:* Confusion of an event that happened to someone else with one that happened to you or a belief that you remember something, when it never actually happened.
38. *Confirmation bias:* The tendency to look for or pay attention only to information that confirms one's own belief.
39. *Confusion:* This state is a more profound deficit that includes disorientation, bewilderment and difficulty following commands. Lethargy consists of severe drowsiness in which the patient can be aroused by moderate stimuli and then drift back to sleep.
40. *Consciousness:* Awareness of oneself and the environment. It is defined as the state of being mentally perceptive, alert and awake. For example, during some phases of deep sleep, the mind is active as it directs respiration, yet consciousness can be absent. So consciousness is that bright spot of alertness within the much larger field of the mind. In this work, with the understanding that there are other uses of the word 'consciousness', when it refers to that quality of alertness as an additional component within the mind, the word 'consciousness' will be capitalized.
41. *Conservation:* The understanding that the physical properties of objects, such as the number of items in a cluster or the amount of liquid in a glass, can remain the same even when their form or appearance changes.
42. *Consolidation:* The process by which a long-term memory becomes durable and stable.
43. *Contact comfort:* In primates, the innate pleasure derived from close physical contact; it is the basis of the infant's first attachment.
44. *Continuous reinforcement:* A reinforcement schedule in which a particular response is always reinforced.
45. *Control condition:* In an experiment, a comparison condition in which subject is not exposed to the same treatment, as in the experimental condition.

46. *Convergence:* The turning inward of the eyes, which occurs when they focus on a nearby object.
47. *Convergent thinking:* The ability to produce responses that are based primarily on knowledge and logic.
48. *Corpus callosum:* The bundle of nerve fibers, connecting the two cerebral hemispheres.
49. *Correlation:* A measure of how strongly two variables are related to one another.
50. *Correlational study:* A descriptive study that looks for a consistent relationship between two phenomena.
51. *Counseling:* It is an accepting, trusting and safe relationship in which clients learn to discuss openly what worries and upsets them, to define precise behavioral goals to acquire essential social skills and to develop the courage and self-confidence to implement the desired new behaviors. Counseling is a process of enabling the individuals to know themselves and their present and possible future situations in order that they may make substantial contributions to the society and to solve own problems through a face-to-face personal relationship with the counselor.
52. *Counter conditioning:* In classical conditioning, the process of pairing a conditioned stimulus with a stimulus that elicits a response that is incompatible with an unwanted conditioned response.
53. *Creative intelligence:* It involves insights, synthesis and the ability to react to novel situations and stimuli. It consists of ability, which allows people to think creatively and adjust creatively and effectively to new situations. Novel tasks or situations are good measures of intellectual ability because they assess an individual's ability to apply existing knowledge to new problems.
54. *Creative process:* The creative process is any process by which something new is produced—an idea or an object including a new form, or arrangement of old elements. The new creation must contribute to the solution of some problem.
55. *Creative thinking:* It means that the predictions and/or inferences for the individual are new, original, ingenious and unusual. The creative thinker is one who explores new areas and makes new observation, new predictions, and new inferences. This type of thinking is chiefly aimed at creating something new. It is in

search of new relationships and associations to describe and interpret the nature of things, events and situations. It is not bound by any pre-established rules. The individual himself/herself usually formulates the problem and is free to collect evidence and invent tools for its solution. The thinking of the scientists or inventors is an example of creative thinking.

56. *Creativity:* It is the capacity of a person to produce compositions, products or ideas, which are essentially new or novel and previously unknown to the producer.
57. *Critical thinking:* The ability and willingness to assess claims and make judgments on the basis of well-supported reasons and evidence, rather than emotion or anecdote. It is a higher order, well-disciplined thought process, which involves the use of cognitive skills like conceptualization, interpretation, analysis, synthesis and evaluation for arriving at an unbiased, valid and reliable judgment of the gathered or communicated information or data as a guide to one's belief and action.
58. *Cross-sectional study:* A study in which subjects of different ages are compared at a given time.
59. *Crystallized intelligence:* Cognitive skills and specific knowledge of information acquired over a lifetime; it is heavily dependent on education and tends to remain stable over the lifetime.
60. *Cue-dependent forgetting:* The inability to retrieve information stored in memory, because of insufficient cues for recall.
61. *Culture:* A program of shared rules that govern the behavior of members of a community or society and a set of values, beliefs and attitudes shared by most members of that community.

D

1. *Dark adaptation:* A process by which visual receptors become maximally sensitive to dim light.
2. *Decay theory:* The theory that information in memory eventually disappears if it is not accessed; it applies better to short-term than the long-term memory.
3. *Declarative memories:* The memories of facts, rules, concepts and events ('knowing that'); they include semantic, and episodic memories.

4. *Deductive reasoning:* A form of reasoning in which a conclusion follows necessarily from certain premises; if the premises are true, the conclusion must be true.
5. *Deep processing:* In the encoding of information, the processing of meaning rather than simply the physical or sensory features of a stimulus.
6. *Defense mechanisms:* Methods used by the ego to prevent unconscious anxiety or threatening thoughts from entering consciousness. It is a pattern of adjustment through which an individual relieves or decreases anxieties caused by an uncomfortable situation that threatens self-esteem. Ego defense mechanism is consciously or unconsciously operating device to keep confliction issues out of consciousness of the individual to bring some protective measures.
7. *Deindividuation:* In groups or crowds, the loss of awareness of one's own individuality.
8. *Delusional projection:* Grossly, Frank delusions about external reality are usually of a persecutory nature. This defense mechanism is common feature of psychotic mental illnesses like schizophrenia, delusional disorder, etc. These delusions are the false beliefs of the person, which are not shared by race, age, educational background, etc. For example, a man says that his family members are planning to kill him very soon.
9. *Dendrites:* A neuron's branches that receive information from other neurons and transmit it toward the cell body.
10. *Denial:* It is protecting self from unpleasant reality by refusal to perceive it or face it. It is a defense mechanism in which a person is faced with a fact that is too painful to accept and reject it. The individual may deny the reality of the unpleasant fact altogether, admit the fact, but deny its seriousness or admit both the fact and seriousness, but denies responsibility. The concept of denial is particularly important to the study of addiction.
11. *Deoxyribonucleic acid (DNA):* The chromosomal molecule that transfers genetic characteristics by way of coded instructions for the structure of proteins.
12. *Dependent variable:* A variable that an experimenter predicts will be affected by manipulations of the independent variable.
13. *Depressants:* Drugs that slow down activity in the central nervous system.

14. *Descriptive methods:* The methods that yield descriptions of behavior but not necessarily causal explanations.
15. *Descriptive statistics:* The statistical procedures that organize and summarize research data.
16. *Dialectical reasoning:* A process in which opposing facts or ideas are weighed and compared, with a view to determining the best solution or resolving differences.
17. *Difference threshold:* The smallest difference in stimulation that can be reliably detected by an observer when two stimuli are compared; also called just noticeable difference (JND).
18. *Differential aptitude test:* It was developed by USA Psychological Corporation. It has proved more successful in predicting academic success and found especially useful for providing educational and vocational guidance to secondary school children.
19. *Diffusion of responsibility:* In organized or anonymous groups, the tendency of members to avoid taking responsibility for actions or decisions, assuming that others will do so.
20. *Discriminative stimulus:* A stimulus that signals when a particular response is likely to be followed by a certain type of consequence.
21. *Display rules:* Social and cultural rules that regulate when, how and where a person may express (or must suppress) emotions.
22. *Dissociation:* A split in consciousness in which one part of the mind operates independently of others.
23. *Dissociative identity disorder:* A controversial disorder, marked by the apparent appearance within one person of two or more distinct personalities, each with its own name and traits; commonly known as multiple personality disorder (MPD).
24. *Distortion:* A gross reshaping of external reality to meet internal needs. For example, mentally ill patients have no intact contact with reality. These patients are suffering with psychosis.
25. *Doctrine of specific nerve energies*: The principle that different sensory modalities exist because signals received by the sense organs stimulate different nerve pathways leading to different areas of the brain.
26. *Double-blind study:* An experiment in which neither the subjects nor the individuals running the study know, which subjects are in the control group and which are in the experimental group until after the results are tallied.

27. *Drive:* A drive is a tendency initiated by shifts in physiological balance, tissue tension, sensitivity to stimuli of certain class, and response in any of the variety of ways that are related to the attainment of certain goals.

E

1. *Echoic memory:* A momentary sensory memory of auditory stimulus. If attention is elsewhere, sounds and words can still be recalled within 3 to 4 seconds. It would playback auditory information and gives time to recognize sounds as words.
2. *Eclectic counseling:* In eclectic counseling, the strategy arises out of the appropriate knowledge of individual behavior and a combination of directive and other approaches. Irrespective of the differences, all approaches should have developmental, preventive and remedial values.
3. *Educational guidance:* It helps the students to get maximum benefit out of education and to solve their problems related to education. The emphasis is on providing assistance to students to perform satisfactorily in their academic work, choose the appropriate course of study, overcome learning difficulties, foster creativity, improve levels of motivation, utilize institutional resources optimally such as library, laboratory, etc.
4. *Educational psychology:* In this branch of psychology, we try to study the behavior of the learner in relation to educational environment. As a science of education, the subject matter of this branch helps in improving all the processes and products of education. The teachers can teach well and the students can learn well with the help of the knowledge, and skills gained through the study of this subject. It also helps the teachers in gaining proper insight for bringing desirable modification in the behavior and seeking an all-round harmonious development of the personality of the students.
5. *Effect size:* The amount of variance among scores in a study accounted by the independent variable.
6. *Ego:* In psychoanalysis, the part of personality that represents reason, good sense and rational self-control.
7. *Egocentric thinking:* Seeing the world from only his/her own point of view; the inability to take another person's perspective.

8. *Elaborative rehearsal:* Association of new information with already stored knowledge and analysis of the new information to make it memorable.
9. *Electroconvulsive therapy (ECT):* A procedure used in cases of prolonged and severe major depression, in which a brief brain seizure is induced.
10. *Electroencephalogram (EEG):* A recording of neural activity detected by electrodes.
11. *Emotion:* A state of arousal involving facial and bodily changes, brain activation, cognitive appraisals, subjective feelings and tendencies toward action, all shaped by cultural rules.
12. *Emotion work:* Expression of an emotion that the person does not really feel, often because of a role requirement.
13. *Emotional intelligence:* The ability to identify one's own and others' emotions accurately, express the emotions clearly and regulate them in oneself and others.
14. *Emotional quotient (EQ):* The concept of EQ in understanding and measuring one's level of emotional intelligence in the same way, and as we utilize the concept of intelligence quotient (IQ) in understanding, utilizing and measuring one's level of intelligence or intellectual potential. As a result, the term EQ represents a relative measure of one's emotional intelligence potential in the same way as IQ does for the measurement of one's intellectual potential.
15. *Emotionality:* It has a powerful role to play in personality. The emotional stability and the maturity is required for healthy personality.
16. *Empirical:* Relying on or derived from observation, experimentation or measurement.
17. *Endocrine glands:* Internal organs that produce hormones and release them into the bloodstream.
18. *Endogenous:* Generated from within rather than by external cues.
19. *Endorphins:* Chemical substances in the nervous system that are similar in structure and action to opiates; they are involved in pain reduction, pleasure and memory and are known technically as endogenous opioid peptides.
20. *Entrainment:* The synchronization of biological rhythms with external cues, such as fluctuations in daylight.

21. *Entrapment:* A gradual process in which individual's escalates their commitment to a course of action to justify their investment of time, money or effort.
22. *Environment:* The totality of conditions within and surrounding the organism, that serves to stimulate behavior or act to bring about change of behavior.
23. *Environmental psychology:* Field of psychology focuses on the effects of environmental setting on an individual's feeling and behavior.
24. *Episodic memories:* The memories of personally experienced events and the contexts in which they occurred.
25. *Episodic memory:* It concerns information specific to a particular context such as a time and place. It is used for more personal memories such as sensations, emotions and personal associations of a particular place.
26. *Equilibrium:* The sense of balance.
27. *Ethnic identity:* A person's identification with a racial, religious or ethnic group.
28. *Ethnocentrism:* The belief that one's own ethnic group, nation or religion is superior to all others.
29. *Etiology:* Identification of the cause of a problem. The cause may be direct or a contributing factor in the development of client's problem or need.
30. *Evaluation:* It is the determination of the worth or the value of an event, object or individual in terms of a specified criterion. Educators evaluate student progress by comparing student performance to the criteria of success based on instructional objectives. They evaluate a program in terms of how well children progress compared to how they might do in an alternative program.
31. *Evolution:* A change in gene frequencies within a population over many generations; a mechanism by which genetically influenced characteristics of a population may change.
32. *Evolutionary psychology:* A field of psychology emphasizing evolutionary mechanisms that may help to explain human commonalities in cognition, development, emotion, social practices and other areas of behavior. The branch of psychology, which seeks to identify behavior patterns that result from genetic inheritance from our ancestors.

33. *Existential therapy:* A form of therapy designed to help clients explore the meaning of existence and face the great questions of life, such as death, freedom, free will, alienation and loneliness.
34. *Experiment:* A controlled test of a hypothesis in which the researcher manipulates one variable to discover its effect on another.
35. *Experimenter effects:* Unintended changes in subjects' behavior due to cues inadvertently given by the experimenter.
36. *Explicit memory:* Conscious, intentional recollection of an event or an item of information.
37. *Exposure (flooding):* In behavior therapy, a method in which a person suffering from an anxiety disorder such as a phobia or panic attacks, is taken directly into the feared situation until the anxiety subsides.
38. *External environment:* The environment afterbirth is more complex and powerful. It involves variety of physical and social contacts.
39. *Extinction:* The weakening and eventual disappearance of a learned response. In classical conditioning, it occurs when the conditioned stimulus is no longer paired with the unconditioned stimulus; in operant conditioning, it occurs when a response is no longer followed by a reinforcer.
40. *Extrinsic motivation:* The pursuit of an activity for external rewards such as money or fame. It comes from outside the individual. Common extrinsic motivations are rewards like money and grades, coercion and threat of punishment. Competition is generally extrinsic because it encourages the performer to win and beat others, not to enjoy the intrinsic rewards of the activity. A crowd cheering on the individual and trophies are also extrinsic motivation.
41. *Extrinsic reinforcers:* Reinforcers that are not inherently related to the activity being reinforced.

F

1. *Facial feedback:* The process by which the facial muscles send messages to the brain about the basic emotion being expressed.
2. *Factor analysis:* Statistical methods for analyzing the intercorrelations among various measures or test scores; clusters of measures or scores that are highly correlated are assumed to measure the same underlying trait, ability or aptitude (factor).

3. *Family-systems perspective:* An approach to doing therapy with individuals or families by examining, how each member forms part of a larger, interacting system.
4. *Fear:* It is a basic survival mechanism or emotional response to a threat or specific stimuli. The stimuli or the threat may be that of pain or danger of losing one's life. Fear is generally experienced by an individual with respect to a particular worsening situation.
5. *Feature detectors:* Cells in the visual cortex that is sensitive to specific features of the environment.
6. *Feminist psychology:* A psychological approach that analyzes the influence of social inequities on gender relations and on the behavior of the two sexes.
7. *Field research:* Descriptive or experimental research conducted in a natural setting outside the laboratory.
8. *Fixed-interval schedule:* An intermittent schedule of reinforcement in which a reinforcer is delivered for the first response made after a fixed period of time has elapsed, since the last reinforcer.
9. *Fixed-ratio schedule:* An intermittent schedule of reinforcement in which reinforcement occurs only after a fixed number of responses.
10. *Fluid intelligence:* The capacity for deductive reasoning and the ability to use new information to solve problems; it is relatively independent of education and tends to decline in old age.
11. *Formative evaluation:* It can be defined as the designing and using the tests for only one specific purpose—to promote learning. Formative evaluation enables teachers to monitor their instruction, so they can keep it on course. Also, if any student cannot learn excellently from the original instruction, the student can learn excellently from one or more correctives. While most teachers agree that going over test answers in class can help some students to learn more about the material. It is essential that there be a much more systematic use of evaluation, separate from grading and aimed only at promoting learning.
12. *Fraternal (dizygotic) twins:* The twins that develop from two separate eggs fertilized by different sperm; they are no more alike genetically, than are like any other pair of siblings.
13. *Free association:* In psychoanalysis and other psychodynamic therapies, the process of saying freely, whatever comes to mind in connection with dreams, memories, fantasies or conflicts.

14. *Frequency distribution:* A summary of how frequently each score in a set occurred.
15. *Frequency polygon (line graph):* A graph showing a set of points obtained by plotting score values against score frequencies; adjacent points are joined by straight lines.
16. *Frontal lobes:* The lobes at the front of the brain's cerebral cortex; they contain areas involved in short-term memory, higher-order thinking, initiative, social judgment and (in the left lobe, typically) speech production.
17. *Functionalism:* An early psychological approach that emphasized the function or purpose of behavior and consciousness.
18. *Fundamental attribution error:* The tendency, in explaining other people's behavior, to overestimate personality factors and underestimates the influence of the situation.

G

1. *g factor:* A general intellectual ability assumed by many theorists to underlie specific mental abilities and talents.
2. *Ganglion cells:* Neurons in the retina of the eye, which gather information from receptor cells (by way of intermediate bipolar cells); their axons make up the optic nerve.
3. *Gate control theory:* The theory states that the experience of pain depends in part on whether pain impulses get past a neurological 'gate' in the spinal cord and thus, reach the brain.
4. *Gender identity:* The fundamental sense of being male or female; it is independent of whether the person conforms to the social and cultural rules of gender.
5. *Gender schema:* A cognitive schema (mental network) of knowledge, beliefs, metaphors and expectations about what it means to be male or female.
6. *Gender typing:* The process by which children learn the abilities, interests, personality traits and behaviors associated with being masculine or feminine in their culture.
7. *General adaptation syndrome:* According to Hans Selye, a series of physiological responses to stressors that occur in three phases: alarm, resistance and exhaustion.
8. *General aptitude test battery:* Developed by the Employment Service Bureau of the United States of America (USA) has 12 tests, eight of which are paper-pencil tests as for name comparison,

computation, vocabulary, arithmetic reasoning, form matching, test matching, three-dimensional spaces, etc. The other four require the use of simple equipment in the shape of moving pegs on boards, assembling and dissembling rivets and washers.

9. *Generalized anxiety disorder:* A continuous state of anxiety marked by feelings of worry and dread, apprehension, difficulties in concentration and signs of motor tension.
10. *Genes:* The functional units of heredity; they are composed of DNA and specify the structure of proteins. The parts of the chromosomes through which genetic information is transmitted.
11. *Genetic marker:* A segment of DNA that varies among individuals has a known location on a chromosome and can function as a genetic landmark for a gene involved in a physical or mental condition.
12. *Genome:* The full set of genes in each cell of an organism (with the exception of sperm and egg cells).
13. *Gestalt principles:* The principles that describe the brain's organization of sensory information into meaningful units and patterns.
14. *Glia:* Cells that support nurture and insulate neurons, remove debris when neurons die, enhance the formation and maintenance of synapses and modify neuronal functioning.
15. *Graph:* A drawing that depicts numerical relationships.
16. *Graphic art test:* It requires the subject to produce sketches from given patterns of lines and figures. The created sketches of the subject are then evaluated according to the standard given by the author of this test.
17. *Group:* Two or more people who, for longer than a few moments, interact with and influence one another and perceive and another as 'us'.
18. *Group counseling:* This form of counseling is sometimes successful with clients, who have not responded well to individual counseling. This group interaction helps the individual to gain insight into the problems by listening to others discussing their difficulties. Group counseling often not only helps the individual to change but also enhances his/her desire and ability to help others faced with distressing life circumstances.
19. *Groupthink:* In close-knit groups, the tendency for all members to think alike for the sake of harmony and to suppress disagreement.

20. *Guidance:* It is the assistance made available by qualified and trained person to an individual of any age, to help that individual to manage own life activities, develop own point of view, make own decision and carry on own burden. In educational context, guidance means assisting students to select courses of study appropriate to their needs and interests, achieve academic excellence to the best possible extent, derive maximum benefit of the institutional resources and facilities, inculcate proper study habits and satisfactorily participate in curricular and extracurricular activities.
21. *Guilt:* It is the emotional or cognitive experience, which succeeds the realization that one has violated a moral standard. The concept of remorse and guilt are closely related to each other.

H

1. *Hallucinations:* False sensory perception not associated with real external stimuli. Hallucinations may involve any of the five senses.
2. *Health:* Dynamic state in which an individual adapts to internal and external environments so that there is a state of physical, emotional, intellectual, social and spiritual well-being.
3. *Health behavior:* Activities through which a person maintain, attains or regains behavior as an expression of personal health beliefs.
4. *Health guidance:* It implies the assistance rendered to students for maintaining sound health. Sound health is a prerequisite for participating in curricular and co-curricular activities. This type of guidance focuses on enabling students to appreciate conditions for good health and take steps necessary for ensuring good health, maintaining sound physical and mental health.
5. *Health promotion:* Activities directed towards maintenance or enhancing the health and well-being of clients.
6. *Health promoting behavior:* Considered a third subcategory of health behavior and through assessment, reveal needs for vehicular safety, home safety, domestic violence recognition, recreational safety, occupational safety and health.
7. *Hereditary:* Genetic transmission of characteristics from parents to their children or the totality of biologically transmitted factors that influence the structure of the body and thus limit behavior.

8. *Heritability:* A statistical estimate of the proportion of the total variance in some trait that is attributable to genetic differences among individuals within a group.
9. *Heuristic:* A rule of thumb that suggests a course of action or guides problem solving, but does not guarantee an optimal solution.
10. *Higher-order conditioning:* In classical conditioning, a procedure in which a neutral stimulus becomes a conditioned stimulus through association with an already established conditioned stimulus.
11. *Hindsight bias:* The tendency to overestimate one's ability to have predicted an event once the outcome is known; the 'I knew it all along' phenomenon.
12. *Hippocampus:* A brain structure involved in the storage of new information in memory.
13. *Histogram (bar graph):* A graph in which the heights (or lengths) of bars are proportional to the frequencies of individual scores or classes of scores in a distribution.
14. *Holistic health:* A system of comprehensive or total care that considers the physical, emotional, social, economical and spiritual needs of the person, the response to the illness and the effect of the illness on the person's ability to meet self-care needs.
15. *Hormones:* Chemical substances, secreted by organs called glands that affect the functioning of other organs. A secretion of a specific organ, often an endocrine gland, into the bloodstream, where it is carried to various organs of the body to have an effect, a chemical messenger.
16. *Hue:* The dimension of visual experience specified by color; names and related to the wavelength of light.
17. *Hypochondriasis:* The transformation of negative feelings toward others into negative feelings toward self, pain, illness and anxiety. Hypochondrias (or hypochondria), sometimes referred to as health phobia, refers to an excessive preoccupation or worry about having a serious illness. Often, hypochondria persist even after a physician has evaluated a person and reassured him/her that his/her concerns about symptoms do not have an underlying medical basis.
18. *Hypothalamic pituitary adrenal (HPA) axis:* A system activated to energize the body to respond to stressors. The hypothalamus sends chemical messengers to the pituitary, which in turn prompts adrenal cortex to produce cortisol and other hormones.

19. *Humanist psychology:* A psychological approach that emphasizes personal growth, resilience and the achievement of human potential, rather than the scientific understanding and assessment of behavior.
20. *Humanist therapy:* A form of psychotherapy based on the philosophy of humanism, which starts from the assumption that people seek self-actualization and self-fulfillment; it emphasizes people's free will to change, not past conflicts.
21. *Hypnosis:* A procedure in which the practitioner suggests changes in the sensations, perceptions, thoughts, feelings or behavior of the subject.
22. *Hypothalamus:* A brain structure involved in emotions and drives vital to survival such as fear, hunger, thirst and reproduction; it regulates the autonomic nervous system.
23. *Hypothesis:* A statement that attempts to predict or to account for a set of phenomena; scientific hypotheses specify relationships among events or variables and are empirically tested.

I

1. *Iconic memory:* A form of sensory memory that holds visual information for almost quarter of a second or more. It makes visual world appear smooth and continuous despite frequent blinks and an eye movements.
2. *Id:* In psychoanalysis, the part of personality containing inherited psychic energy, particularly sexual and aggressive instincts.
3. *Identical (monozygotic) twins:* They develop when a fertilized egg divides into two parts that develop into separate embryos.
4. *Identification test:* The identification test includes a wide variety of test situations representing various degree of realism. In some cases, a student may simply be asked to identify a tool or piece of equipment and to indicate its function. A more complex test situation might present the students with a particular performance task (e.g. locating a short in an electrical circuit) and ask them to identify the tools, equipment and procedures needed in performing the task.
5. *Images:* As mind pictures consist of personal experiences of olects, persons or scenes; once actually seen, heard or felt. These mind pictures symbolize the actual objects, experiences

and activities. In thinking, we usually manipulate the images instead of actual objects, experiences or activities.

6. *Implicit learning:* The learning that occurs when you acquire knowledge about something without being aware of how you did so and without being able to state exactly what it is you have learned.
7. *Implicit memory:* Unconscious retention in memory, as evidenced by the effect of a previous experience or previously encountered information on current thoughts or actions.
8. *Independent variable:* A variable that an experimenter manipulates.
9. *Individual counseling:* This is a one-to-one helping relationship between the counselor and the counseled. It is focused upon the individual's need for growth and adjustment, problem solving and decision-making. This type of counseling requires counselors with the highest level of training and professional skills. In addition, it also requires that they have a certain personality type as well; counseling will be rendered ineffective unless counselors exhibit such personality traits as understanding, warmth, humaneness and positive attitudes toward the client.
10. *Individualist cultures:* The culture in which the self is regarded as autonomous and individual goals and wishes are prized above duty and relations with others.
11. *Induction:* A method of child rearing in which the parent appeals to the child's own resources, abilities, sense of responsibility and feelings for others in correcting the child's misbehavior.
12. *Inductive reasoning:* A form of reasoning in which the premises provide support for a conclusion, but it is still possible for the conclusion to be false.
13. *Inferential statistics:* The statistical procedures that allow researchers to draw inferences about how statistically meaningful a study's results are.
14. *Influenceability:* Most personality traits are not related to the ease with which someone is persuaded. A person's general personality profile will be of little use in predicting whether a given message will be persuasive. It is known, however, that some people are more easily influenced than others and that some people are downright gullible. The latter, bombarded with conflicting viewpoints, will believe the one they heard most recently. As might be expected, there are group differences in

this trait. Obviously, children are more easily influenced than adults and poorly educated people are more easily influenced than the well-educated.

15. *Insight learning:* In a typical insight situation a problem is passed, a period follows during which no progress is made and then the solution comes suddenly. A learning curve of insight learning would show no evidence of learning for a time and then suddenly learning would be almost complete.
16. *Instinct:* It is usually defined as a faculty acting in such a way as to produce certain ends, without foresight of the ends and without previous education in the performance.
17. *Intelligence:* An inferred characteristic of an individual, usually defined as the ability to profit from experience, acquire knowledge, think abstractly, act purposefully or adapt to changes in the environment. It is capacity of an individual to learn and to solve problems, and adjust to relatively new and changing conditions. There are individual differences, but it is desired from well-balanced personality in which intelligence is supplemented by healthy social being. It is the aggregate or global capacity of the individual to think rationally, to act purposefully and to deal effectively with the environment. Intelligence consists of an individual's those mental or cognitive abilities, which help in solving their actual life problems and leading a happy and well-contented life.
18. *Intelligence quotient (IQ):* A measure of intelligence, originally computed by dividing a person's mental age by his/her chronological age and multiplying the result by 100; it is now derived from norms provided for standardized intelligence tests. It is a measure of intelligence obtained by dividing the individual's mental age as determined by his/her performance on standardized test items, by his/her chronological age and multiplied by 100. It can be defined as the ratio between mental age and chronological age multiplied by 100.
19. *Interest:* It is a tendency to give selective attention to one activity or activities rather than giving interest to others.
20. *Internal environment:* The internal environment refers to the prenatal environment.
21. *Intrinsic motivation:* The pursuit of an activity for its own sake. It refers to motivation that is driven by an interest or enjoyment in the task itself and exists within the individual rather than

relying on any external pressure. Intrinsic motivation occurs when people are internally motivated to do something because it either brings them pleasure, they think it is important or they feel that what they are learning is significant. It has been shown that intrinsic motivation for education drops from grades 3 to 9 though the exact cause cannot be ascertained.

22. *Intrinsic reinforcers:* The reinforcers that are inherently related to the activity being reinforced.
23. *Introspection:* It means looking within, looking into the working of our own minds and reporting what we find there.

J

1. *Just-world hypothesis:* The notion that many people need to believe that the world is fair and that justice is served; that bad people are punished and good people rewarded.
2. *Justification of effort:* The tendency of individuals to increase their liking for something that they have worked hard or suffered to attain a common form of dissonance reduction.

K

1. *Kinesthesia:* The sense of body position and movement of body parts; also called kinesthesia.

L

1. *Language:* A system that combines meaningless elements such as sounds or gestures to form structured utterances that convey meaning. It is the most efficient and developed vehicle used for carrying out the process of thinking. When one listens or reads or writes words, phrases or sentences, or observes gestures in any language, the person is stimulated to think. Reading and writing of the written documents and literature also helps in stimulating and promoting our thinking process. The language broadens our thinking.
2. *Language acquisition device:* According to many psycholinguists, an innate mental module that allows young children to develop language, if they are exposed to an adequate sampling of conversation.

3. *Latent learning:* A form of learning that is not immediately expressed in an overt response; it occurs without obvious reinforcement.
4. *Lateralization:* Specialization of the two cerebral hemispheres for particular operations.
5. *Learned motives:* The learned motives are those, which the person develops after the birth. They are learnt from the environment such as family and society. Learned motives include the need to be with others, to be approved by others, to be secure, to achieve success or social prestige.
6. *Learning:* A relatively permanent change in behavior (or behavioral potential) due to experience. It is the process by which an activity originates or is changed through reacting to an encountered situation provided that the characteristics of the change in activity cannot be explained on the basis of native responses, tendencies and maturation or temporary states of the organism like fatigue or effect of drugs. It is the process by which an activity originates or is changed through reacting to an encountered situation, provided that the characteristics of the change in activity cannot be explained on the basis of native response, tendencies, maturation or temporary states of the organism.
7. *Learning perspective:* A psychological approach that emphasizes, how the environment and experience affect a person's or animal's actions; it includes behaviorism and social-cognitive learning theories.
8. *Libido:* In psychoanalysis, the psychic energy that fuels the life or sexual instincts of the Id.
9. *Limbic system:* A group of brain areas involved in emotional reactions and motivated behavior.
10. *Linkage studies:* The studies that look for patterns of inheritance of genetic markers in large families in which a particular condition is common.
11. *Lithium carbonates:* A drug frequently given to people suffering from bipolar disorder.
12. *Localization of function:* Specialization of particular brain areas for particular functions.
13. *Locus of control:* A general expectation about, whether the results of your actions are under your own control (internal locus) or beyond your control (external locus).

14. *Long-term memory (LTM):* In the three-box model of memory, the memory system involved in the long-term storage of information. It has the unlimited capacity to store information for days, months, years and even for a lifetime. LTM codes information according to meaning, pattern and other characteristics. With the help of LTM we can store, retain and remember most of the things in our life at record notice and thus make things quite easy.
15. *Long-term potentiation:* A long-lasting increase in the strength of synaptic responsiveness, thought to be a biological mechanism of long-term memory.
16. *Longitudinal study:* A study in which subjects are followed and periodically reassessed over a period of time.
17. *Loudness:* The dimension of auditory experience related to the intensity of a pressure wave.
18. *Lucid dream:* A dream in which dreamer is aware of dreaming.

M

1. *Magnetic resonance imaging (MRI):* A method for studying the body and brain tissue, using magnetic fields and special radioreceivers.
2. *Maintenance rehearsal:* Rote repetition of material in order to maintain its availability in memory.
3. *Major depression:* A mood disorder involving disturbances in emotion (excessive sadness), behavior (loss of interest in one's usual activities), cognition (thoughts of hopelessness) and body function (fatigue and loss of appetite).
4. *Mastery (learning) goals:* The goals framed in terms of increasing one's competence and skills.
5. *Maturation:* Produces an increase in competence, an ability to function at a higher level depending on the child's heredity. It is the changes in behavior of an organism resulting from physiological growth, the blueprints of which are provided by hereditary. It is a developmental process within a person, from time to time manifests different traits, the 'blueprints' for which have been carried in his/her cells from the time of one is conception.
6. *Measure of central tendency:* A number intended to characterize an entire set of data.
7. *Measure of variability:* A number that indicates how dispersed scores are around the mean of the distribution.

8. *Mechanical aptitude:* It is not a single unitary function, it is a combination of sensory and motor capacities plus perception of spatial relations, the capacity to acquire information about the mechanical matters and the capacity to comprehend mechanical relationships.
9. *Median:* A measure of central tendency; the value at the midpoint of a distribution of scores, when the scores are ordered from highest to lowest.
10. *Memory:* The power that we have to 'store' our experiences and to bring them into the field of consciousness sometime after experiences have occurred is termed as memory.
11. *Menopause:* The cessation of menstruation and of the production of ova; it is usually, a gradual process lasting up to several years.
12. *Mental age:* It is the average age of an individual who achieve a particular level of performance test. A measure of mental development expressed in terms of the average mental ability at a given age.
13. *Mental disorder:* Any behavior or emotional state that causes an individual great suffering or worry is self-defeating or self-destructive or is maladaptive and disrupts the person's relationships or the larger community.
14. *Mental health:* It is a sound, efficient mind and controlled emotions. It is the total and harmonious functioning of the whole personality of an individual for optimum functioning with maximum realization. A positive mental health shows an individual's ability to cope with the present and to adjust satisfactorily in future. It is a state of compromise and adaptation to a situation in the life leading to better adjustment. Individuals with positive mental health fulfill their responsibilities, function effectively and are satisfied with their interpersonal relationships and themselves.
15. *Mental hygiene:* It is an art and science, which includes application of scientific principles and practices for the promotion, preservation and maintenance of mental health, and prevention of mental disorders; and enjoys healthy practices to lead productive, happy and contended life.
16. *Mental image:* A mental representation that mirrors or resembles the thing it represents; mental images occur in many and perhaps all sensory modalities.

17. *Mental retardation:* It is having significantly below average intellectual functioning and limitations in at least two areas of adoptive functioning.
18. *Mental set:* A tendency to solve problems using procedures that worked before on similar problems.
19. *Meta-analysis:* A procedure for combining and analyzing data from many studies; it determines how much of the variance in scores across all studies can be explained by a particular variable.
20. *Metacognition:* The knowledge or awareness of one's own cognitive processes.
21. *Minnesota multiphasic personality inventory (MMPI):* A widely used objective personality test.
22. *Mnemonics:* Strategies and tricks for improving memory, such as the use of a verse or a formula.
23. *Mode:* A measure of central tendency; the most frequently occurring score in a distribution.
24. *Monochronic cultures:* The cultures in which time is organized sequentially; schedules and deadlines are valued over people.
25. *Monocular cues:* Visual cues to depth or distance, which can be used by one eye alone.
26. *Motivation:* An inferred process within a person or animal that causes movement, either towards a goal or away from an unpleasant situation.
27. *Motive:* It is a state within the individual, which under appropriate circumstances initiates or regulates behavior in relation to a goal.
28. *Myelin sheaths:* A fatty insulation that may surround the axon of a neuron.

N

1. *Narcissistic personality disorder:* A disorder characterized by an exaggerated sense of self-importance and self-absorption.
2. *Narcolepsy:* A sleep disorder involving sudden and unpredictable daytime attacks of sleepiness or lapses into rapid eye movement (REM) sleep.
3. *Natural selection:* The evolutionary process in which individuals with genetically influenced traits that are adaptive in a particular environment tend to survive and to reproduce in

greater numbers than do other individuals; as a result, their traits become more common in the population.

4. *Need:* A need is the lack of something, which if present, will tend for the further welfare of the organism or for the species, or to facilitate its usual behavior.
5. *Need for achievement:* A learned motive to meet personal standards of success and excellence in a chosen area.
6. *Need for affiliation:* The motive to associate with other people, as by seeking friends, companionship or love.
7. *Negative correlation:* An association between increase in one variable and decrease in another.
8. *Negative reinforcement:* A reinforcement procedure in which a response is followed by the removal, delay or decrease in intensity of an unpleasant stimulus; as a result, the response becomes stronger or more likely to occur.
9. *Nerve:* A bundle of nerve fibers (axons and sometimes dendrites) in the peripheral nervous system.
10. *Neurobiology:* The science of the nervous system includes neuroanatomy, neurophysiology, neurochemistry, neuropharmacology, neuroembryology, physiological psychology and other disciplines concerned with the structure, function and development of the nervous system.
11. *Neurogenesis:* The production of new neurons from immature stems cells.
12. *Neuron:* A cell that conducts electrochemical signals; the basic unit of the nervous system; also called nerve cell.
13. *Neurotransmitter:* A chemical substance that is released by a transmitting neuron at the synapse and that alters the activity of a receiving neuron. A chemical substance stored in vesicles and released into synaptic clefts or neuromuscular junction to excite or inhibit neurons or muscle fibers.
14. *Non-conscious processes:* Mental processes occurring out of conscious level and not available to conscious awareness.
15. *Non-shared environment:* It is a unique aspects of a person's environment and experience that are not shared with family members.
16. *Normal curve:* A symmetrical, bell-shaped frequency polygon representing a normal distribution.
17. *Normal distribution:* A theoretical frequency distribution having certain special characteristics. For example, the distribution is

symmetrical; the mean, mode and median all have the same value and the further a score is from the mean, the less the likelihood of obtaining it.

18. *Nursing:* It is an art, science and profession by which we render, serve to human being to help to regain or to keep a normal state of body and mind and when it cannot accomplish this, it help patients for the relief from physical pain, mental anxiety or spiritual discomfort.

O

1. *Object permanence:* The understanding, which develops throughout the 1st year that an object continues to exist even when you cannot see it or touch it.
2. *Object-relations school:* A psychodynamic approach that emphasizes the importance of the infant's first 2 years of life and the baby's formative relationships, especially with the mother.
3. *Objective tests (inventories):* Standardized questionnaires requiring written responses; they typically include scales on which people are asked to rate themselves.
4. *Observational learning:* A process in which an individual learns new responses by observing the behavior of another (a model), rather than through direct experience; sometimes called vicarious conditioning.
5. *Observational study:* A study in which the researcher carefully and systematically observes and records behavior without interfering with the behavior; it may involve either naturalistic or laboratory observation.
6. *Obsessive-compulsive disorder (OCD):* An anxiety disorder in which a person feels trapped in repetitive, persistent thoughts (obsessions) and repetitive, ritualized behaviors (compulsions) designed to reduce anxiety.
7. *Obtundation:* It is a state similar to lethargy in which the patient has a lessened interest in the environment, slowed responses to stimulation and tends to sleep more than normal with drowsiness in between sleep states.
8. *Oedipus complex:* In psychoanalysis, a conflict occurring in the phallic (oedipal) stage, in which a child desires the parent of the other sex and views the same-sex parent as a rival.

9. *Operant conditioning:* The process by which a response becomes more likely to occur or less so, depending on its consequences. It refers to a kind of learning process, where, a response is made more probable or more frequently by reinforcement. It helps in the learning of operant behavior, the behavior that is not necessarily associated with known stimuli.
10. *Operational definition:* A precise definition of a term in a hypothesis, which specifies the operations for observing and measuring the process or phenomenon being defined.
11. *Operations:* In Piaget's theory, mental actions that are cognitively reversible.
12. *Opiates:* Drugs, derived from the opium poppy that relieve pain and commonly produce euphoria.
13. *Opponent-process theory:* A theory of color perception that assumes that the visual system treats pairs of colors as opposing or antagonistic.

P

1. *Panic attacks:* The periods of intense anxiety, fear, physiological arousal, discomfort and stomach problems, etc. which occur suddenly and are discrete in nature, are termed as panic attacks. The panic attacks are associated with a variety of cognitive and somatic symptoms.
2. *Panic disorder:* An anxiety disorder in which a person experiences recurring panic attacks, periods of intense fear and feelings of impending doom or death, accompanied by physiological symptoms such as rapid heart rate and dizziness.
3. *Paper-and-pencil performance:* A paper-and-pencil performance test differs from the more traditional paper-and-pencil test by placing greater emphasis on the application of the knowledge and skill in a simulated setting. These paper-and-pencil applications might result in desired terminal learning outcomes or they might serve as an intermediate step to performance that involves a higher degree of realism (e.g. the actual use of equipment).
4. *Parallel distributed processing (PDP) model:* A model of memory in which knowledge is represented as connections among thousands of interacting processing units, distributed in a vast network and all operating in parallel.

5. *Parapsychology:* The study of purported psychic phenomena such as ESP and mental telepathy.
6. *Parasympathetic nervous system:* The subdivision of the autonomic nervous system that operates during relaxed states and that conserves energy.
7. *Pattern recognition:* The identification of a stimulus on the basis of information already contained in long-term memory.
8. *Percentile scores:* A score that indicates the percentage of people, who scored at or below a given raw score; also called percentile rank.
9. *Perception:* The process by which the brain organizes and interprets sensory information. A process of organizing environmental stimuli into some meaningful patterns of wholes.
10. *Perceptual constancy:* The accurate perception of objects as stable or unchanged, despite changes in the sensory patterns they produce.
11. *Perceptual learning:* The child gets sensation through organs of sense and he/she attaches meaning to each sensation. The earliest sensations of the infant are undifferentiated to the extent that he/she cannot differentiate between one object and another. In course of time, he/she recognizes specific objects and perceives these separately.
12. *Perceptual or concrete thinking:* It is the simplest form of thinking. The basis of this type of thinking is perception, i.e. interpretation, of sensation according to one's experience. It is also named as concrete thinking, as it is carried by the perception of actual or concrete objects and events. It is thinking of a lower order. Such type of thinking is present in animals and children.
13. *Perceptual set:* A habitual way of perceiving; based on expectations.
14. *Performance goals:* The goals framed in terms of performing well in front of others, being judged favorably and avoiding criticism.
15. *Peripheral nervous system (PNS):* All portions of the nervous system outside the brain and spinal cord; it includes sensory and motor nerves.
16. *Personal guidance:* It refers to the guidance offered to students for enabling them to adjust themselves to their environment, so that they become efficient citizens. Adolescent behavior to a great extent depends upon the moods and attitudes of the adolescent.

Emotional instability is a characteristic of adolescents and this is often the cause of many of their personal problems. Personal guidance will help them to solve these problems.

17. *Personality:* A distinctive and relatively stable pattern of behavior, thoughts, motives and emotions that characterizes an individual throughout life. It is the distinctive patterns of behavior, thought and emotions that characterize an individual's adaptation to the situations of his/her life. Personality is the individual's characteristic (and relatively enduring) organization (or integration) of ways of behaving (or traits, interests, abilities, attitudes), and modes of adjustment to others, and to his/her total environment.
18. *Personality disorders:* Rigid, maladaptive personality patterns that cause personal distress or an inability to get along with others. The personality disorders are psychological disorders characterized by lifelong maladaptive behavior patterns, antisocial personality disorder, schizotypal personality disorder, compulsive personality disorder and histrionic personality.
19. *Personality dynamics:* It includes the following:
    a. The interactions among personality characteristics, especially motives.
    b. The behavioral expression of personality characteristics in the process of adjusting to the environment.
    c. In psychoanalysis, the management of the personality's energy system through the interactions of the Id, ego and superego.
20. *Personality structure:* In general, the unique organization of traits, motives and ways of behaving that characterizes a particular person; in psychoanalytic theory, the conception of the personality in terms of Id, ego and superego.
21. *Personality tests:* Tests to measure the characteristic ways a person behaves, thinks and feels. Compare ability tests, achievement tests. Personalized system of instruction (PSI), an educational application of instrumental conditioning/operant conditioning in which the material in a course is divided into small units, each of which must be mastered at a high level of proficiency before the next unit is attempted.
22. *Phobia:* An exaggerated, unrealistic fear of a specific situation, activity or object.

23. *Phrenology:* The discredited theory that different brain areas account for character and personality traits, which can be 'read' from bumps on the skull.
24. *Pitch:* The dimension of auditory experience related to the frequency of a pressure wave; the height or depth of a tone.
25. *Pituitary gland:* A small endocrine gland at the base of the brain, which releases many hormones and regulates other endocrine glands.
26. *Placebo:* An inactive substance or fake treatment used as a control in an experiment or given by a medical practitioner to a patient.
27. *Placebo affects:* The apparent success of a medication or treatment due to the patient's expectations or hopes rather than to the drug or treatment itself.
28. *Polychronic cultures:* The cultures in which time is organized horizontally; people tend to do several things at once and value relationships over schedules.
29. *Pons:* A structure in the brainstem involved in among other things, sleeping, waking and dreaming.
30. *Positive correlation:* An association between increase in one variable and increase in another or decrease between the in one and the other.
31. *Positive reinforcement:* A reinforcement procedure in which a response is followed by the presentation of, or increase in intensity of a reinforcing stimulus; as a result, the response becomes stronger or more likely to occur.
32. *Positron-emission tomography (PET):* A method for analyzing biochemical activity in the brain, using injections of glucose, like substance containing a radioactive element.
33. *Postdecision dissonance:* In the theory of cognitive dissonance, tension that occurs when you believe you may have made a bad decision.
34. *Post-traumatic stress disorder (PTSD):* An anxiety disorder in which a person who has experienced a traumatic or life-threatening event has symptoms such as psychic numbing, reliving of the trauma and increased physiological arousal.
35. *Power assertion:* A method of child rearing in which the parent uses punishment and authority to correct the child's misbehavior.
36. *Practical intelligence:* It is the intelligence, which operates in the real world. People with this type of intelligence can adapt to or

shape their environment. It is influenced not only by mental skills but also by attitudes and emotional factors.

37. *Precognition:* It is the perception of a future event. Precognition is psychic knowledge of something in advance of its occurrence. In other words it is the knowledge; a person may have of another person's future thoughts.
38. *Primary controls:* An effort to modify reality by changing other people, the situation or events; a fighting back philosophy.
39. *Primary emotions:* These are considered to be universal and biologically based; they generally include fear, anger, sadness, joy, surprise, disgust and contempt.
40. *Primary motives:* The primary motives are those, which are necessary for survival. These are caused by the needs of the body. The main primary motives are hunger, thirst, avoidance of pain, needs for air, sleep and elimination of wastes and regulation of body temperature.
41. *Primary punisher:* A stimulus that is inherently punishing; an example is electric shock.
42. *Primary reinforcer:* A stimulus that is inherently reinforcing, typically satisfying a physiological need; an example is food.
43. *Priming:* A method for measuring implicit memory in which a person reads or listens to information and is later tested to see, whether the information affects performance on the same or another type of task.
44. *Principle of falsifiability:* The principle that a scientific theory must make predictions that are specific enough to expose the theory to the possibility of disconfirmation, i.e. the theory must predict not only what will happen but also what will not happen.
45. *Proactive interference:* Forgetting that occurs when previously stored material interferes with the ability to remember similar, more recently learned material.
46. *Procedural memories:* The memories for the performance of actions or skills (knowing how).
47. *Professional aptitude:* The aptitude related to the activities of various professions and occupations are included in this category. These aptitudes are able to predict the future success of an individual in the field or profession related to these aptitudes.
48. *Projective tests:* Psychological tests used to infer a person's motives, conflicts and unconscious dynamics on the basis of the person's interpretations of ambiguous stimuli.

49. *Proposition:* A unit of meaning that is made up of concepts and expresses a single idea.
50. *Prototype:* An especially representative example of a concept.
51. *Psi (pronounced 'sigh'):* It is a term commonly used by parapsychologist to refer to both extrasensory perception (ESP) and psychokinesis taken together. The term was coined by BP Weisner and recommended by RH Thousless.
52. *Psychedelic drugs:* Consciousness-altering drugs that produce hallucinations, change thought processes or disrupt the normal perception of time and space.
53. *Psychoactive drug:* A drug capable of influencing perception, mood, cognition or behavior.
54. *Psychoanalysis:* A theory of personality and a method of psychotherapy, originally formulated by Sigmund Freud, which emphasizes unconscious motives and conflicts.
55. *Psychoanalytic theory:* Freud's theory that all human behavior is dominated by instinctual biological urges that must be controlled; it is the conflict between the urges and the efforts to control them that leads to emotional problems.
56. *Psychodrama:* A method of therapy in which one acts out scenes in order to bring out their emotional significance of behavior.
57. *Psychodynamic perspective:* A psychological approach that emphasizes unconscious dynamics within the individual, such as inner forces, conflicts or the movement of instinctual energy.
58. *Psychodynamic theories:* The theories that explain behavior and personality in terms of unconscious energy dynamics within the individual.
59. *Psychodynamic therapy:* They share the goal of exploring the unconscious dynamics of personality such as defenses and conflicts.
60. *Psychogenic amnesia:* The partial or complete loss of memory (due to non-organic causes) for threatening information or traumatic experiences.
61. *Psychokinesis (PK):* Whereby a mental operation affects a material body or an energy system, e.g. wishing for a number, affects what number comes up in the throw of dice.
62. *Psychological tests:* Procedures used to measure and evaluate personality traits, emotional states, aptitudes, interests, abilities and values.

63. *Psychology:* The discipline concerned with behavior and mental processes and how they are affected by an organism's physical state, mental state and external environment; the term is often represented by ψ, the Greek letter psi (usually pronounced 'sy'). It is a study of systematic and scientific study of human and animal behavior. It has its own special methods, which help us in gathering and organizing its subjective matter or the essential facts about it.
64. *Psychometrics:* The measurement of mental abilities, traits and processes. It is a branch of psychology dealing with the development and application of statistical and other mathematical procedures to psychology.
65. *Psychoneuroimmunology (PNI):* The study of the relationships among psychology, the nervous and endocrine systems and the immune system.
66. *Psychophysiological:* It is pertaining to processes that have both bodily or material and psychological or mental aspects.
67. *Psychosis:* An extreme mental disturbance involving distorted perceptions and irrational behavior; it may have psychological or organic causes (plural: psychoses). A severe mental disorder characterized by disorganization of the thought process, disturbances in emotion, disorganization as to time, place and person in some cases.
68. *Psychosocial:* It is pertaining to social relationships involving psychological factors.
69. *Psychosocial development:* Development of individual's interactions, understanding of each other and of their knowledge and understanding of themselves as members of society.
70. *Psychosomatic:* A reference to the influence of the mind or higher functions of the brain (emotions, fears, desires, etc.) upon the functions of the body; especially, in relation to body disorders or disease.
71. *Psychosomatic disorder:* A disorder caused by a combination of organic and psychological factors. In psychosomatic disorders there may be tissue changes, as with peptic ulcers.
72. *Psychosurgery:* Any surgical procedure that destroys selected areas of the brain; believed to be involved in emotional disorders or disturbed behavior.
73. *Psychotechniques:* The practical application of psychological principles to the control and management of behavior.

74. *Psychotherapy:* The application of specialized techniques to the treatment of mental disorders or to the problems of everyday adjustment. The major techniques employed by psychotherapists include depth interviews, conditioning, suggestion and interpretation.
75. *Psychotic:* Characterizing a state of psychosis or resembling the behavior of an individual who has a psychosis.
76. *Puberty:* The age at which a person becomes capable of sexual reproduction. The period, during which the capability for sexual reproduction is attained, it is marked by changes in both primary and secondary sexual characteristics and is dated from menarche in girls and the emergence of pigmented public hair in boys.
77. *Punishment:* The process by which a stimulus or event weakens or reduces the probability of the response that it follows.

R

1. *Random assignment:* A procedure for assigning people to experimental and control groups in which each individual has the same probability, as any other of being assigned to a given group.
2. *Randomized controlled trials:* Research designed to determine the effectiveness of a new medication or form of therapy in which people with a given problem or disorders are randomly assigned to one or more treatment groups or to a control group.
3. *Range:* A measure of the spread of scores, calculated by subtracting the lowest score from the highest score.
4. *Rapid eye movement (REM) sleep:* The sleep periods characterized by eye movement, loss of muscle tone and dreaming.
5. *Rational analysis:* Involves the careful weighing of evidence for and against a particular attitude. The nurse giving health education to slum people will influence their attitude for personal hygiene when informing about rationale of unhygienic conditions.
6. *Rational emotive behavior therapy (REBT):* A form of cognitive therapy devised by Albert Ellis, designed to challenge the client's unrealistic or irrational thoughts.
7. *Reasoning:* The drawing of conclusions or inferences from observations, facts or assumptions.
8. *Recall:* The ability to retrieve and reproduce from memory, previously encountered material.

9. *Reciprocal determinism:* In social-cognitive theories, the two-way interaction between aspects of the environment and aspects of the individual in the shaping of personality traits.
10. *Recognition:* The ability to identify previously encountered material.
11. *Reflective thinking or logical thinking:* It aims at solving complex problems rather than simple problems. It requires reorganization of all the relevant experiences and finding new ways of reacting to a situation. Mental activity in reflective thinking does not undergo any mechanical trial and error type of effort. There is an insightful cognitive approach in reflective thinking. It takes logic into account in which all the relevant facts are arranged in a logical order, in order to get to the solution of the problem in hand.
12. *Registration:* It is the short-term storage of the sensory input. Most of the information briefly held in the sensory register is lost. However, we pay special attention to some of the information in the sensory register. When we do this, the attended information is passed on to the short-term storehouse. The sensory register holds information for such a brief time that some psychologists prefer to discuss it as related to perception rather than memory.
13. *Reinforcement:* The process by which a stimulus or event strengthens or increases the probability of the response that it follows. It is a collective term meaning either reward or punishment. It is often used when a principle is stated, which applies to both reward and punishment for instance, "reinforcement is most effective when it occurs immediately after the response."
14. *Relearning method:* A method for measuring retention that compares the time required to relearn material with the time used in the initial learning of the material.
15. *Reliability:* In test construction, the consistency of scores derived from a test, from one time and place to another. It is concerned with the consistency, stability and dependability of the results. In other words, a reliable result is one that shows similar performance at different times or under different conditions. If a student takes a test several times and has not grown in the area, the test measures, he/she should earn a similar score each time.

16. *Representative sample:* A group of subjects, selected from a population for study, which matches the population on important characteristics such as age and sex.
17. *Repression:* In psychoanalytic theory, the selective and involuntary pushing of threatening or upsetting information into the unconscious.
18. *Resistance to change/persuasion:* Attitudes socialized early in life and to which the person is highly committed, do not change very much in adulthood. They are largely unaffected by mass communications or life changes like aging, geographical mobility and social mobility.
19. *Retention:* It refers to a permanence of what was learnt. When the active process of learning ceases, a comparatively passive process of retaining takes place. The material is retained when we are not thinking about it. People differ in their retentive capacity, which is largely due to genetic constitution.
20. *Reticular activating system (RAS):* A dense network of neurons found in the core of the brainstem; it arouses the cortex and screens incoming information.
21. *Retina:* Neural tissue lining the back of the eyeball's interior, which contains the receptors for vision.
22. *Retinal disparity:* The slight difference in lateral separation between two objects as seen by the left eye and the right eye.
23. *Retroactive interference:* Forgetting that occurs when recently learned material interferes with the ability to remember similar material stored previously.
24. *Retrocognition:* It is a type of clairvoyance involving knowledge of something after its occurrence through psychic menaces.
25. *Rods:* Visual receptors that respond to dim light.
26. *Role:* A given social position that is governed by a set of norms for proper behavior.
27. *Rorschach inkblot test:* A projective personality test that requires respondents to interpret abstract, symmetrical inkblots.

S

1. *Saturation:* Vividness or purity of color; the dimension of visual experience related to the complexity of light waves.
2. *Schizophrenia:* A psychotic disorder or group of disorders marked by positive symptoms (e.g. delusions, hallucinations,

disorganized and incoherent speech and inappropriate behavior) and negative symptoms (e.g. emotional flatness and loss of motivation).

3. *Seasonal affective disorder (SAD):* A controversial disorder in which a person experiences depression during the winter and an improvement of mood in the spring.
4. *Secondary control:* An effort to accept reality by changing the attitudes, goals or emotions; a 'learn to live with it' philosophy.
5. *Secondary emotions:* The emotions that develop with cognitive maturity and vary across individuals and cultures.
6. *Secondary punisher:* A stimulus that has acquired punishing properties through association with other punishers.
7. *Secondary reinforcer:* A stimulus that has acquired reinforcing properties through association with other reinforcers.
8. *Selective attention:* The focusing of attention on selected aspects of the environment and the blocking out of others.
9. *Self-esteem:* A person's overall self-evaluation or the sense of self-worth.
10. *Self-efficacy:* A person's belief that he/she is capable of producing desired results such as mastering new skills and reaching goals. A sense that one is competent and effective, distinguished from self-esteem, one's sense of self-worth. A bombardier might feel high self-efficacy and low self-esteem.
11. *Self-fulfilling prophecy:* An expectation that comes true because of the tendency of the person holding it to act in ways that bring it about.
12. *Self-perception theory:* The theory that when we are unsure of our attitudes, we infer them much as would someone observing us, by looking at our behavior and the circumstances under which it occurs.
13. *Self-serving bias:* The tendency, in explaining one's own behavior, to take credit for one's good actions and rationalize one's mistakes.
14. *Selective attention and interpretation:* Whether a message will influence a recipient depends upon how it is perceived and interpreted. Most important, it depends upon whether the message is attended in the first place.
15. *Semantic memory:* It is the accumulation of facts and experiences gained over a lifetime. Semantic memory is used for remembering everyday types of facts and informations. It is also called

knowledge. Unlike other forms of memory, we usually do not remember where or when we learned the information in semantic memory.

16. *Semantic memories:* The memories of general knowledge, including facts, rules, concepts and propositions.
17. *Semicircular canals:* Sense organs in the inner ear that contribute to equilibrium by responding to rotation of the head.
18. *Sensation:* The detection of physical energy emitted or reflected by physical objects; it occurs when energy in the external environment or the body stimulates receptors in the sense organs.
19. *Sense receptors:* Specialized cells that convert physical energy in the environment or the body to electrical energy that can be transmitted as nerve impulses to the brain.
20. *Sensory adaptation:* The reduction or disappearance of sensory responsiveness, when stimulation is unchanging or repetitious.
21. *Sensory defect:* Defect in the function of one or more of the senses, resulting in visual, auditory or olfactory impairments.
22. *Sensory deprivation:* The absence of normal levels of sensory stimulation.
23. *Sensory memory:* A memory system that momentarily preserves extremely accurate images of sensory information.
24. *Separation anxiety:* The distress that most children develop, at about 6 to 8 months of age, when their primary caregivers temporarily leave them with strangers.
25. *Serial-position effects:* The tendency for recall of the first and last items on a list to surpass recall of items in the middle of the list.
26. *Set point:* The genetically influenced weight range for an individual, maintained by biological mechanisms that regulate food intake, fat reserves and metabolism.
27. *Sex hormones:* The hormones that regulate the development and functioning of reproductive organs and that stimulate the development of male and female sexual characteristics; they include androgens, estrogens and progesterone.
28. *Sexual scripts:* Sets of implicit rules that specify proper sexual behavior for a person in a given situation, varying with the person's age, culture and gender.
29. *Shaping:* An operant-conditioning procedure in which successive approximations of a desired response are reinforced.

30. *Short-term memory (STM):* In the three-box model of memory, a limited-capacity memory system involved in the retention of information for brief periods; it is also used to hold information retrieved from long-term memory for temporary use. It holds a relatively small amount of information about seven items for a short period of time (15–30 second) though not nearly as short-lived as the immediate memory.
31. *Signal-detection theory:* A psychophysical theory that divides the detection of a sensory signal into a sensory process and a decision process.
32. *Significance tests:* Statistical tests that show, how likely it is that a study's results occurred merely by chance.
33. *Single-blind study:* An experiment in which subjects do not know, whether they are in an experimental or a control group.
34. *Skill learning:* Right from the birth, the child acquires skill. His/her bodily organs learn to handle the things. He/she moves legs and begins to crawl. In course of time, he/she learns other motor skills like walking, speaking, drawing, writing, reading, playing music, cycling, swimming, etc.
35. *Skills training:* In behavior therapy, an effort to teach the client skills that he/she may lack, as well as new, more constructive behaviors to replace self-defeating ones.
36. *Sleep apnea:* A disorder in which breathing briefly stops during sleep, causing the person to choke and gasp and momentarily awaken.
37. *Social cognition:* An area in social psychology concerned with social influences on thought, memory, perception and other cognitive processes.
38. *Social comparison:* Evaluating one's abilities and opinions by comparing oneself to others.
39. *Social exchange theory:* The theory that human interactions are transactions that aims to maximize one's rewards and minimize one's costs.
40. *Social guidance:* It enables the student to make substantial contributions to the society, assume leadership, confirm to the social norms, work as team members, develop healthy and positive attitudes, appreciate the problems of society, respect the opinions and sentiments of fellow human beings, acquire traits of patience, perseverance and friendship. Its main purpose is to enable the student to become an efficient citizen.

41. *Social identity:* The part of a person's self-concept that is based on his/her identification with a nation, culture or ethnic group or with gender or other roles in society.
42. *Social intelligence:* It is the ability of an individual to react to social situations in daily life. It includes the ability to understand people and to act wisely in human relationships. Persons having this type of intelligence know the art of winning friends and influence them. For example, leaders, ministers, salesmen, diplomats, etc. are socially intelligent.
43. *Social learning theory:* The theory that we learn social behavior by observing and imitating and by being rewarded and punished.
44. *Social loafing:* A group-produced reduction in individual output on easy tasks where contributions are pooled.
45. *Social neuroscience:* The study of the relationship between neural and social processes.
46. *Social norm:* A general rule of conduct reflecting standards of social approval and disapproval.
47. *Social perception:* A general term for the processes by which people come to understand one another.
48. *Social psychology:* This branch of psychology studies the human behavior in relation to their social environment, one's behavior as a member of the group, the process of communication and interpersonal relationship. Group dynamics and social relationship, etc. form the subject matter of this branch. The scientific study of how people think, influences and relate to one another.
49. *Social representations:* Socially shared beliefs, and widely held ideas and values, including our assumptions and cultural ideologies. Our social representations help us make sense of our world.
50. *Social role theory:* The theory that small gender differences are magnified in perception by the contrasting social roles occupied by men and women.
51. *Social support:* The helpful coping resources provided by friends and other people.
52. *Social-cognitive theories:* The theories that emphasize how behavior is learned and maintained through observation and imitation of others, positive consequences and cognitive processes such as plans, expectations and beliefs.

53. *Socialization:* The processes by which children learn the behaviors, attitudes and expectations required of them by their society or culture.
54. *Sociobiology:* An interdisciplinary field that emphasizes evolutionary explanations of social behavior in animals, including human beings.
55. *Sociocultural perspective:* A psychological approach that emphasizes social and cultural influences on behavior.
56. *Somatic nervous system:* The subdivision of the peripheral nervous system that connects to sensory receptors and to skeletal muscles; sometimes called the skeletal nervous system.
57. *Source amnesia:* The inability to distinguish what you originally experienced from what you heard or were told about an event later.
58. *Space relations:* It is the ability to visualize a constructed object from a picture of a pattern and an ability to imagine how an object would appear, if rotated in various ways for measurement of space perception. It means that these tests require mental manipulation of objects in three-dimensional spaces.
59. *Spinal cord:* A collection of neurons and supportive tissue running from the base of the brain down the center of the back, protected by a column of bones (the spinal column).
60. *Spontaneous recovery:* The reappearance of a learned response after its apparent extinction.
61. *Standard deviation (SD):* A commonly used measure of variability that indicates the average difference between scores in a distribution and their mean; more precisely, the square root of the average squared deviation from the mean.
62. *Standardize:* In test construction, to develop uniform procedures for giving and scoring a test.
63. *State-dependent memory:* The tendency to remember something when the remembered is in the same physical or mental state as during the original learning or experience.
64. *Statistically significant:* A term used to refer to a result that is extremely unlikely to have occurred by chance.
65. *Stem cells:* Immature cells that renew themselves and have the potential to develop into mature cells; given encouraging environments, stem cells from early embryos can develop into any cell type.

66. *Stereotype:* A summary impression of a group, in which a person believes that all members of the group share a common trait or traits (positive, negative or neutral).
67. *Stereotype threat:* A burden of doubt a person feels about his or her performance, due to negative stereotypes about his/her group's abilities.
68. *Stimulants:* Drugs that speed up activity in the central nervous system.
69. *Stimulus:* These are inborn, but not necessary for survival. They include activity, curiosity, exploration, manipulation and physical contact. An occurrence or event, which produces some effect on some organism.
70. *Stimulus discrimination:* The tendency to respond differently to two or more similar stimuli. In classical conditioning, it occurs when a stimulus similar to the conditioned stimulus fails to evoke the conditioned response; in operant conditioning, it occurs when an organism learns to make a response in the presence of other, similar stimuli that differ from it on some dimension.
71. *Stimulus generalization:* After conditioning, the tendency to respond to a stimulus that resembles one involved in the original conditioning. In classical conditioning, it occurs when a stimulus that resembles the conditioned stimulus elicits the conditioned response; in operant conditioning, it occurs when a response that has been reinforced (or punished) in the presence of one stimulus occurs (or is suppressed) in the presence of other similar stimuli.
72. *Stress:* It may be defined as "an adjustive demand placed on the organism. The condition or force or object giving rise to this demand may be internal or external and is designated as the stressor." It is an unpleasant state of arousal in which people perceive the demands of an event as taxing or exceeding their ability to satisfy or alter those demands.
73. *Structuralism:* An early psychological approach that emphasized the analysis of immediate experience into basic elements.
74. *Student performance:* It emphasizes proper procedure. The student is typically expected to perform the same motions as those required in the actual performance of the task, but the conditions are simulated. In physical education, e.g. swinging a bat at an imaginary ball, shadow boxing and demonstrating various swimming strokes out of water are simulated performances.

75. *Stupor:* It means that only vigorous and repeated stimuli will arouse the individual and when left undisturbed, the patient will immediately lapse back to the unresponsive state.
76. *Subconscious mind:* Consciousness does not have access to the entire body/mind; thus the term subconscious. The subconscious mind has access on all parts of the body/mind that consciousness mind does not have. Because the body and mind cannot be separated, it is more accurate to call this as the subconscious mind/body. This long phrase has been shorted in this work to simply the subconscious.
77. *Subconscious processes:* Mental processes occurring outside of conscious awareness, but accessible to consciousness when necessary.
78. *Successive approximations:* In the operant-conditioning procedure of shaping, behaviors that are ordered in terms of increasing similarity or closeness to the desired response.
79. *Superego:* In psychoanalysis, the part of personality that represents conscience, morality and social standards. According to Freud, the part of the personality that acquires the values and ideals of the parents and society and imposes constraints on the id and ego, the conscience.
80. *Surveys:* Questionnaires and interviews that ask people directly about their experiences, attitudes or opinions.
81. *Suggestion:* Advertisers and propagandists often rely on suggestion, the uncritical acceptance of a statement. They design their messages in hopes that people will accept a belief, form an attitude or be incited to action by someone else's saying so, without requiring facts.
82. *Summative evaluation:* Teachers have been using tests almost exclusively for determining grades, it may be assumed that with all that practice, teachers are systematic in the way they convert raw scores into letter grades. But this is not so. Each teacher seems to have an individual system and many teachers use a different system in each grading period. It is so because most teachers never find a system, with which they are satisfied. There is no single system that is right for all classes. Once the strengths and weaknesses of various grading systems are known, the choice can be exercised with greater wisdom.
83. *Sympathetic nervous system:* The subdivision of the autonomic nervous system that mobilizes bodily resources and increases the output of energy during emotion and stress.

84. *Synapse:* The site, where transmission of a nerve impulse from one nerve cell to another occurs; it includes the axon terminal, the synaptic cleft and receptor sites in the membrane of the receiving cell.
85. *Synesthesia:* A condition in which stimulation of one sense also evokes another.
86. *Systematic desensitization:* In behavior therapy, a step-by-step process of desensitizing a client to a feared object or experience; it is based on the classical-conditioning procedure of counter conditioning.

T

1. *Tacit knowledge:* Strategies for success that are not explicitly taught, but that instead must be inferred.
2. *Taste buds:* Nests of taste-receptor cells.
3. *Telegraphic speech:* A child's first word combinations, which omit (as a telegram did) unnecessary words.
4. *Telepathy:* It is the perceptions of objects or events not influencing the senses.
5. *Temperaments:* Physiological dispositions to respond to the environment in certain ways; they are present in infancy and are assumed to be innate.
6. *Temporal lobes:* The lobes at the sides of the brain's cerebral cortex, just above the ears; they contain areas involved in hearing, memory, perception, emotion and (in the left lobe, typically) language comprehension.
7. *Testing:* A test is a set of specified, uniform tasks to be performed by students. These tasks are appropriate samples from the knowledge or skills in a broader field of content. From the number of tasks performed correctly in the sample, the teacher makes an assumption of how the student is likely to perform in the total field.
8. *Thalamus:* A brain structure that relays sensory messages to the cerebral cortex.
9. *Thematic apperception test (TAT):* A projective test that asks respondents to interpret a series of drawings, showing scenes of people; usually scored for unconscious motives, such as the need for achievement, power or affiliation.

10. *Theory:* An organized system of assumptions and principles that purports to explain a specified set of phenomena and their interrelationships.
11. *Theory of mind:* A system of beliefs about the way one's own mind and the minds of others work and how cognitions and feelings affect behavior.
12. *Therapeutic alliance:* The bond of confidence and mutual understanding established between therapist and client, which allows them to work together to solve the client's problems.
13. *Thinking:* It is a complex mental activity. It is symbolic in character, initiated by a problem, which the individual is facing, involves the response of the individual to this problem. Thinking is a problem-solving process in which we use ideas or symbols in places of overt activity.
14. *Timbre:* The distinguishing quality of a sound; the dimension of auditory experience related to the complexity of the pressure wave.
15. *Tolerance:* Increased resistance to a drug's effects accompanying continued use; as tolerance develops, larger doses are required to produce effects, once brought about by smaller ones.
16. *Trait:* A characteristic of an individual, describing a habitual way of behaving, thinking and feeling.
17. *Tranquilizers:* Drugs commonly, but often inappropriately prescribed for patients who complain of unhappiness, anxiety or worry.
18. *Transcranial magnetic stimulation (TMS):* A method of stimulating brain cells, using a powerful magnetic field produced by a wire coil placed on a person's head; it can be used by researchers to temporarily inactivate neural circuits and is also being used therapeutically.
19. *Transference:* In psychodynamic therapies, a critical process in which the client transfers unconscious emotions or reactions, such as emotional feelings about his/her parents, onto the therapist.
20. *Triarchic theory of intelligence:* A theory of intelligence that emphasizes information-processing strategies, the ability to creatively transfer skills to new situations and the practical application of intelligence.
21. *Trichromatic theory:* A theory of color perception that proposes three mechanisms in the visual system, each sensitive to a

certain range of wavelengths; their interaction is assumed to produce all the different experiences of hue.

22. *Two-factor theory of emotion:* The theory that emotions depend on both physiological arousal and a cognitive interpretation of that arousal.

U

1. *Unconditional positive regard:* According to Carl Rogers, love or support given to another person with no conditions attached.
2. *Unconditioned response (UR):* The classical-conditioning term for a reflexive response, elicited by a stimulus in the absence of learning.
3. *Unconditioned stimulus (US):* The classical-conditioning term for a stimulus that elicits a reflexive response in the absence of learning.
4. *Unconscious motivation:* Some attitudes are held because they serve some unconscious function for an individual. For example, a person who is threatened by his/her homosexual feelings, may employ the defense mechanism of reaction formation and become a crusader against homosexuals.

V

1. *Validity:* The ability of a test to measure what it was designed to measure.
2. *Validity effect:* The tendency of people to believe that a statement is true or valid simply because it has been repeated many times.
3. *Variable-interval schedule:* An intermittent schedule of reinforcement in which a reinforcer is delivered for a response made after a variable period of time has elapsed, since the last reinforcer.
4. *Variable-ratio schedule:* An intermittent schedule of reinforcement in which reinforcement occurs after a variable number of responses.
5. *Variables:* Characteristics of behavior or experience that can be measured or described by a numeric scale.
6. *Verbal reasoning:* It is a measure of ability to understand concepts framed in words. It is aimed at evaluation of the student's ability to abstract or generalize and to think constructively, rather than simple, fluency or vocabulary recognition. The words used

in these items may come from history, geography, literature, science or any other content area.

7. *Visual memory:* It is part of memory preserving some characteristics of our senses pertaining to visual experience. We are able to place in memory information that resembles objects, places, animals or people in sort of a mental image.
8. *Vocational guidance:* It is the assistance provided for selection of a vocation and preparation for the same. It is concerned with enabling students to acquire information about career opportunities, career growth and training facilities.
9. *Volunteer bias:* A shortcoming of findings derived from a sample of volunteers instead of a representative sample; the volunteers may differ from those who did not volunteer.
10. *Vulnerability-stress models:* Approaches that emphasize; how individual vulnerabilities interact with external stresses or circumstances to produce mental disorders.

W

1. *Wernicke's area:* An area in the temporal lobe of cerebrum, which is necessary for the recognition of speech sounds and therefore, for the comprehension of language, also plays a part in the formulation of meaningful speech.
2. *Withdrawal symptoms:* Physical and psychological symptoms that occur when someone addicted to a drug, stops taking it.
3. *Working memory:* In many models of memory, a memory system comprising short-term memory plus the mental processes that control retrieval of information from long-term memory and interpret that information appropriately for a given task.

Z

1. *z-score (standard score):* A number that indicates, how far a given raw score is above or below the mean, using the SD of the distribution as the unit of measurement.

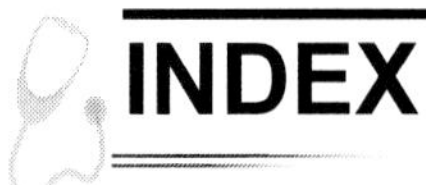

INDEX

Page numbers followed by '*f*' and '*t*' indicate figures and tables respectively.

D

E

N

Q

R

S